# LIVING WITH
# CHRONIC PAIN

To Katharine—
I hope you don't
need this information for
many years!
Love
Jennifer
10-4-04

# LIVING WITH CHRONIC PAIN

*The Complete Health Guide
to the Causes and Treatment
of Chronic Pain*

JENNIFER P. SCHNEIDER, M.D., Ph.D.

**healthy**living**books**

*New York • London*

LIVING WITH CHRONIC PAIN

Healthy Living Books
Hatherleigh Press
5-22 46th Avenue, Suite 200
Long Island City, NY 11101
www.healthylivingbooks.com

DISCLAIMER
This book does not give legal or medical advice.
Always consult your doctor, lawyer, and other professionals.
The names of people who contributed anecdotal material have been changed.

Names of medications are typically followed by TM or ® symbols, but these symbols are not stated in this book.

The ideas and suggestions contained in this book are not intended as a substitute for consulting with a physician. All matters regarding your health require medical supervision.

Library of Congress Cataloging-in-Publication Data

Schneider, Jennifer P.
 Living with chronic pain / Jennifer P. Schneider.
    p. cm.
 Includes bibliographical references and index.
 ISBN 1-57826-175-9
 1. Chronic pain--Popular works. I. Title.
 RB127.S365 2004
 616'.0472--dc22

                              2004011232

All Hatherleigh Press titles are available for bulk purchase, special promotions, and premiums. For information about reselling and special purchase opportunities, please call 1-800-528-2550 and ask for the Special Sales Manager.

Cover and interior design by Deborah Miller

10 9 8 7 6 5 4 3 2 1
Printed in Canada

# DEDICATION

To my daughter, Jessica Grace Wing, 1971–2003.

Cancer brought her pain and suffering
Yet she lived her life fully until the end
Death freed her
She will always be with me in spirit.
Her music will keep her alive in the hearts of many.


To my son, Benjamin Patai Wing,

He showed me up close that chronic pain can take away a person's life
and that good pain management can restore it.

# CONTENTS

# PREFACE

## Why Another Book on Chronic Pain?

*Dr. Richard A. Gardner, a [noted] psychiatrist and psychoanalyst
. . . died on May 25 at his home in Tenafly, NJ. He was 72. . . . The
cause was suicide, said Dr. Gardner's son, Andrew, who said his father
had been distraught over the advancing symptoms of reflex sympathetic dystrophy, a painful neurological syndrome.*
                    —NEW YORK TIMES, JUNE 9, 2003, P. A29.

P AIN CAN KILL. PATIENTS WITH CHRONIC PAIN ATTEMPT SUICIDE M O R E
often than people without pain, and they are two to three times
more successful than suicide attempts in the general population.
Some of these suicide attempts are caused by depression, which is very
common in people with chronic pain. But others occur in people who are
not clinically depressed but who simply are no longer able to tolerate their
undertreated pain. What most people who request assistance to die really
want is help in ending their pain.

Unfortunately, chronic pain, especially chronic pain unrelated to cancer,
is notoriously undertreated. In 1999, the American Pain Society surveyed
805 people with chronic pain about the adequacy of treatment they
received from their physicians.[1] More than 50 percent of the survey
respondents had been in pain for more than five years, and more than 40
percent of respondents with moderate to severe pain could not find
adequate relief. For most sufferers, the cause was arthritis or back disorders.
Almost half of the 805 patients had changed doctors at least once. The most

common reasons were too much pain (42 percent), the perception that their last physician did not know a lot about pain management (31 percent), the belief that the doctor didn't take their pain seriously enough (29 percent) and the doctor's unwillingness to treat their pain aggressively (27 percent). Only 26 percent of those respondents with "very severe" pain reported taking opioids (narcotics, the strongest painkillers available) at the time of the survey. Responding to the survey results, Dr. Russell Portenoy, a pioneer in treating cancer and non-cancer pain, said, "This survey shows the stigma associated with opioid drugs. Although these drugs can clearly benefit some patients with chronic pain, patients, caregivers, and physicians overestimate the risks and fail to use the drugs appropriately."

Dr. Portenoy has been one of my heroes for many years, ever since I began learning about appropriate treatment of chronic pain. For many years I was an internal medicine physician, treating adults with diabetes, hypertension, heart disease, and other nonsurgical problems. I knew no more about treating pain than do most internists, which is to say I knew very little. But then a family problem led me to become interested in addiction medicine and that, in turn, led to requests by other primary care doctors to consult on their patients who kept asking for more pain medicine for their chronic pain. "Please evaluate his drug-seeking behavior," they would request. So I began learning about treating chronic pain, about available medications and nondrug modalities, and about differentiating drug addicts from chronic pain patients. Eventually, I gave up primary care, and these days I limit my practice to pain management and addiction medicine. I also travel around the country giving talks to other health professionals on treating chronic pain. And, coincidentally, in the past few years both of my children have personally experienced chronic pain and its treatment, which made me more committed than ever to promote its better treatment.

Recently, I decided to write about what I have learned. There are already hundreds of books on chronic pain available! So why did I decide to write another? Because despite the extensive number of books already out there, many questions are still unanswered and many subjects misunderstood.

One area in which this is particularly true is the role of opioids in the treatment of chronic pain. Morphine and its related drugs are the most powerful painkillers available, and they are now routinely prescribed to patients dying of cancer. But fear and lack of knowledge of these drugs prevent many doctors from prescribing them for people whose pain is caused by anything other than cancer. The "War on Drugs," which has been waged unsuccessfully against drug dealers and addicts by the government of the United States, has spilled over into the practice of prescribing painkillers by physicians. The result is that even those physicians who might otherwise recommend painkillers for their suffering patients are hesitant because they are in fear of risking their medical license. Although a few physicians have indeed been unfairly targeted, most doctors' concerns are overinflated and unwarranted. Regulatory agencies and professional medical associations have recently issued guidelines to physicians regarding the appropriate prescribing of opioids for chronic pain. Physicians need only to be educated about these guidelines.

But educating doctors is not enough. An editorial titled "When will adequate pain treatment be the norm?" published in 1995 in the *Journal of the American Medical Association (JAMA)* explained,

> Bringing about significant change may, in reality, depend on empowering patients to demand adequate pain treatment, regardless of what that treatment may require. If so, this empowerment will not come easily, especially if opioids [narcotics] must be used for pain relief and if the pain is of a nonmalignant origin.[2]

To be effective advocates for themselves, patients also need education about painkillers and their proper use. This book will help you understand these drugs better so that you can work with your physician to obtain better relief for your chronic pain.

Another area of particular interest to me is the interaction between personality and pain. Chronic pain is more than just pain signals going into your brain. Your perception of pain is influenced by your expectations, your emotions (you probably already know that depression makes any pain worse), your cultural background, and your personality. Understanding yourself better can lead to more effective responses to the problems that your chronic pain condition has caused you.

In this book I will introduce you to a powerful system of personality typing, the enneagram. Once you determine which of nine personality types you are, a whole new world of understanding yourself will open up to you, and you will see the particular challenges that your personality creates for you in living with your chronic pain. You will be better able to meet those challenges.

The areas I will cover in *Living with Chronic Pain* include an explanation of chronic pain, new research about its causes, new strategies for its prevention, descriptions of various medications, and information about various pain-relieving procedures, operations, and psychological approaches. A whole section is devoted to enhancing your understanding of opioid analgesics. Personality and pain is addressed in another section, along with information on how to better understand your own personality. Another chapter explains how you can more effectively work with your doctor in alleviating your pain and improving your day-to-day life. And last, but not least, I will describe the challenges of the spouse or significant other (or partner) of the pain patient. All too often this person is neglected— despite the extremely important role that the partner often plays in the life of the patient with chronic pain.

I hope this book will make *you* a more educated consumer so that you can better help yourself and be a more effective team member in treating and living with your chronic pain.

# PART I

# UNDERSTANDING CHRONIC PAIN

# 1

# INTRODUCTION TO CHRONIC PAIN

## *What It Is*

ALL OF US HAVE EXPERIENCED PAIN AT SOME time in our lives—all of us except for those rare unfortunate people who were born with an inability to feel pain. Pain is the most common reason people seek medical attention; about 80 percent of doctor visits are primarily because of some pain problem. The International Association for the Study of Pain defines pain as "an unpleasant sensory and emotional experience arising from actual or potential tissue damage or described in terms of such damage."[1] This definition makes it clear that pain is more than just a chemical or electrical signal. Pain can include diverse unpleasant sensations such as aching, tightness, burning, and numbness.

Pain also has adverse effects on the body beyond the perception of pain. The physical effects of pain can include:
- poor wound healing, weakness, and muscle breakdown.
- decreased movement of the affected body parts, resulting in an increased risk of blood clots in the veins (thromboembolism) and in the lungs (pulmonary embolism).
- shallow breathing and cough suppression, which can increase the risk of pneumonia.
- increased sodium and water retention in the kidneys.

- decreased gastrointestinal motility.
- increased heart rate.
- increased blood pressure.
- Weakening of the body's immune system, causing decreased natural killer cell counts.
- insomnia.
- loss of appetite and weight loss.
- fatigue.

Fatigue is an important consequence of pain. This was documented in a recent review of 23 reports about the association between pain and fatigue, which found overwhelmingly that they are related and suggested that there may be a cause-and-effect relationship.[2]

Unrelieved pain also has adverse psychological effects. It causes anxiety, depression, fear, stress, loss of enjoyment of life, and difficulty relating to other people. It can increase marital conflict, reduce sexual desire, and cause feelings of anger and resentment.

Pain also has a major economic impact. A recent telephone survey of working adults found that during one 2-week period, 13 percent of the total workforce in the United States lost productive time because of pain. The lost productive time attributed to common pain conditions, if extrapolated to the long term, costs about 61.2 billion dollars per year! Most of the pain-related lost productive time resulted from reduced performance on the job rather than from time away from work.[3]

Pain is generally thought of as being either *acute* or *chronic*. Acute pain results from some trauma to the body—an injury, an operation, or an illness. It usually resolves when the underlying injury has healed or the cause has been treated. Although it is uncomfortable, acute pain serves a useful function: It signals that there is something wrong and motivates the person to get help. Because of the pain caused by an inflamed appendix, most people manage to undergo surgery before the appendix bursts, which constitutes a much more serious surgical problem. Because a heart attack usually causes severe chest pain, an increasing number of people with coronary artery disease are hospitalized early enough to benefit from procedures that prevent further damage to the heart. Acute pain is beneficial.

Acute pain usually has a clear cause. The same is true for postoperative pain (pain following surgery). Doctors are much less reluctant to treat pain whose origin is well understood; but even now postoperative pain is often undertreated. A random sample of 250 adults who had undergone surgical procedures were recently surveyed about their pain experience.[4] Approximately 80 percent of the patients experienced acute pain after surgery; of these, 86 percent had moderate, severe, or extreme pain, with more patients experiencing pain after being discharged from the hospital than before discharge. Experiencing postoperative pain was the most common concern (59 percent) of patients. The study concluded that many patients continue to experience intense pain after surgery.

## How Does Chronic Pain Differ from Acute Pain?

About 9 percent of the U.S. population suffers from persistent moderate to severe chronic pain. Several surveys in Europe show that about 18 percent of people have chronic pain, and the prevalence increases with age.[5] Chronic pain is not just acute pain that lasts longer than a week or a month. It differs from acute pain in several respects. It has become clear that acute and chronic pain are processed differently in the brain. The severity and extent of chronic pain may be out of proportion to the original injury and may continue long past the period in which the damaged tissue has healed. Chronic pain is pain that has outlived its usefulness and is no longer beneficial.

Acute and chronic pain have different treatment goals. The primary goals of acute pain treatment are to diagnose the source and remove it. With chronic pain, the main goals are to minimize the pain and maximize the person's functioning. Diagnosis is, of course, a first step, but frequently the source is either already clearly understood (for example, multiple unsuccessful back operations or osteoarthritis of the knee) or else very poorly understood and unlikely to be better understood (for example, fibromyalgia or chronic pelvic pain). In either case, the pain persists and must be treated in its own right. With chronic pain, however, treatment goals must be realistic. Complete relief of the pain is rare. A more realistic goal is to decrease the level of pain to a tolerable level that allows the person to focus on everyday activities. Returning to work is clearly a desirable goal, but in fact, only about 50 percent of patients who undergo comprehensive multidisciplinary pain rehabilitation are able to return to work.[6]

## What Is Breakthrough Pain?

We define chronic pain as pain that has lasted for more than a few months and has outlived its usefulness. But this doesn't mean that the pain is the same 24/7. Most people with chronic pain experience good times and bad times. Sometimes you can predict when the pain will get worse—if you suddenly increase your physical activity, or when it rains, or if you twist or turn a certain way. At other times, you may not have a clue as to why you're hurting so much more at that moment. The medications that you take for your chronic pain may not be enough for those times when you have additional, or *breakthrough*, pain. It's helpful for many chronic pain patients to have a plan of action for dealing with breakthrough pain—to lie down, use a heating pad, or have available a fast-acting pain medication.

## Chronic Pain: Nociceptive Versus Neuropathic

*My knees gradually ached more and more. It wasn't too bad in the morning, although they were pretty stiff when I first got up, but as the day progressed my knees would develop a deep ache that made it hard for me to walk. With each step I'd feel them grinding as though the bone was rubbing against bone. It got so that I avoided low chairs because I couldn't get up from them without help.*

—RUTHANN

*When the rash and blisters on the right side of my chest resolved I thought I was finished with the shingles I'd had for three weeks. Turns out that was only the beginning of my troubles! Although my skin now looked normal, I had a burning stinging pain in the area of the rash. Not only that, but even the slightest touch was excruciating. I gave up wearing a bra, and could only wear large shirts which barely touched my skin. The pain went on for months.*

—JOAN

Different types of pain have different treatments, so if you're going to be an educated consumer, you need to have an understanding of the two major types of chronic pain. *Nociceptive* pain and *neuropathic* pain originate in different structures in the body. Nociceptive pain arises from injury to muscles, tendons, and ligaments (somatic pain) or in the internal organs (visceral pain). Nerve cells called nociceptors transmit information about the pain via electrical and chemical signals to the spinal cord, from which it travels up to the brain. The quality of nociceptive pain is described as deep and throbbing. In nociceptive (also called somatic) pain, undamaged nerve fibers are responding to an injurious stimulus outside of themselves. Somatic pain is usually fairly well localized, whereas visceral pain is more diffuse. Examples of chronic nociceptive pain are chronic low back pain, osteoarthritis, rheumatoid arthritis, fibromyalgia, osteomyelitis (chronic bone infection), headaches, interstitial cystitis, or chronic pelvic pain. Interstitial cystitis and chronic pelvic pain are examples of visceral pain (a second type of nociceptive pain), which comes from the internal organs and is more diffuse and less localized than pain in muscles or joints.

The second type of pain—neuropathic pain—results from abnormal nerve function or direct damage to a nerve. Nerves are cells that transmit information from one part of the body to another by means of chemicals and electric current. Nerves in the brain and spinal cord constitute the *central nervous system*, whereas nerves in the arms, legs, and the rest of the body are the *peripheral nervous system*. Pain-detecting nerves (nociceptors) in the periphery can suffer direct damage, resulting in peripheral neuropathic pain. The brain itself has no nociceptors. When the brain is injured, for example by a stroke, pain results from disruption in the processing of pain-related information. This type of pain is called *central neuropathic pain*. The following are examples of neuropathic pain.

## PERIPHERAL NEUROPATHIC PAIN
- Post-herpetic neuralgia (shingles)
- Peripheral diabetic neuropathy
- Complex regional pain syndrome (reflex sympathetic dystrophy [RSD])
- Tic douloureux (trigeminal neuralgia)
- Phantom limb pain
- Carpal tunnel syndrome
- Alcoholic polyneuropathy
- Radiculopathy (cervical[neck], lumbosacral [low back])

## CENTRAL NEUROPATHIC PAIN
- Nerve compression from spinal stenosis
- Multiple sclerosis–related pain
- Parkinson's disease–related pain
- Post-stroke pain
- Posttraumatic spinal cord injury pain

Nerve fibers that have been damaged by injury or disease can fire (discharge) spontaneously, both at the site of the injury and at other places along the nerve pathway. Automatic firing can continue indefinitely, resulting in chronic pain, even after the source of injury has stopped sending pain messages. Automatic firing can result in a feeling of pain in a part of the body that is numb or even missing (as in phantom limb pain).

Neuropathic pain can be constant or intermittent, burning, aching, shooting, or stabbing (like a knife or a needle), and it sometimes radiates down the arms or legs. Most patients have both—a constant burning pain plus a shooting or electric shocklike intermittent pain. In neuropathic pain, the damaged nerves react abnormally. For this reason, neuropathic pain, more than nociceptive pain, has a tendency to involve exaggerated responses to painful stimuli (hyperalgesia), spread of pain to areas that were not initially painful, and sensations of pain in response to normally nonpainful stimuli such as light touch (allodynia). It also involves abnormal sensations such as tingling, pins and needles, and intense itching.

Neuropathic pain is often worse at night. Its location is often characteristic, as it follows nerve pathways. This is why some neuropathic pain syndromes can be diagnosed just from their location. For example, pain that goes in a band that stretches from one side of the abdomen to the middle of the back is most likely postherpetic neuralgia, especially if it was preceded by a rash involving the same area.

Some pain syndromes can have elements of both types of pain. For example, when a pinched nerve causes back pain that radiates down the leg ("sciatica") you are likely to be experiencing both somatic and neuropathic pain.

The value of identifying the category of pain is that in addition to the usual analgesics, neuropathic pain can also be alleviated by groups of drugs that are usually used for other medical problems.

A group of pain specialists recently came up with a list of recommended first-line medications for neuropathic pain.[7] These are gabapentin (Neurontin), an anticonvulsant used originally for seizure disorders; a 5-percent lidocaine (a local anesthetic) patch (Lidoderm); opioid (narcotic) painkillers; tramadol (Ultram, a narcoticlike painkiller); and tricyclic antidepressants, which used to be the primary treatment for depression but have since been replaced by newer drugs. Tricyclic antidepressants have an analgesic effect that is separate from their antidepressant action. Neuropathic pain, like nociceptive pain, can also be treated effectively with narcotics (opioids). Chapter 4 will discuss in detail the various medications that are useful for chronic pain.

Although painkillers derived from opium are commonly referred to as "narcotics," this term has become associated with drug abuse. For medical use, opium derivatives are termed *opiates*. Synthetic or semi-synthetic drugs that have opiumlike structures are termed *opioids*. The term opioids commonly refers to all drugs, whether natural or synthetic, that act like morphine. This subject is discussed more fully in chapter 5.

## Common Chronic Pain Syndromes

Although this is not a comprehensive textbook of different types of chronic pain, below are brief descriptions of some of the most common syndromes seen in a chronic pain practice.

CHRONIC LOW BACK PAIN. Chronic low back pain often results from a combination of contributing factors and is the most common chronic pain in the United States, affecting some 60 percent of adults during their lifetime.[8] Treating back pain costs Americans 26 billion dollars a year, and that's not including lost wages.[9]

Back pain has several causes, related to the back's various structures. Some of these causes are listed below.
- Ligaments: strain
- Cartilage: degeneration of an intervertebral disk
- Nerves: compression of a spinal nerve or nerve root
- Bone: compression fracture of vertebral body due to osteoporosis or trauma

- Joints: degenerative joint disease (DJD) of spine, causing bone over-growth, resulting in spinal stenosis; DJD of the hip; sacroiliac joint disease
- Muscles: fibromyalgia, myofascial pain syndrome, piriformis muscle strain
- Other spinal cord infection, herpes zoster (shingles), cancer

The most common causes of back pain are muscle and ligament strains and arthritic changes in the spine. If nerve roots in the spine are compressed, the pain can radiate down the legs. Although a person can develop back pain at any time, it is most likely to begin in people age 30 to 50, and it is the most common cause of work-related disability in people younger than 45. Unfortunately, in most cases it's not possible to say why a person's back hurts. About 85 percent of people can't be given a precise anatomic diagnosis.[10] People with back pain often have normal X-rays and other imaging studies, whereas people with abnormal CT scans or MRIs often have no symptoms. In a well-known study, 50 percent of people *without* back pain had abnormal CT scans of the back, which showed such diagnoses as herniated discs, facet degeneration, and spinal stenosis.[11]

Fortunately, most people who have nonspecific back pain improve rapidly, with or without medical treatment. The symptoms resolve in one-third of patients in less than one month, in one-third at one to five months, and the rest in six months or longer.[12] Low back pain is also likely to recur. After the initial resolution, the symptoms are likely to return in 70 to 90 percent of cases.[13] In other words, most patients with significant back pain have a chronic relapsing disorder.

In people whose back pain begins past the age of 65, other diagnostic possibilities need to be checked out. Spinal stenosis (nerve compression secondary to abnormal bone growth related to DJD [osteoarthritis]), compression fractures of the spine (usually secondary to osteoporosis [bone thinning]), aortic aneurysms (ballooning of the aorta due to arteriosclerosis), and cancer are possible causes in senior citizens.

As for the best treatment for nonspecific back pain without neurologic symptoms, such as numbness and tingling in the leg, this is often very uncertain. Studies have shown that patients who continue with their usual activities do at least as well as those who spend days in bed. Usually an exercise program, stretching exercises, an anti-inflammatory drug, and maybe a muscle relaxer may suffice. If not, then steroid injections into the back and/or strong painkillers can help. Surgery is a last resort and, even then, sometimes the pain recurs. In difficult, recurring cases, a formal program of several weeks of training in strength, flexibility, and endurance can improve the person's functioning even if the pain is not fully eliminated. Studies have shown that intensive exercise decreases pain and improves function in patients with chronic pain. For people with recurring back pain, studies have also shown that exercise programs that combine aerobic conditioning with specific strengthening exercises for the back and legs can decrease the frequency of recurrence of low back pain.

OSTEOARTHRITIS. Osteoarthritis (OA), wear and tear of the joints, is the most common joint disease in the world. By age 75, 85 percent of Americans have symptoms and/or X-ray abnormalities of OA.[14] People with OA have pain in their joints, which typically worsens with weight bearing and movement, and which improves with rest. They also have morning stiffness and gelling of the involved joint after periods of inactivity. On examination, the affected joints are often tender, the bones are enlarged, the knees crackle when they move (crepitus), and joint motion may be limited.

Osteoarthritis is primarily a disease of cartilage. It usually affects the fingers, base of the thumb, knees, hips, neck, and lower back. You are more likely to develop OA if you have a previous joint injury, overuse, obesity, weakness in supporting muscles, congenital bone abnormalities (for example, hip dysplasia), or a family history of OA. Most people older than 65 have some X-ray signs of OA, but many of them have no symptoms. About 60 percent of people who are older than 60 but have no back pain have degeneration of their lumbar spine shown on MRI scanning.[15] The main treatments are weight loss (especially for OA of the knees), physical therapy, exercise, and drugs for pain relief, primarily anti-inflammatory drugs (NSAIDs) and acetaminophen. Surgery and local injections in the knee are additional options.

RHEUMATOID ARTHRITIS. Between 1 and 3 percent of Americans have rheumatoid arthritis (RA), which is an autoimmune disease primarily affecting the small joints of the hands, wrists, ankles, and feet, although other joints can be involved. It also frequently affects the skin, eyes, lungs, heart, and other organs. Although the cause is not known, what is clear is that the immune system attacks the body, causing inflammation and destruction. Unlike osteoarthritis, in which the primary goal is pain management, treatment for RA focuses on early aggressive therapy with multiple drugs, with the goal of preventing or minimizing damage. Pain medications include NSAIDs, which serve a dual role of relieving pain and reducing inflammation, acetaminophen, tramadol (Ultram), steroids, and opioids. Local injections, physical therapy, and surgery are other options.

FIBROMYALGIA. One of the questions physicians most frequently ask about the use of strong painkillers in chronic pain management is, "Do you treat fibromyalgia with opioids?" What they're really saying is, "I'm not sure that fibromyalgia is real, so I'm uncomfortable prescribing strong painkillers for it." Of all the chronic pain conditions that make physicians uncomfortable, fibromyalgia (FM) probably heads the list. The reason is that it's so poorly understood, and physicians are understandably happier to treat diseases we understand. Even more troubling is that patients with FM often also have sleep problems, irritable bowel syndrome, chemical sensitivities, headaches, fatigue, and depression. It's hard for doctors to figure out what came first, what is physical, what is psychological, and what is "real" and what isn't.

Fibromyalgia affects about 2 percent of the U.S. population, and is about seven times as prevalent in women than men. The American College of Rheumatology lists criteria for FM, which include a history of widespread pain of at least three months' duration and pain in at least 11 of 18 sites that are tender to palpation (touch). The cause of FM is an active subject of research. People with FM have lower pain thresholds than individuals without this disorder. They experience pain on palpation at multiple sites (and not only at the classic fibromyalgia tender points), whereas people without FM do not experience these pain sensations. This is true of children with FM as well as adults. In experimental studies, people with FM have been found to be significantly more sensitive to heat pain than are the people in the control groups.[16] It appears that one underlying cause of FM is increased pain sensitivity.

Fibromyalgia patients may also have qualitative differences in their pain perception. There is also some evidence that patients with FM have abnormal activity of their sympathetic nervous system, and that they have abnormalities in their autonomic nervous system (which regulates sleep, breathing, temperature, and automatic body functions). New drugs based on these presumed causes are being tried, and success with some drugs has been reported.

But even though the cause of FM has not yet been clarified, what is clear is that fibromyalgia patients are truly in pain, that many were highly functioning people before fibromyalgia took over their bodies, and that they are not benefiting from having their many symptoms.

Fibromyalgia patients seem to process pain signals differently from people without FM. The FM patients experience pain from stimuli that would not be painful to others. That is, they have *hyperalgesia*. When people with FM immersed a hand in an ice-water bath to test their pain tolerance, they pulled out their hand significantly earlier than non-FM patients, showing they have a lower pain tolerance. Their brain and spinal cord may be more reactive to pain stimuli; that is, they demonstrate *central sensitization*. This phenomenon in fibromyalgia patients may result from prior chronic pain. Most FM patients have had some injury, work-related pain, or other painful condition such as rheumatoid arthritis, low back pain, systemic lupus erythematosis, and osteoarthritis. Persons who are destined to develop fibromyalgia appear to be either genetically predisposed or have had events or experiences that favor its development. These findings suggest that FM patients may be helped by medications that work on the brain, such as tricyclic antidepressants and opioids. This study doesn't suggest a cure for FM, but it does provide evidence that FM is indeed a type of nerve disorder.

MIGRAINE  HEADACHES—NEUROVASCULAR  DISORDER.  Migraine headaches, which affect about 12 percent of the general population of the United States, usually consist of severe headaches on one side of the head, often accompanied by nausea and vomiting, sensitivity to light and sound, sinus stuffiness, and sometimes neck-muscle pain. In about 20 percent of migraine patients, the headaches are preceded by an aura, which usually consists of such visual changes as zigzag lines. Migraines also tend to run in families. Doctors used to think that migraines were caused by vascular abnormalities—that is, by blood vessels in the brain that would first constrict, then dilate (widen). But migraines are now believed to be caused by a neurological event in the brain stem, the base of the brain. The nerves and blood vessels in the brain then interact to cause pain.[17] Migraine patients have elevated levels of a neuropeptide (a small molecule) termed calcitonin gene–related peptide (CGRP) that is normally found in certain nerve cells in the brain. This chemical is a potent dilator of blood vessels in the brain and its surrounding membrane. When the nerves are activated, this chemical is released, causing inflammation, widening of the blood vessels, and pain. Scientists have synthesized an antagonist of CGRP and have shown that it is an effective and well-tolerated treatment for migraine headaches.[18] The drug is still in the research phase, but may eventually result in a whole new class of useful migraine drugs.

POST-HERPETIC NEURALGIA. Herpes zoster, commonly known as shingles, is a painful rash caused by varicella zoster, the same virus that causes chicken pox. It is easy to recognize because it affects only one side of the body, involving the skin overlying one or more nerves, most often on the trunk or the face. The rash and pain usually resolve after two to four weeks, but about 9 to 34 percent of patients then develop post-herpetic neuralgia, a severe, ongoing neuropathic pain condition. The herpes zoster virus lives in nociceptor nerve cells. As you get older and your T-cell immunity declines, or if you are immunosuppressed because of illness or medications, the virus increases its production and produces the zoster rash. The virus damages not only the peripheral nerve underlying the skin, but also the section of the nerve that travels through the spinal cord and into the central nervous system. The nerve damage is the cause of the pain.

Current effective treatments include a lidocaine patch and the anti-seizure drugs gabapentin (Neurontin) and carbamazepine (Tegretol). Tricyclic antidepressants and opioids are also commonly used (see chapters 4 and 5).

## Assessing Chronic Pain

Until recently, in hospitals, nursing homes, and other health-care organizations, pain assessment and management took second place to disease management. That changed in the year 2000 when the Joint Commission on Accreditation of Health Care Organizations (JCAHO) published guidelines for assessment and management of both acute and chronic pain.[19] To maintain their accreditation, hospitals and other health-care organizations must adhere to these guidelines. The guidelines include making pain the "Fifth Vital Sign," which must be regularly assessed, along with your pulse and blood pressure, temperature, and respiratory rate.

The main goal of treating acute pain is to diagnose and treat the cause. Alleviating the pain is secondary. It's very different with chronic pain. A workup for the cause is clearly necessary, but it may be very time-consuming and often nonproductive. Sometimes the cause is obvious, at other times there may never be a clear answer. At some point it makes no sense to continue prescribing more tests. A more effective approach is to consider the chronic pain a primary disorder in itself, and to consider relieving the pain (rather than diagnosing its cause) as the main goal. A second important goal of chronic pain treatment is to improve function. This means being able to do physical things you could not do before, such as walking the dog, puttering about in the garden, having sex, or returning to work.

Assessment of chronic pain is difficult. The physical exam, lab tests, and imaging studies such as X-rays, CT scans, and MRIs often do not correlate with the patient's symptoms. A few years ago I had so much pain in my right thumb that I could no longer lift a glass. When it became severe enough that I couldn't even write prescriptions, it was time for a workup. X-rays showed severe osteoarthritis of the thumb, a very common area of osteoarthritis in middle-aged women. My left thumb looked even worse than the right on the X-rays, but interestingly, I had no pain in my left thumb. Undoubtedly this is because I'm right-handed, so that for years I'd stressed the right hand but not the left. In the four years since I had surgery on the right thumb, I have continued to have no pain in the left. Two years ago, I mysteriously fractured my femur (thigh bone) without an injury. It turned out I'd been walking around for two months with an undiagnosed stress fracture of the middle of the largest bone in the body. Then one day, when I stepped hard on that leg while in a moving subway train, the bone shattered. When I first arrived in the hospital, the doctors thought I must have had some abnormal weakness in the bone, probably due to cancer. I had CT scans done from head to toe, in search of an undiagnosed malignancy (fortunately, none was found, and we never figured out how I got the stress fracture in the first place). The CT of my low back showed severe osteoarthritis, but I rarely have back pain.

The opposite situation is equally common. Many people have severe back pain but unimpressive back X-rays or CT scans, and patients with migraine headaches have normal imaging studies of their head. Fibromyalgia patients appear normal on all the usual tests, yet their muscle aches can incapacitate them. Neuropathic pain is notoriously difficult to "see" on testing, and patients with chronic pelvic pain usually have not only normal CT scans, but also normal laparoscopic exams. Yet the pain is real.

This is why the gold standard for assessing chronic pain is the patient's word. Pain management physicians are taught to believe the patient, unless we have reason not to. A good way to convey an idea of how severe the pain is is to grade it on a scale of 0 to 10. Imagine the worst pain you've ever had, or could imaging having, and assign that pain the number 10. Then think about the pain you're having now, and assign it a number. If it's mild, it might be a 2 or 3; if moderately severe, a 7 or 8.

Another aspect of assessing pain is to look at its effects on your life. What was your life like before you had your chronic pain? What are you still able to do? What parts of your life have you had to give up?

When you think about what your life might be like if your pain were relieved, what would you do again? It helps to have some goals for yourself, but recognize that complete relief of your pain is usually not an attainable goal. A more realistic goal might be "to get enough pain relief that I can return to work," ". . . walk my dog again," ". . . get on a plane and visit my parents."

The next chapter will describe how pain signals are transmitted from the source of pain to the brain, how the brain responds, what mechanisms the body has for fighting pain, and what factors can either alleviate or worsen your pain.

# 2

# THE CAUSES
# OF CHRONIC PAIN

## *Why It Happens*

ONSIDER THE FOLLOWING SCENARIO: YOU ARE in the kitchen preparing a salad, and suddenly your hand slips and the sharp knife you are holding slices your thumb. Your hand will pull itself away from the knife blade even before you are aware of the pain. You will "feel" the sensation of pain very quickly, but by the time you look at your finger it will probably already be bleeding. The mechanism of this straightforward pain event is well understood.

### *An Introduction to the Body's Pain Processing System*

Very few physicians understand how the body's pain processing system works because much of what is known has been only recently discovered. If you find it difficult to understand or remember the explanation below, don't worry—just recognize how complex the process is, how amazingly well it functions in the human body, and how many mechanisms the body has for influencing your final pain experience.

Step one in pain transmission is the *nociceptive* (pain-producing) event, which in the above case is the injury induced by the knife cutting your thumb. There are specialized receptors (nerves called *nociceptors)* in the thumb and throughout your body that recognize heat, cold, pressure, and pain. When stimulated, these receptors send electrical signals to the part of the spinal cord called the *dorsal horn*. (See Figure 1.) There the signals are *modulated*, meaning acted upon and either increased or decreased in intensity. They then race upward to the brain, which responds with an instant command to jerk away your hand and recognition that your thumb hurts. The brain also triggers the release of the body's own painkillers.

Pain signals between the body and the brain are of two types—chemical and electrical. Tissue injuries trigger the release of chemicals that give rise to an inflammatory reaction at the site of injury. The inflammation produces other chemicals, such as prostaglandins, which cause nearby sensory neurons termed *C-fiber nociceptors* to fire. These neurons fire not only in response to chemicals but also in response to mechanical stretching or compression. Activation of the C-fiber nociceptors triggers electrical pain signals that travel relatively slowly along the nerve fibers to other neurons in the dorsal horn of the spinal cord. From the dorsal horn, the pain signal is transmitted via a nerve pathway called the *spinothalamic tract* to the cerebral cortex of the brain. There it is analyzed, processed, and acted upon. Interestingly, the signals end up in two different areas of the brain—one that is involved with the sensation

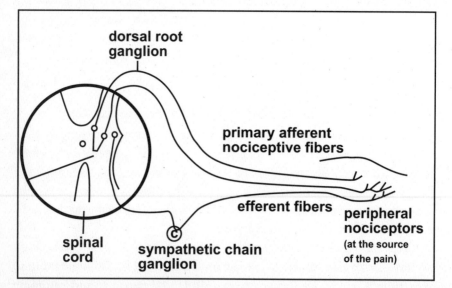

**Figure 1.** *Nociceptive nerve fibers. Pain pathway between source of pain and spinal cord.*

of pain, and the other with the emotional response to pain. The *somatosensory* cortex and associated areas mediate the sensory aspects of pain, whereas the *ventral medial nucleus* of the hippocampus and the central nucleus of the amygdala are brain regions involved in the affective (feeling) response to pain. The responses to the incoming (afferent) pain signals travel downward through the midbrain *periaqueductal gray,* which modulates the descending (efferent) impulses that result in pain and suffering. In other words, the pain and suffering you experience in response to an injury depend on input from many parts of the nervous system, not just the initial injury.

Tissue damage, inflammation, or injury to the nervous system can modify (modulate) the response of the nociceptor nerves. For example, when they are repeatedly stimulated, sensory fibers that normally transmit only messages of "light touch," can begin to send out signals that cry "pain!" The original injury may have healed, but to you it feels like the pain is continuing. What has happened is that your central nervous system (CNS) has become more excitable. Non-painful stimuli have become painful. People who have migraine headaches experience this when they complain of scalp or muscle pain during the headaches. Hypersensitivity explains why people with irritable bowel syndrome feel pain from normally painless stretching of the intestines during digestion, and why people with myofascial pain or fibromyalgia complain of diffuse muscle aches.

To add to the complexity of the body's processing of pain, our pain-producing (nociceptive) system is balanced by an equally complex antinociceptive (pain-relieving) system. Pain signals arriving from peripheral tissues stimulate the release of the body's own pain-relieving morphinelike chemicals: *endorphins* in the periaqueductal gray matter of the brain, and *enkephalins* in the *nucleus raphe magnus* (one of the identifiable structures) of the brainstem. Endorphins and enkephalins bind to the same receptors in the periphery and in the dorsal horn of the spinal cord, releasing chemicals that dampen pain signals. The effect is similar to what happens when you take a pill or shot of morphine, but the pain-relieving chemicals are produced by your own body.

Notice that the entire process involves both incoming (afferent) signals, which go up to the brain from the periphery, and outgoing (efferent) signals, those that travel downward from the brain to the spinal cord and the periphery. Pain signals can also be modulated at several places along the way. One of the most important discoveries about the modulation of pain signals was made by two researchers in 1965.[1] They described a spinal cord mechanism that regulated the transmission of pain sensations between the periphery and the brain. Their "gate control" model offered the possibility of various interventions to decrease pain. For example, transcutaneous (through the skin) electrical nerve stimulation (TENS), sends mild electric shocks that stimulate the large sensory fibers in the spinal cord by means of pads applied to painful areas in the back or other places. Transmission of impulses by those fibers competes with pain signals going up to the brain, closing the gate. Acupuncture and rubbing may work similarly. These manipulations may also work by stimulating the production of the body's endorphins.

The natural pain-relieving system may be as important to normal functioning as the pain-signaling system. Because of it, minor injuries such as a cut finger or stubbed toe make us upset and dysfunctional for only a few minutes—not for days, as might be if the pain persisted until the injury completely healed.

What happens if the pain-relieving (antinociceptive) system doesn't function normally? It's been suggested that this is exactly what happens in people with fibromyalgia. Recent studies show that people with fibromyalgia have altered pain processing in the spinal cord and a decreased ability to inhibit pain signals from going down from the brain. Their descending pain-inhibitory pathways have become impaired.

## The Causes of Chronic Pain

To summarize the above discussion, it is now clear that chronic pain is not just a prolonged version of acute pain. As pain signals are repeatedly generated, nerve pathways undergo changes that make them hypersensitive to the pain signals and resistant to the body's pain-relieving mechanisms. Like a painful memory, the abnormal processing can persist in the spinal cord.

Chronic pain often begins with an injury that causes inflammation, but persists after the original injury has healed. For some reason, the nervous system continues to send pain signals to muscles as though the original injury was still present. In chronic pain, a temporary peripheral injury results in permanent changes in the spine and the brain. These changes include:

- *allodynia*—normally such non-painful simuli as touch or vibration are perceived as pain.
- widening of the painful area so that areas that were not inner-vated (stimulated) by the originally injured nerve transmit pain signals.
- *hyperalgesia*—a lowered pain threshold, so that a mild pain stimulus is perceived as severe pain.

The ability of the nervous system to permanently change in response to ongoing pain signals is called *neuronal plasticity*, and this characteristic of the nervous system helps explain how pain can persist long after any cause is identified or even treated. These changes are more likely to occur in the presence of undertreated pain. When peripheral pain nerves are repeatedly activated, there is a progressive buildup of electrical impulses in the dorsal horn, with resulting increases of the intensity of the pain messages sent to the brain. This phenomenon is referred to as *windup*. The windup phe-nomenon may explain how persistent stimulation of peripheral nerves can lead to upregulation (increased reactivity to pain stimuli) of the CNS, resulting in hyperalgesia, allodynia, and persistent pain.

## A Bad Player in the Alphabet Soup of Pain: NMDA

So far we haven't discussed the nature of the "words" by which nerve cells communicate. These are chemicals called *neurotransmitters*. The main neurotransmitter used by nociceptor nerve cells to transmit messages to the dorsal horn of the spinal cord is *glutamate*. This chemical is released by the nociceptor at its boundary (synapse) with the dorsal horn cells. Glutamate can bind to several different classes of receptors, like a key fitting into a lock. When a key fits the lock, it can open a door. When a neurotransmitter such as glutamate binds to a receptor on the surface of a neuron in the dorsal horn, that cell is then activated to release other chemicals and to send electrical pain signals upward through the spinal cord to various parts of the brain. (See Figure 2 on page 21.)

Following an injury, glutamate binds primarily to AMPA (alpha-amino-3-hydroxy-5-methyl-isoxazole-4-propionic acid) receptors in the dorsal horn. When AMPA receptors in the spinal cord are repeatedly activated by large quantities of glutamate, they expose another set of receptors that are involved in chronic pain. When this second type of receptor, NMDA (N-methyl-D-aspartate) receptors, are activated by glutamate, they begin the process of hypersensitization of the central nervous system (CNS). The onset of hypersensitization marks the transition from acute to chronic pain. A further effect of NMDA receptor activation is that it causes nociceptors to release another neurotransmitter, *substance P*, which further amplifies the pain signal.

All you need to remember is that stimulation of NMDA receptors is undesirable, because it increases pain perception. Activation of NMDA receptors causes spinal neurons carrying pain to be stimulated by reduced amounts of pain (a phenomenon known as windup), less glutamate to be required to transmit the pain signal, and more pain-relieving medication to be required to stop it. Endorphins and other natural painkillers can't keep up with the demand, and lose their effectiveness. So do opioids at the usually prescribed dosage.

The cascade of pain-increasing steps can be stopped at various stages. Chapter 4 will describe various types of pain medications, but the following are a few other possibilities.

## Interconnections: "The Thigh Bone's Connected to the Knee Bone . . . "

Now that you have some understanding of the interconnectedness of the biochemical and neurologic pathways that affect pain perception, let's look at the big picture—the interconnectedness of the body and how it affects pain.

After I broke my femur (thigh bone) in the New York subway some years ago, I was hospitalized, had surgery, and lay on my back for two weeks. I was then sent to physical therapy for the leg, but I was unable to participate at first because of severe back pain. Understand, I had not injured my back, but the two weeks of lying in bed had so deconditioned my back muscles that just standing was painful. Eventually, I overcame the weakened back, but then came another problem. When I walked with my newly acquired walker, my gait was abnormal. I held my body differently, trying to protect the injured leg. This stressed new muscles, causing added back pain. Throughout my recovery, my worst problem was my back! Added to this was the emotional depression over the difference between my formerly active life and my current pain and disability. Depression worsens pain. Also, I used to sleep soundly and restfully. But my body was hurting too much to turn, sleep was hard in coming, and I awakened frequently. Disturbed sleep also increases pain.

It is easy to see how chronic pain originating in one part of the body can spread to others and can worsen, all in the absence of original injury to those other parts. It is also easy to see why

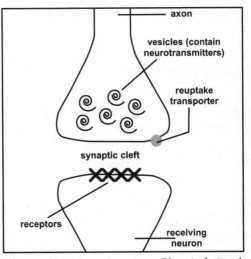

**Figure 2.** *Nerve junction. Chemical signals (neurotransmitters) travel across the synaptic cleft and are taken up by the receptors on the receiving neuron.*

chronic pain management is not just pills and needles; it's equally important to pay attention to your body mechanics, your sleep, and your emotional state.

## What About the Role of Muscles?

As you know, muscles surround and provide a protective framework for deeper structures in the body. When an injury occurs, the surrounding muscles, whether or not they themselves were injured, tend to tighten and go into spasm to protect the injured part. Unfortunately, their response can become a part of the problem.

Almost 30 years ago, speaking at the First World Congress on Pain, Dr. Janet Travell explained the role of muscles in chronic pain:

... Chronic painful states of obscure causes often depend on feedback cycles from myofascial trigger points .... Symptoms long outlast precipitating events, owing to perseverating [ongoing] reflex patterns and continuing mechanical stresses on affected somatic structures. When injured, most tissues heal, but skeletal muscles "learn"; they readily develop habits of guarding that limit movement and impair circulation. Chronic pain, stiffness, and dysfunction of muscles result.[2]

This is why physical therapy and exercises are such an important part of recovering from most pain syndromes.

## Other Factors that Affect Pain

Pain begins with a physical stimulus which, as we have seen, is processed through a complex neurological and biochemical system in the body. But there are numerous other factors that influence how we experience and respond to pain. Pain can be decreased or increased by a number of factors, both innate—gender, age, and temperament—and situational—emotional state, previous experience with pain, context or meaning of the pain, the presence of drugs (prescribed or recreational) in the body, and the doctor's and patient's attitudes about pain and its treatment. This section describes the influence of some of these factors.

A study of the effects of gender and age on how patients are medicated for pain after surgery found that women were given pain medications less frequently than men. Doctors and nurses saw women as prone to exaggerating their pain complaints. Both men and women younger than age 61 received more frequent pain medication than their elders; younger men were medicated more frequently, and older women least frequently.[3] You might wonder, "Do women and older people receive fewer pain medications because of prejudice, or do age and gender actually influence the perception of pain?" Let's address these two factors separately.

## Gender and Hormones

Women are more likely than men to have several chronic pain conditions, including migraine and tension headaches, temporomandibular joint (TMJ) disorders, fibromyalgia, and irritable bowel syndrome. In the United States, women visit their physicians more often than men. There are several reasons for this, including cultural expectations. For example, men are afraid of being perceived as whiners and tend to endure more pain before consulting a physician. Until recently, this was believed to be the primary reason for the gender difference in utilization of medical care. Men and women were assumed to respond similarly to treatments, and most studies of new treatments used only men as subjects, to make the patient population more uniform.

In recent years, however, it has become apparent that men and women differ in their physiology (the body's functions and processes) in some ways. New studies have found differences when comparing men and women's responses. In the area of pain perception, for example, women have lower pain thresholds and lower pain tolerance than men.[4] The pain threshold is the point at which a stimulus is experienced as painful. Pain tolerance is the point at which the pain becomes intolerable. For a given pain stimulus, women feel pain sooner than men, and they can tolerate a smaller amount of pain. It isn't just that women report more pain. Studies of the involuntary pain responses, such as pain-related muscle reflexes, dilation of the pupil of the eye, and brain responses, have shown that women are actually more sensitive to pain. Women also experience windup pain sooner than men.[5] This was shown in a study in which healthy young volunteers had a hot probe of increasing temperature repeatedly touch their skin. The women had a significantly lower pain threshold and pain tolerance to the repeated stimuli, but not to a single, discrete stimulus. Positron-emission tomography (PET) scans were also done of young healthy men and women who were subjected to the same painful stimulus (an injection of saline [salt solution] into a muscle), and their degree of opioid receptor activation was determined. The activation of opioid receptors works to relieve pain. The men showed relatively greater opioid system activation in several brain regions believed to be involved in pain control (that is, anterior thalamus, ventral basal ganglia, and amygdala), indicating that men obtain greater pain relief than women.[6] Many research studies have confirmed gender differences in responsiveness to various pain medications including clonidine, morphine, and oxycodone.[7] One exception to this bad news for women is that in contrast to their poorer pain relief from pure opioids, in response to opioids that are mixed agonist-antagonists, such as butorphanol (Stadol), pentazocine (Talwin), and buprenorphine (see Chapter 5, Opioids), women get significantly better pain relief than men.[8]

These differences are probably in large part due to the differences in sex hormones of males and females. In support of the role of female hormones is the finding that postmenopausal women on hormone replacement therapy (HRT) had lower pain thresholds (that is, they experienced more pain with smaller stimuli) than did women who were *not* on HRT; men also had higher pain thresholds than women on HRT.[9] Along the same lines, women with fibromyalgia who are still menstruating have increased pain during the last days of each cycle, a time when progesterone levels are high.[10]

As to the pattern of pain during the menstrual cycle, most studies have shown the greatest sensitivity to painful stimuli during the luteal phase—that is, just before menstruation, when hormone levels are high.[11] This is particularly true with migraine headaches. About 60 percent of women with migraine headaches experience worsening of headaches around the time of menstruation;[12] about 6 percent of women with migraine have headaches *only* at the time of menstruation. The most likely cause of menstrual migraines is a drop in estrogen levels. As these levels fall, levels of serotonin, a neurotransmitter that stabilizes pain receptors in the brain, also decline. At the same time, the levels of endorphins in the brain also drop.

Another reason why women experience more pain than men may be their greater prevalence of anxiety and depression. Both of these psychological problems are associated with increased pain and other physical symptoms. Interestingly, however, in a recent population survey of pain and depression in 70-year-olds living in the community (that is, not living in nursing homes), although a higher percentage of the women had pain than did men (79 percent versus 53 percent), men with pain were more likely to also have depression than women with pain.[13] The authors of the study point out that both physical illness and pain can contribute to loss of autonomy, and they speculate that the response to such loss may be more pronounced in men. (The association between pain and depression will be discussed in greater detail in chapter 11).

## Children and Pain

Patients at either end of the age spectrum—children and the elderly—are often undertreated for pain because of myths about how they experience pain. Until recently, children were thought to feel less pain than adults because their nervous system is not fully developed; this was further compounded by the fact that most children have no memory of their early years. Surprisingly, new studies have shown just the opposite—infants and young children most likely experience more pain than adults because children have a more intense inflammatory reaction to pain and less-developed descending neurologic pathways for inhibiting pain signals. Pain

# Types of Studies

IN THIS BOOK, reference is made to several types of published studies. Here are some definitions to help you understand the ways these studies were performed.

*Double-blind study:* Two or more groups of subjects are given different treatments, but neither the patients nor the researchers are told which treatment is being given to which subject. The purpose of this "blinding" is to prevent possible biases caused in assessment by a researcher who knows which treatment is being given, or by a patient who knows which treatment he or she is receiving.

*Meta-analysis:* A study that combines the results of several other published studies of a type of treatment. Its value is that it can report the experiences of a much larger sample of subjects than each separate study.

*Placebo-controlled study:* The group or groups of subjects given the study treatments are compared with a control group that gets a dummy treatment. The reason for this is that people often get better with dummy treatments if they believe they are getting the "real" drug.

*Prospective study:* Subjects are chosen in advance, are given one or another treatment, and then their response to that treatment is studied.

*Randomized study:* Subjects are divided at random into each of the two or more study groups, as opposed to being allowed to choose which group they want to be in. The purpose of this is to make the different groups more comparable.

*Retrospective study:* Subjects are asked about past treatments or experiences, or a series of charts are reviewed. The information is collected and subjected to statistical analysis. The weaknesses of this approach include (1) relying on people's memories (if the study design consists of questionnaires or interviews), and (2) uncertainty about whether groups who received different treatments are comparable.

signals in newborns may reach the baby's brain without modulation, leading to more pronounced pain sensations than in older children and adults.[14]

Compared to an adult, a newborn's nervous system is much more sensitive to such sensory stimuli as touch, heat, and cold. A newborn's nervous system processes pain much differently than an adult's. Repeated or sustained painful and even non-painful stimuli can make them even more sensitive to pain.[15] Earlier in this chapter, the concept of neuronal plasticity, the ability of the nervous system to permanently change in response to ongoing pain signals, was discussed. In young children, the nervous system is still developing and it has even more ability to be permanently altered in response to pain.[16] This is all the more reason that infants and children should be adequately treated for pain. Otherwise they may be at risk for developing chronic pain in later years.

Nonetheless, because they can't easily communicate their pain to adults, children are often under-medicated for such procedures as circumcision or needle sticks in the heel (where blood samples are frequently drawn from infants) which would certainly warrant pain medication in adults. This is particularly true of newborns. In a recent article titled "Do We Still Hurt Newborn Babies?" researchers studied 151 ill newborns admitted to several neonatal intensive care units (NICUs). On average, each baby was subjected to 14 procedures per day, most of them painful (for example, injections, blood draws, insertion of tubes, spinal taps, and so on). Unfortunately, 40 percent of the babies did not receive any pain medication throughout their stay in the NICU.[17]

Even more disturbing is evidence that painful experiences in early childhood can have lasting effects, actually lowering the child's pain tolerance for months after a painful procedure. Compared with newborns who received a local anesthetic when circumcised, those who underwent this procedure without any anesthesia showed more distress four to six months later when they were given routine immunizations.[18] Similarly, children with cancer whose first bone marrow aspiration or spinal tap was done without adequate analgesia later showed more severe distress when they had other similar procedures (this time *with* adequate analgesia) than did children who were given a strong opioid painkiller for the first procedure.[19] Even years later, children who experienced painful procedures in infancy may have increased risk of pain. Adolescents 12 to 18 years of age who were born prematurely had significantly more tender points (assessed with thumb pressure) and lower tender thresholds (as measured by a pressure-producing instrument called a dolorimeter) than did adolescents who were born at full term.[20] The authors of this study concluded that the preterm-born adolescents have higher somatic pain sensitivity and may be prone to developing pain syndromes in the future.

According to a report titled "Current Status of Pain Management in Children" in the *Journal of the American Medical Association (JAMA)* "Pain and its treatment may have consequences beyond the normal period of recovery, and there is a substantial population of children who endure long-term pain and would benefit from better access to pain management."[21] This population includes children with such well-understood diseases as juvenile rheumatoid arthritis or sickle cell anemia. Recurrent headaches are common in adolescents. Many children have chronic musculoskeletal pain or abdominal pain that is poorly understood, and others have other "idiopathic pain syndromes" (pain whose origin is uncertain). Some of these children fully recover, but others go on to develop significant chronic pain and disability.[22] Rather than assuming that most children will outgrow their pain problems, it would make more sense to treat the pain aggressively, with the goal of preventing future chronic pain and physical and emotional disability. There is no reason to avoid painkillers in children. For children with chronic pain, acetaminophen, aspirin, and anti-inflammatory drugs are available. For those with severe chronic pain, sustained-release morphine, oxycodone pills, and transdermal fentanyl patches are useful, as well as methadone elixir or tablets.

## The Elderly and Pain

Up to one-half of community-dwelling (that is, not living in nursing homes) adults more than 65 years of age report pain severe enough to interfere with normal function, and between 60 and 80 percent of nursing home residents have persistent pain.[23] Among 70-year-old men and women living in the community, 79 percent of women and 53 percent of men reported pain within the prior two weeks. Back pain was the most common type of pain in both men and women.[24] This study showed how common pain is in older people. Cancer patients, age 70 and older, were reported less likely to receive adequate outpatient pain relief than a younger group of patients.[25] Elderly people are frequently undertreated for their chronic pain. There are several reasons for this, which include:

- under-reporting of pain by patients, based on their mistaken belief that pain is inevitable with aging.
- concern by patients about the cost or pain of additional tests, or that the pain indicates worsening of some disease.
- the belief by patients and doctors that older people experience less pain.
- cognitive decline in older patients can make it harder for physicians to assess their pain.
- difficulty in diagnosing the cause because older people often have multiple sources of pain.
- concerns by physicians that elderly patients are more sensitive to pain medications (and to all medications in general).

There is no physiological basis for the belief that injury or disease in older people causes less pain than in younger people. Older patients do indeed report less pain intensity and less suffering from their pain; conditions that produce pain in younger people may instead cause confusion, restlessness, aggressiveness, or fatigue in the elderly. The result can be a delay in diagnosis and treatment. Although older adults do perceive less pain, these changes aren't significant enough to reduce the need for pain management.

Patients who can't communicate that they hurt are only half as likely to have pain diagnosed as those who can. Consequently, patients with cognitive impairments (those who have Alzheimer's disease or other forms of dementia) are significantly less likely to be given pain medications than other older patients.[26] This is why if you have a relative who can't describe her pain problems, it's crucial that you or another friend or family member accompany her as an advocate and explain her situation.

## Smoking

Many chronic pain specialists are reluctant to treat smokers with strong pain medications. They believe that smoking makes people more likely to have pain, worsens the intensity of their pain, and makes them less responsive to pain medications. Several epidemiologic studies support a connection between smoking and increased pain. For example, questionnaires about back pain were sent out to a random sample of adults in a British community, and more than 34,000 questionnaires were returned; one-quarter of this group reported having had back pain the previous 12 months. One of the interesting findings was that current smokers were 50 percent more likely to have back pain than were nonsmokers. Among smokers, those who smoked at least 15 cigarettes per day were more likely to have back pain than those who smoked fewer cigarettes.[27] Eight years later, in 2003, another survey involving 13,000 people, showed that current and ex-smokers had higher risks than lifetime nonsmokers for back, neck, and limb pain; the prevalence of pain severe enough to limit activities was 60 percent higher in current smokers.[28]

In another study of a random sample of almost 2,000 people in Sweden, men and women who were current smokers reported increased pain in the low back, neck, and widespread areas. Smokers were 60 percent more likely to have chronic musculoskeletal pain than were nonsmokers. The greater the number of cigarettes smoked, the greater the prevalence of chronic low back pain.[29] A study in Norway found that among 4,490 adults who had chronic musculoskeletal pain, smokers experienced more intense pain than did nonsmokers.[30] All these studies show that smokers are more likely to experience pain than are nonsmokers. This is even true for secondhand smoke! Children with sickle cell disease who are exposed to secondhand tobacco smoke at home are at significantly greater risk for painful sickle cell crises that require hospitalization—more than twice the risk as children not exposed to tobacco smoke at home.[31]

Although the mechanism by which smoking may raise pain levels or lower pain threshold is not clear, it's possible that nicotine affects the way the brain processes pain signals. There are nicotine receptors in the nucleus accumbens of the brain, a region that is involved in addiction and pain relief. An experimental study of laboratory animals also showed that nicotine interacts with the effects of opioids.[32]

Another possible reason why smokers experience more pain is that they deplete their bodily stores of vitamin C faster than nonsmokers. A recently reported study compared pain levels in smoking and nonsmoking men and women who had osteoarthritis of the knee. The highest pain scores were in male smokers, who also had the lowest vitamin C levels in their bodies.[33]

## Genetic Factors

Are you one of those people who seem to be able to tolerate pain better than most people? Or, on the contrary, like the Hans Christian Anderson fairy tale about the princess and the pea, are you aware of even the slightest pain input? You may actually have an array of genes that explain your reaction to pain. Genetic background affects pain sensitivity in animals and may influence susceptibility to the development of persistent pain.[34]

Almost 40 people have been found who have a congenital insensitivity to pain. They can feel pressure, heat and cold, but not pain. They are also unable to sweat. This strange disorder is now known to be caused by an alteration in a single gene.[35] Without the warning signals that pain provides, these unfortunate people are constantly getting injured. Their life is very difficult.

Among a group of people who received morphine after they had a tooth pulled (dental pain is often used for research on pain medications), some were clearly "responders" and others were "non-responders" when given several doses of the painkiller.[36] It is likely that these differences were caused by genetic variation in responsiveness to morphine.

In humans, the mu-opioid system (see box below) becomes activated during pain and acts to reduce the pain and stress response. An enzyme called COMT (catechol-0-methyltransferase) induces activation of the mu-opioid system, which then produces neurotransmitters which relieve pain, lessen anxiety, and dampen the physical responses to pain such as increased heart rate and blood pressure. People with two copies of a variant of the usual COMT gene have diminished ability to produce this enzyme. This results in increased pain and blood pressure compared to the reactions of people with the normal genes.[37]

---

## Mu receptors

MU RECEPTORS are areas in the body that interact with opioids in the same way as do a lock and key. When opioids attach to the mu receptor, pain is relieved. These opioids can be either *exogenous* (introduced into the body from the outside) or *endogenous* (produced by the body itself).

## Trauma History

Adults who have chronic pain syndromes are more likely to report some type of childhood abuse than are people who don't have chronic pain. A number of studies have reported a history of child abuse among patients with fibromyalgia and among adult women with chronic pelvic pain. But in an illuminating study, researchers obtained reports from 1967 to 1971 of 676 children who were physically or sexually abused or neglected, and then interviewed them as young adults (from 1989 to 1995). The children were younger than 11 years old at the time of the court-substantiated abuse or neglect. Compared with non-abused children, the likelihood of any type of chronic pain problem was *not* increased in the abused group compared with the controls. This was also true for the group who'd been sexually abused as children.[38] It seems that although adults with chronic pain report more childhood abuse, this was not confirmed when children with documented abuse were followed up years later.

Most studies of childhood trauma and its effects focus on women. In an interesting retrospective study, 73 adults with chronic pain, 50 percent male and 50 percent female, were given a questionnaire about a history of all types of trauma both in childhood and adulthood. This included not only childhood sexual and physical abuse, but also any other subsequent traumatic events such as being robbed or mugged, experiencing a disaster, or witnessing death. The results showed no correlation between severity of pain or activity level and previous trauma. Moreover, women who'd experienced any type of trauma had no more distress in response to their pain than did women who hadn't. Surprisingly, however, male chronic pain patients who had a trauma history showed more anxiety and depression and more general emotional distress than did men with chronic pain but no trauma history. It appears that men and women differ in the way in which a history of trauma affects their adjustment to pain.

## Weather

Have you ever heard your elderly relative complain that his arthritis pain is acting up so it must be about to rain? Or have you yourself found that your chronic pain is worse when the weather is cold? In Cordoba, Argentina, a city where there are significant weather changes throughout the year, patients with rheumatoid arthritis (RA) and osteoarthritis (OA) kept a record of their daily pain ratings for one year. Patients with both OA and RA reported more pain when the temperature was low and humidity high. In addition, patients with RA had more pain when the barometric pressure was high. However, none of the patient groups were able to predict changes in the weather based on their pain. The results support the belief that weather influences rheumatic pain.[39] Another study found that fibromyalgia patients are more sensitive to cold than to heat.[40] So if you find that the weather affects your pain symptoms, recognize that this is common and try to avoid the most troublesome weather conditions.

## Sleep Disorders

Sleep disorders and pain are closely related. In some disorders, such as fibromyalgia, poor sleep is considered a possible causative factor. At the very least, it worsens fibromyalgia pain. When you have pain of any type, a good night's sleep is harder to attain, and the bad sleep is likely to make you feel more fatigued and achy during the day. Depression, which many people with chronic pain experience, is a major cause of insomnia.

# 3

# DECIDING ON A DOCTOR

## *Working with the Specialist of Your Choice*

HAVE YOU EVER HAD TO VISIT AN EMERGENCY room because of a broken bone, car accident, or sliced finger? It's quite likely that you don't remember much about the doctor who took care of you, other than whether she did a good job. Most likely you never saw that physician again. In that setting, your personal relationship with the emergency room doctor was not all that important. But when dealing with chronic pain, it's a whole other story. Your pain doctor becomes an important part of your life. In a study of treatment of chronic non-cancer pain, Drs. Russell Portenoy and Kathleen Foley concluded that the most important treatment factor contributing to a satisfactory outcome was "the intensive involvement of a single physician."[1] You undoubtedly hope to have such a relationship with a caring, knowledgeable physician.

Yet everyone knows a person whose chronic pain was undertreated. It seems at times that physicians just don't care. It's certainly true that many health care providers don't like treating chronic pain, and that many undertreat it. For example, a survey in 2001 of primary care physicians in California found that only 15 percent liked treating patients with chronic pain, and that 41 percent did not prescribe pain medication unless the patient first asked for it.[2] The same survey of California doctors found that 35 percent of them *never* prescribe Schedule II opioids (that is, potent painkillers such as morphine, oxycodone, or fentanyl) for chronic pain. The main barriers to prescribing painkillers were concerns about physical dependence, tolerance, and addiction to such drugs. This is a shocking finding, as it would be unusual for a primary care physician *not* to have in his or her practice at least several patients who could benefit from such drugs. Even more shocking is that many physicians are uncomfortable using opioids (narcotics) to treat patients with cancer pain, a scenario that is much less controversial than treating non-cancer pain. A survey published in 1993 found that one-third of physicians waited until a cancer patient had six months or less to live before initiating treatment with strong painkillers.[3]

Most physicians who undertreat pain do so not because they are uncaring, but because they are afraid and lack knowledge. Many physicians subscribe to erroneous beliefs about the use of opioids, such as that most patients become addicted to them or that most patients need ever-increasing doses, and many physicians are afraid that prescribing strong painkillers will cost them their license. Some doctors think that "no pain is strong enough to require morphine" or that patients who want strong painkillers are likely to abuse them.

Part of the reason physicians so often fail to appreciate the need to alleviate patients' suffering is that many of them are young and don't have personal experience with pain and suffering, a major loss, illness, or the death of a loved one.[4] Lacking this experience, they can acquire empathy toward the suffering of others only by being actively taught. Unfortunately, little attention is provided in medical education to suffering or caring for the whole person. Physicians are taught to treat the body rather than the person.

But some do care, and those who are knowledgeable about treating pain feel frustrated when they see that patients are getting inadequate pain management. A survey of more than 1,000 members of the American Pain Society and the American Academy of Pain Medicine, two well-known professional associations for pain specialists, found that physicians had less training in the ethical issues of pain management, compared with nurses and psychologists. The respondents expressed the greatest concern about inappropriate pain management, especially at the end of life, closely followed by general undertreatment of pain, and specifically, undertreatment of pain in the elderly and in children. The respondents complained that "both family practitioners and specialists tend to pass their own judgment on patients' pain, undertreat pain, and worse, label some patients with reasonable and justified reasons for having pain as 'addicts.' This label becomes part of the medical record and can be ruinous to patients. Practitioners have a tendency to be very cynical and ignorant in their dealing with patients who have persistent pain problems."[5]

A survey of 1,912 physicians across the United States found significant differences in the prescribing of opioids by various specialties. Rheumatologists reported significantly greater long-term prescribing of opioids than any other specialty group, probably because their practice is largely made up of painful conditions such as osteoarthritis, rheumatoid arthritis, and fibromyalgia.[6] No one specialty was more concerned than others about the side effects of opioids, but there were significant differences among the specialties in their view of the negative effects of tolerance, addiction, and physical dependence on this type of painkiller. The surgeons were the most concerned about these negative effects and were also the most concerned about regulatory pressures. Rheumatologists were the least concerned about these issues.

Very few physicians are truly uncaring, although many are afraid to prescribe strong painkillers. In an article entitled, "Treat Pain, Avert Suicide," Dr. Daniel Brookoff, a Memphis oncologist who also treats non-cancer patients for pain, was quoted to say, "I have had people come to me who have tried to kill themselves because they have unremitting pain that nobody could treat. The people who are in despair have not been appropriately treated for their ailments."[7] Some people do commit suicide because of undertreated pain.

In the Preface, I also spoke of patients who commit suicide because of undertreated pain. Yet pain is not the only cause of patients' suffering. Patients with amyotrophic lateral sclerosis (ALS, or Lou Gehrig's disease) gradually lose all muscle function and often die because they can't move their chest muscles well enough to breathe. A study of ALS patients seeking assisted suicide showed that their motivation in many cases was not pain but rather distress at being a burden to others or suffering from some discomfort other than pain.[8] Insomnia, nausea, depression, loss of hair, disfigurement resulting from surgery, and total dependence on others all can cause suffering.

## Which Professional to Choose?

How, then, do you work with your doctor? First, you need to find an empathetic doctor who's not afraid to care for chronic pain patients. Second, professionals in several different specialties treat chronic pain, but with very different approaches. You need to understand the focus of that professional's practice. The following is a list of various specialists who treat chronic pain. Some may have training in more than one of these areas.

PHYSICAL MEDICINE AND REHABILITATION (PM&R) PHYSICIANS. These are medical doctors who are also called physiatrists. They are trained in improving the patient's functioning. They take a functional and "whole body" approach to chronic pain. Because much of chronic pain involves the musculoskeletal system (that is, muscles, tendons, ligaments, joints, and bones), physiatrists focus on these structures. They frequently utilize physical modalities, such as ultrasound, electrical stimulation and therapeutic massage to decrease pain and swelling. They also perform different types of injections, including trigger point injections and cortisone injections into some joints, and prescribe medications to decrease pain, relax the muscles, and reduce inflammation.

Much chronic pain is associated with severe weakness of the muscles and tendons, and this weakness causes further problems, because if the muscles and tendons are not strong and flexible they can't support your joints. Physiatrists combat muscle/tendon weakness and stiffness and seek to reverse the problems associated with immobility, inactivity, and deconditioning by ordering specific flexibility and strengthening exercises. They work with patients to help modify their posture and may train patients to adjust the way they walk, bend, or lift. Physiatrists often prescribe assistive devices (such as walkers, canes, or specialized tools) to help patients perform their daily activities and may suggest modifications to a patient's work and home environments. Their goal is to maximize flexibility, strength, and endurance thereby maximizing function at the same time they are reducing pain.

ANESTHESIOLOGIST/PAIN SPECIALISTS. These doctors specialize in procedures to relieve pain. Like physiatrists, they can inject local anesthetics and steroids into painful areas, but they also can inject materials directly into the spinal canal. They can destroy damaged nerves using heat or chemicals. They can implant electrical stimulators into the spinal canal or pumps that keep releasing painkillers into the body. Although some anesthesiologists do prescribe medications for chronic pain, most prefer to have other physicians deal with medications.

INTERNISTS/PAIN SPECIALISTS AND NEUROLOGIST/PAIN SPECIALISTS. These physicians prescribe pain medications and adjunctive drugs, but most do not do procedures except for local injections. They have broad training in general medicine, so they are also able to provide primary care. Neurologists are also skilled at evaluating whether the pain has a neurologic basis.

PSYCHIATRISTS. Psychiatrists are medical doctors who specialize in treating emotional and psychiatric disorders. Most present-day psychiatrists focus on prescribing medications rather than doing "talk therapy," which is left to psychologists, counselors, and other psychotherapists. However, because many chronic pain patients are anxious and depressed, and many anxious and depressed patients have pain as a symptom of their psychological distress (see chapter 11), patients who seek psychiatric help often have pain problems. Because of this, some psychiatrists have become proficient at treating chronic pain.

PSYCHOLOGISTS. These health care professionals are "doctors of the mind." They have a Ph.D. in psychology and their emphasis is on some aspect of the mind. Some psychologists specialize in biofeedback, others in hypnosis, and still others in cognitive-behavioral therapy or other types of psychotherapy. Because they are not medical doctors, they do not provide medications.

CHIROPRACTORS. Chiropractors specialize in manipulating various parts of the body, especially the spine, to relieve pain. Their degree, a Doctor of Chiropractic, does not permit prescribing medications.

PHYSICAL THERAPISTS. These caregivers are trained to provide physical modalities to relieve pain. They can assess your muscle strength, joint stability, mobility, and gait. They can design an exercise program for you, apply heat, massage, and electrical stimulation, improve your gait and the way you stand, and recommend various assistive devices such as canes, crutches, or walkers and show you the correct way to use them. They do not prescribe medications.

OCCUPATIONAL THERAPISTS. These therapists focus on teaching the patient skills for returning to the workplace or maneuvering in an environment. They can show a patient in a wheelchair how to transfer in and out of it. They can teach a disabled person how to get in and out of the bathtub or an automobile or how to get dressed. They do not prescribe medications.

The above list is only a starting point. Other pain specialists may have training in some particular procedure, such as acupuncture or various types of massages. Some pain specialists will concentrate on the particular modality that is their specialty. Others will look at the big picture, and may recommend physical therapy, acupuncture, counseling, and other treatments. Some are willing to prescribe opioids for chronic pain, others aren't. Some will ask you about your emotional state and your family life, whereas others will be more narrowly focused. Just knowing the professional's specialty won't necessarily tell you whether the specialist's perspective is narrow or broad.

I recommend that you begin by asking your primary care doctor—or surgeon if that's whom you've been seeing for your pain problem—for a recommendation as to which type of pain practitioner is best for you. Support groups, either local or on the Internet, are another source of recommendations. But sometimes the only way to find out if a particular pain specialist is right for you is a face-to-face meeting.

## Preparing for Your First Appointment with the Pain Specialist

Even before your first appointment, you will have some work to do. Unless your pain is new and has not previously been evaluated, you will probably be asked to provide the specialist with your medical records. It's very helpful for the specialist to have reports of operations, consultations with other specialists, the results of laboratory tests and imaging studies, and office notes that describe what treatments have already been tried, what medications prescribed, and what were the results. Many chronic pain patients are very knowledgeable about their disease, and you may be able to provide the specialist with a great deal of useful information. Nonetheless, it is highly desirable to have written records of your prior care.

At your first appointment you should bring with you a list of all the medications you are taking, including the doses and frequency. Even more desirable is for you to bring all your medication bottles with you. That way, the physician can learn not only what drugs you are taking, but also how many of each you have left.

You should also bring with you, preferably in writing, the following information:

- **The name of the physician who referred you and why you were referred**. If you don't know why, then ask your referring physician before your new appointment.
- **The history of the pain problem for which you are being seen**. When did it start and how? What treatments have you already had (including procedures, operations, alternative treatments, and medications)? What was the result of those treatments?
- **Your remaining medical history**. What other medical problems do you have or have you had in the past? What operations have you had?
- **The names of any medications to which you are allergic**. Also a description of the allergic reaction caused by the medication.
- **Any of your medical records that you have**. The doctor's office can make copies of them and return your records to you.

## What Happens at the First Appointment?

Your first appointment will consist of an interview and a physical exam. The doctor will usually begin by asking you why you are here and what is your goal. You will then be asked to describe your pain problem and its history. You will also be asked to describe specifically what your pain feels like. Important questions are listed below.

- **Location of the pain**: Where does it hurt? For example, is it only in your lower back, or does it also radiate down your legs? If it's a headache, what part(s) of the head does it involve?
- **Intensity of the pain**: How bad is it? I usually ask, "On a scale of zero to ten, where zero is no pain and 10 is the worst pain you've ever had or could imagine, what number would you give to your pain right now? What number is it most of the time?" If you have pain in several areas, you will be asked about the intensity in each of the locations.
- **Character of the pain**: Is it sharp, dull, burning, throbbing, constant, or like an ice pick?
- **Duration of the pain**: Is it always present? Is it worse in the morning or in the evening? Is it a sharp twitch that's gone in seconds, only to recur unexpectedly?
- **Precipitating and alleviating factors**: What makes the pain better or worse? Does weather affect it? Does exercise help or make it worse? Is the intensity greater when you're upset about something or when you haven't slept well? Do medications help? Which ones?

As explained in earlier chapters, chronic pain can affect many aspects of your life. The physician will ask you about these aspects, including how well you sleep; if your ability to work has been affected; how your ability to exercise, travel, participate in sports, or enjoy sex has changed; and if your psychological well being has taken a downturn. Many chronic pain patients are depressed, and treating the depression may help reduce the pain.

The doctor will also ask for information about your past medical history, your medications and medication allergies, your family's medical history, your living situation and marital status, and whether you are working and, if so, what type of work you do. It is important for the physician to be aware of your use of tobacco and alcohol, and whether you have used recreational drugs in the past (or present) or have any history of drug or alcohol addiction. This information will help your doctor plan the best medication strategy for safely alleviating your pain. Finally, the doctor will do a "review of systems," meaning she or he will ask you about possible problems with your heart, lungs, kidneys, intestines, and other parts of your body.

At your initial consultation, the physician will also welcome the presence of your spouse or significant other or someone who is actively involved in your care. Sometimes they can provide additional input into your situation, and they may have questions regarding the treatment plan.

Next comes a physical exam, which will usually be focused on the areas involved with your chronic pain. There will be an examination for scars relating to prior operations. A rubber hammer will be used to check the deep tendon reflexes in your arms and legs. You will be asked to move parts of your body in various directions, and the physician will also passively move your arms or legs. If you have back pain, the examiner will push on various parts of your back to see where there is pain or tenderness. Overall, the exam depends on the particular medical problems you have. Some problems, for example, require an extensive neurological exam.

The visit will conclude with a discussion of treatment options. The physician may tell you that more information is needed before a decision can be reached about the best treatment. In that case, a follow-up appointment will be scheduled and you may be asked to sign additional releases to other hospitals or doctors for more records. You might be referred to another specialist for further diagnostic tests or consideration of other treatment options such as surgery. For example, if you have gradually worsening knee pain caused by osteoarthritis, you might be referred to an orthopedic surgeon to see whether arthroscopic surgery of the knee might relieve the pain or whether you might benefit from a total knee replacement.

Alternatively, the physician may begin a particular treatment regimen. Usually it takes several visits before the most effective treatment is determined and implemented. Treatment may consist of a combination of medications, physical therapy, exercise, referral to another specialist, and recommendation to see an alternative practitioner for hypnosis, biofeedback, or acupuncture.

## Working with Your Doctor on an Ongoing Basis

How often you need a follow-up appointment regarding your chronic pain depends on several factors. For example:

- You will need more frequent visits if your pain problem requires a diagnostic workup or evaluation by a specialist.

- You will need fewer visits if the pain problem is stable and well understood.
- While your medications are being adjusted, you will need more frequent visits than after you are on a regimen that gives you adequate pain relief.
- If you are on certain types of medications, such as opioids, your prescribing physician will want to see you at least once every two months for as long as you are on these medications.
- If you are not on opioids, and your treatment regimen is effective and your pain intensity is stable, then two visits a year might suffice.

At each follow-up visit, you will be asked about your pain level, what you are able to do physically, medication side effects, and your mood. If you are having increased pain, or if your medication is simply not sufficiently effective, your doctor may adjust the treatment. If you've changed your day-to-day routine, tell your doctor about it. The following scenario, for example, happens all too often and can cause confusion for your doctor.

Mrs. B, who's had three back operations and persistent back pain, comes in at 11 A.M. for a routine follow-up visit. She is being treated with sustained-release oxycodone (OxyContin) for her pain. She usually takes her pills at 7 A.M. and 7 P.M. Here's part of her conversation with Dr. A:

MRS. B: *Wow! Does my back ache today!*
DR. A: *On a scale of zero to 10, how much pain are you having right now?*
MRS. B: *10 out of 10.*
DR. A: *That's a real increase from last time, when your pain was 6 out of 10. Any idea why that might be?*
MRS. B: *I don't know, maybe because it rained yesterday. I haven't changed my activities or anything. . . .*

Dr. A. does a physical exam, but finds no reason for the increased pain.

DR. A: *Well, let's leave your medication dose as it is for now. If the increased pain persists by your next visit, we might have to increase the*

*dose and order a new CT scan to see if anything has changed with your*
*back. By the way, where's Mr. B today? He's usually with you.*
MRS. B: *He isn't feeling so good, so I drove here myself. But don't worry,*
*I didn't take my pain pills this morning.*

Dr. A groans as she realizes she's been on the wrong track. Mrs.
B doesn't need more medication or a CT scan—she needs to take
her medications more consistently.

DR. A: *Mrs. B, you've never mentioned before that your pills make you*
*feel foggy or sleepy or affect your mental alertness.*
MRS. B: *They don't—I feel normal on them, just less pain.*

Dr. A explains to Mrs. B that if she feels mentally clear it's okay
to take her pills even if she plans to drive.

## Follow the Doctor's Instructions—"Compliance"

The above conversation is an example of the difficulties that can result
when a patient changes her routine without letting the doctor know. If
you feel you need to increase your dose of medication because you need
more pain relief, or if you decide to decrease the dose or stop the medication because of side effects or other reasons, talk it over first with your
doctor. It's a good idea to discuss with her early on how she wants to
handle problems that come up between appointments. Most physicians
want you to phone them during office hours and leave a message. Hopefully, they will return your call in a short time.

If you are on opioid medications, your physician will undoubtedly
express reluctance to fill your medications early if you run out without
having first obtained his permission to increase the dose. And when it
comes to requests for early refills that result from having lost your medication, you need to understand that we physicians have heard it all: The
pills fell down the toilet; a guest stole them; the dog ate them; or a bird
flew in the window and made off with the pill bottle. We want to be
your advocate, not your judge: We do not relish having to decide
whether a patient is telling the truth or lying. Part of your responsibility
if you are taking strong pain medications is to safeguard them and to use
them responsibly. If there is risk of someone in your home taking your

medications, you need to hide them or keep them in a lock box or elsewhere. Don't carry a large amount of medication in your purse or wallet, where they are more vulnerable to theft; keep them in a safe place at home, and take only what you need for the day.

You may not realize that it's illegal to allow someone else to use your scheduled prescription drugs (medications such as opioids and benzodi-azepines [for example, Valium] that have special laws pertaining to use). In my practice, if a patient allows other people to use their drugs, or cannot safeguard their pain medications from theft or loss, I am unwilling to continue prescribing them.

## Don't Wait Until the Last Minute to Request Refills

One of most doctors' pet peeves is the patient who phones for a medication refill on the day it's running out, asking for same-day action. You may not realize that whenever you call the office for a refill, the file clerk must first pull your chart and place it on the doctor's desk, the doctor then looks at the chart and okays the refill if it's time, and finally a nurse phones in the refill or else the doctor writes out the prescription. All this takes time—easily a couple of days, and more so if the doctor is very busy or is out of the office for a day or two each week. It's one thing if a patient needs a new medication urgently, for example, an antibiotic for a new infection. But if the refill you want is for a medication you take daily, then surely you must realize a few days in advance that it will soon be running out. Make your doctor's life a little easier by asking for the refill several days early.

Finally, remember that a significant goal of your treatment for chronic pain is to improve your level of functioning. When your doctor recommends exercise, physical therapy, and more physical activity, part of your responsibility as a patient is to follow through on these recommendations. Living positively with chronic pain is a team effort. Relieving your pain is primarily the physician's responsibility, but improving your function is primarily yours. Part of following through on your agreement with your doctor is to take seriously her recommendations regarding your activity, even if in the short run your pain increases.

## Doctor-Patient Communication: Cultural Issues

To be able to assess and treat your pain, your physician needs to fully understand the extent and consequences of your pain and your treatment goals. Sometimes this process is impeded by the cultural diversity of our nation. Many cultural factors that impair physician-patient communication, including language barriers and culture-based attitudes, can hinder pain assessment and treatment. Studies have shown that African Americans, Hispanics, Asians, and Native Americans are at significant risk for undertreated pain.[9]

Some ethnic groups are uncomfortable discussing body issues, including pain, with the doctor because of modesty. A study of African-American cancer patients found that more than 90 percent wanted to be strong and not "lean on" pain medicines.[10] Because it is culturally unacceptable among Japanese patients to complain about gastrointestinal problems, some might not discuss having opioid-induced constipation or nausea.[11] Among some Asians and Christian African-Americans, pain and suffering are considered necessary for personal redemption or purification.[12]

Health professionals clearly need to be sensitive to cultural issues. At the same time, patients need to understand that optimal pain management requires a team effort, with good communication between physician and patient.

# PART II

## THE TREATMENT OF CHRONIC PAIN

# 4

# AN INTRODUCTION TO MEDICATIONS

## *Their Uses and Side Effects*

*Health care professionals may have inadequate knowledge of analgesic pharmacology and pain therapy, poor pain assessment practices, and ungrounded concern about regulatory oversight. They may also fear the side effects of opioid analgesics—in particular, tolerance and addiction. And they may be more focused on curing the underlying diseases than on treating pain. Individuals may contribute to the undertreatment problem by their reluctance to both report pain and take pain medications. Finally, too few health care systems currently make pain management a high priority.*[1]

—JOINT COMMISSION ON ACCREDITATION
OF HEALTH CARE ORGANIZATIONS

PAIN IS OFTEN UNDERTREATED. THIS IS TRUE DESPITE THE many old and new medications and other treatments available. This chapter will review various non-opioid pain medications and other helpful drugs. The next chapter (chapter 5) will cover information on opioids because these drugs are so important and so misunderstood that they deserve a complete chapter overview.

No matter how else your chronic pain is treated, medications are usually a part of the plan. You probably expect to walk out of your doctor's appointment with a medication prescription, and might consider it the most important part of treating your pain. Don't forget, however, that pills and potions are only a part of the treatment plan. Walking or riding an exercise bicycle or other aerobic device, stretching and weight-bearing exercises, physical therapy, occupational therapy, psychotherapy or counseling, local injections, devices implanted in your body, and other invasive procedures, including surgery, may all be part of the plan, as well as alternative modalities such as acupuncture, hypnosis, and meditation. It's important to follow through on all aspects of treatment; pills alone are unlikely to suffice.

This chapter will describe the types of medications that your doctor is likely to prescribe for pain, their uses, and their side effects. We'll begin by reviewing the most commonly prescribed medications and then go on to specific pain disorders that can benefit from additional drugs. The list below is not exhaustive; I have chosen to describe the drugs you need to know about, and the medications for which there is new evidence of efficacy in pain management.

Most chronic pain patients receive more than one type of drug and end up taking a cocktail of pills. Because some drugs can interact with others and can increase or decrease their efficacy or risk drug toxicity, it's important to tell your doctor *all* the medications you are currently taking, including prescription and over-the-counter medications, supplements, and herbs. Keep a list at all times in case you end up in an emergency room, hospital, or seeking help from another physician.

As you saw in chapter 2, the perception of pain involves a complex pathway that begins with chemical and electrical signals put out by peripheral nociceptors (signals originating from an injury to some part of the body). These signals travel along the spinal cord to the brain, which evaluates the sensory and emotional aspects of the pain and sends signals back down through the spinal cord. Different pain treatments target various sites along this route. Analgesic (pain-relieving) medications specifically affect the different sites. Some of these are listed below.

- **Local anesthetics** are applied on the skin or by injection at the site of the pain source (for example, thumb, around a tooth, on the skin before sewing up a laceration); they numb peripheral nerves and block pain signals from leaving the site of injury. Local anesthetics are also injected directly into the spinal column to prevent further transmission of the pain signals.

- **Anti-inflammatory drugs** (such as steroids, aspirin, NSAIDs, COX-2 inhibitors) are taken orally or by injections; they have effect on the periphery, spinal cord and the brain.
- **Opioids** are taken orally or by injection; they affect the spinal cord and brain.
- **Alpha-2 adrenergic agonists** (such as clonidine) affect the spinal cord and brain. This class of drugs has been taken by mouth for years to treat hypertension, but these sedative drugs are also effective in relieving pain and anxiety. They act at both the spinal cord and brain. When used for pain management, clonidine (Catapres, a member of this class) is effective when injected in small amounts directly into the spinal canal. When injected in combination with opioids, either into the spinal canal or a vein, clonidine can decrease the dose of opioid required to relieve pain. Its main side effects when taken by mouth are fatigue and dry mouth.

Some categories of medications described in this chapter are:
- **Analgesics** (pain relievers) other than narcotics (opioids); examples are acetaminophen, anti-inflammatory drugs, and tramadol.
- **Adjuvant drugs**, drugs whose primary indication is not for pain, but which are useful for pain relief. Examples are antidepressants, alpha-2 adrenergic agonists, and corticosteroids.
- **Drugs particularly useful for neuropathic pain**; examples are anticonvulsants, topical analgesics, and NMDA-receptor antagonists.
- Muscle relaxants
- Sleeping pills

## Non-opioid Pain Medications

ACETAMINOPHEN. Because this drug is so commonly used for pain and is present in so many over-the-counter combination remedies, you may not be fully aware of its benefits and risks. Acetaminophen (Tylenol) is a very effective pain reliever. It's considered the first-line remedy for mild to moderate osteoarthritis pain (acetaminophen is the American College of Rheumatology's recommended first-line therapy for osteoarthritis of the hip and knee), dental pain, and various other types of pain. However, when taken in excess, acetaminophen is toxic to the liver and can even cause death. If you are taking this drug for long-term daily analgesia, read the labels of any other over-the-counter remedy you are considering using, to see whether it also contains acetaminophen. It's easy to exceed the recommended daily limit.

SALICYLATES. The oldest drug of this class, aspirin, was introduced by the Bayer Company in 1899 and has been valued for more than a century for its ability to relieve pain, reduce inflammation, and lower fever. Aspirin also interferes with platelet function (antiplatelet), thereby decreasing the ability of blood to clot. One dose of aspirin will irreversibly inhibit platelet function for the life of the platelet, which is 8 to 10 days. This drug is like a double-edged sword: Its effect on platelets makes aspirin still the drug of choice for preventing heart attacks and strokes. However, if you have any surgical procedure planned, your doctor will most likely ask you to stop taking aspirin a couple of weeks in advance in order to avoid the risk of increased postoperative bleeding. When large doses of aspirin are taken on a regular basis, ulcers and gastrointestinal bleeding can result.

Other salicylates such as choline magnesium trisalicylate (Trilisate) and disalcid differ from aspirin in that their molecular structure lacks the acetyl group. The importance of this feature is that they are much less likely than aspirin to inhibit platelet aggregation or cause bleeding.

## SALICYLATES

| Drug Name | Manufacturer | Generic Name |
|-----------|--------------|--------------|
| aspirin | several | aspirin |
| Disalcid | 3M Pharmaceuticals | salsalate |
| Trilisate | Purdue Frederick | choline magnesium trisalicylate |

STEROIDS. Steroids are potent anti-inflammatory drugs and pain relievers. In chronic pain, steroids such as prednisone, prednisolone, and dexamethasone are used primarily to treat the underlying disorder such as rheumatoid arthritis and lupus. When steroids are used for more than a short time, they have significant side effects such as depression or euphoria, diabetes, and osteoporosis, among others. For this reason steroids are usually given in injections or pills for very short-term treatment of exacerbation of back, joint, and muscle pain. For example, your doctor might give you an injection of a steroid plus local anesthetic every few months in the area of your body (such as a knee or shoulder) that is chronically painful.

NONSTEROIDAL ANTI-INFLAMMATORY DRUGS (NSAIDs). The nonselective nonsteroidal anti-inflammatory drugs (NSAIDs), such as ibuprofen (Motrin, Advil), naproxen sodium (Naprosyn), and diclofenac (Voltaren), have effects similar to aspirin, reducing both pain and inflammation. These are widely used for arthritis pain, headaches, and other pain syndromes. They are excellent painkillers for mild to moderate pain and they do reduce inflammation, but they can also irritate the lining of the stomach and cause bleeding. People who've had ulcers in the past should avoid NSAIDs. As with aspirin, NSAIDs also inhibit platelet aggregation and thin the blood but, unlike aspirin, the effect is reversible and lasts only until the drug is out of your system, usually only a few days. Compared to other NSAIDs, naproxen has a particularly potent antiplatelet effect, although aspirin is even more effective in this regard than naproxen. NSAIDs are well tolerated by most people, but they can cause blood pressure elevation, fluid retention (edema), and some damage to the kidneys. In asthmatics who are sensitive to aspirin, NSAIDs can precipitate an asthma attack. It's not a good idea to take more than one of these drugs at a time. However, they can be safely taken in combination with opioids.

## NSAIDs

| Drug Name | Manufacturer | Generic Name |
|---|---|---|
| Advil | Wyeth | ibuprofen |
| Motrin IB | McNeil Consumer | ibuprofen |
| Naprosyn | Roche Laboratories | naproxen sodium |
| Voltaren | Novartis | diclofenac sodium |

COX-2 INHIBITORS OR COXIBS. Normally, the stomach lining (gastric mucosa) is protected from irritation by chemicals called prostaglandins that are synthesized with the help of the enzyme cyclooxygenase-1 (COX-1). Different prostaglandins, synthesized by the enzyme cyclooxygenase-2 (COX-2), produce pain. Nonselective NSAIDs work by inhibiting COX-2 in the brain and the periphery, thereby turning off the pain-producing prostaglandins, but they also inhibit the COX-1 enzyme, which results in making the lining of the stomach more vulnerable to damage.

A relatively new class of drugs, the COX-2 inhibitors (coxibs), which are second-generation NSAIDS, inhibits COX-2 to a far greater extent than COX-1, meaning that they are as effective as the older NSAIDs in their pain-relieving and anti-inflammatory effect, while having a much less harmful effect on the lining of the stomach. The coxibs that are currently available are celecoxib (Celebrex), rofecoxib (Vioxx), and valdecoxib (Bextra). They have minor differences in the amount of blood pressure elevation and fluid retention they cause. The chief advantage of the coxibs is that they are much less likely to cause gastrointestinal irritation, and they don't inhibit platelet aggregation. Because they don't increase the risk of bleeding, the coxibs (unlike NSAIDs) can be taken right up to the time of surgery.

As stated before, aspirin and some NSAIDs (such as naproxen) reduce the risk of heart attacks by blocking platelet aggregation. Taking COX-2 inhibitors *does not increase* the risk of heart attacks, but it *does not decrease* the risk either. People who have risk factors for heart disease and who are switched from an NSAID to a COX-2 inhibitor for their chronic pain should consider taking an aspirin daily.

## COX-2

| Drug Name | Manufacturer | Generic Name |
|-----------|--------------|--------------|
| Bextra | Pfizer | valdecoxib |
| Celebrex | Pfizer | celecoxib |
| Vioxx | Merck | rofecoxib |

TRAMADOL. It's hard to know where to list tramadol (Ultram), an analgesic that acts in the central nervous system, because it has more than one mechanism of action. It binds to the same receptor as do opioids, the mu receptor, resulting in some morphinelike effects, but these effects are weak enough that the Drug Enforcement Administration (DEA) does not regulate its use.

Tramadol also blocks reuptake of the neurotransmitters norepinephrine and serotonin, thereby relieving pain via a different pathway. Its efficacy in relieving dental pain or cancer pain is similar to that of acetaminophen (Tylenol) with 30 mg of codeine, but in a study of patients who had orthopedic surgery, tramadol was no more effective than a placebo and caused more vomiting than 60 mg of codeine.[2] Tramadol is an expensive, modestly effective analgesic that in some patients can cause seizures.

## Adjuvant Analgesics

ANTIDEPRESSANTS. Pain is so often associated with depression that it is sometimes unclear which came first. Regardless, treating depression not only elevates your mood but also improves your physical functioning. In chapter 11, you will find a detailed discussion about depression and pain. For now, what's important to understand is that antidepressants can relieve pain even in patients who are not depressed. In addition to their antidepressant effect, these drugs seem to have intrinsic analgesic properties. Antidepressants are particularly effective in reducing neuropathic pain and back pain. Many studies have also shown their efficacy in alleviating chronic non-cancer pain.

Antidepressants work by increasing the concentration of one or more of the neurotransmitters dopamine, norepinephrine, and serotonin. They do this by inhibiting the uptake (and destruction) of these chemicals after they are released in the nervous system. The neurotransmitters norepinephrine and serotonin also alleviate pain; thus, the efficacy of some antidepressants in relieving pain may be a direct effect rather than secondary to lifting depression.

The oldest *class* of drugs available to treat depression is the tricyclic antidepressants (TCAs), which inhibit the uptake of both serotonin and norepinephrine. Some tricyclics are amitriptyline (Elavil), doxepin (Sinequan), and imipramine (Tofranil). For depression, you need to take these drugs for about three weeks before your mood will begin to improve, but their analgesic effect begins sooner. It's still not known exactly how they relieve pain. The biggest drawback of tricyclic antidepressants is their side effects. Amitriptyline (Elavil) is particularly prone to cause sedation and dry mouth. This is less a problem in the low doses currently used in pain management than in the much higher doses used for depression. There are also other tricyclics, such as desipramine (Norpramine) and nortriptyline (Pamelor), that are equally effective in pain medicine but have fewer side effects than amitriptyline. Tricyclics are considered first-choice medications for the treatment of neuropathic pain. In a review of randomized controlled trials of analgesic effects of antidepressants, there was significant evidence that tricyclic antidepressants relieve pain. In contrast, pain relief in the trials of selective serotonin reuptake inhibitors (SSRIs) varied. Tricyclics are clearly superior to SSRIs for pain relief.[3] This may be because SSRIs inhibit only serotonin uptake, whereas the tricyclics increase the levels of both serotonin and norepinephrine.

Now widely used for depression because they have such an excellent side effect profile, SSRIs include fluoxetine (Prozac), sertraline (Zoloft), paroxetine (Paxil), fluvoxamine (Luvox), citalopram (Celexa), and escitalopram (Lexapro). Escitalopram is a different molecular configuration of citalopram. Its effects are similar, but it has fewer side effects and no drug-drug interactions. One pain-management alternative would be to combine an SSRI, such as escitalopram, with a low dose of a tricyclic, such as nortriptyline. This combination would inhibit both norepinephrine and serotonin uptake, with minimal side effects.

Might SSRIs be effective for particular types of pain? This was investigated in a review of results from 19 randomized controlled trials of SSRIs in various pain syndromes. The authors of the study found conflicting results for migraine and tension headaches, diabetic neuropathy, and fibromyalgia. They concluded, "Given the evidence for the superiority of antidepressants with mixed mechanisms of action [norepiphrine as well as serotonin uptake inhibition] and the well-documented efficacy of tricyclic antidepressants in the management of various chronic pain syndromes, it seems reasonable to use TCAs first and reserve SSRIs for patients who do not respond to or are intolerant of the tricyclic antidepressants."[4] As for the effect of antidepressants on chronic back pain, a recent review of randomized, placebo-controlled trials found that antidepressants that inhibit norepinephrine reuptake (tricyclic or tetracyclic antidepressants) significantly improved pain, but SSRIs were not beneficial for chronic low back pain.[5]

Venlafaxine (Effexor) is a newer, well-tolerated antidepressant that, like the tricyclics, increases both serotonin and norepinephrine. Venlafaxine alleviates pain in people with chronic low back pain, osteoarthritis, rheumatoid arthritis, and foot ulcers.[6,7] At low doses (less than 150 mg per day), venlafaxine inhibits primarily serotonin uptake; norepinephrine levels are increased only at higher doses. Consequently, low doses of venlafaxine tend to be less effective for pain relief than higher doses.

## ANTIDEPRESSANTS

| DRUG NAME | MANUFACTURER | GENERIC NAME |
|---|---|---|
| Celexa | Forest | citalopram |
| Effexor | Wyeth | venlafaxine |
| Elavil | Merck Sharp & Dohme | amitriptyline |
| Lexapro | Forest | escitalopram |
| Luvox | Sun Pharma | fluvoxamine |
| Norpramin | Aventis | desipramine |
| Pamelor | Mallinckrodt | nortriptyline |
| Paxil | GlaxoSmithKline | paroxetine |
| Prozac | Lilly | fluoxetine |
| Sinequan | Pfizer | doxepin |
| Tofranil | Mallinckrodt | imipramine |
| Zoloft | Pfizer | sertraline |

ALPHA-2 ADRENERGIC RECEPTOR AGONISTS. This class of drugs has been used for years to treat hypertension, but these sedative drugs are also effective in relieving pain and anxiety. They act at both the spinal cord and brain. Clonidine (Catapres), a member of this class, also relieves pain when injected into the spinal canal. Its main side effects are fatigue and dry mouth. When injected in combination with opioids, either into the spinal canal or a vein, clonidine can decrease the dose of opioid required to relieve pain.

Tizanidine (Zanaflex) is better tolerated than clonidine. Both are useful in relieving headache, low back pain, neuropathic pain, and cancer pain. Tizanidine also relieves muscle spasms so it is particularly useful when pain is accompanied by muscle spasticity. Tizanidine has much less effect than clonidine on blood pressure, with only one-fiftieth to one-tenth the effect, so it is much less likely to cause hypotension (low blood pressure). In the treatment of neck and back pain, tizanidine significantly reduces pain and improves function,[8] and is also effective in relieving chronic tension-type headache.[9,10]

## ALPHA-2 ADRENERGIC RECEPTOR AGONISTS

| DRUG NAME | MANUFACTURER | GENERIC NAME |
|---|---|---|
| Catapres | Boehringer Ingelheim | clonidine |
| Zanaflex | Elan | tizanidine |

CORTICOSTEROIDS. Steroids are very potent anti-inflammatory drugs and have widespread use in medicine for both their anti-inflammatory and their pain-relieving effects. In pain management, they are most commonly taken by mouth to relieve the pain of rheumatoid arthritis and other autoimmune diseases, and by injection along with local anesthetics in arthritic joints and in the spinal canal to relieve back pain. Steroids should be used only very judiciously. In high doses given for more than a few days, they can have various adverse effects, including diabetes, osteoporosis, and other damage to bones.

NEUROPATHIC PAIN DRUGS. In the past few years, there has been an explosion of new medications for neuropathic pain. And this is in addition to antidepressants and alpha-2 adrenergic drugs, which were described earlier and are also useful for neuropathic pain.

A team of international experts on pain management regularly reviews randomized controlled trials of drugs for neuropathic pain and has identified five first-line drugs or drug classes that provide significant benefit in neuropathic pain. These are gabapentin, the 5-percent lidocaine patch, opioid analgesics, tramadol, and tricyclic antidepressants.[11]

LOCAL ANESTHETICS. Local anesthetics given by mouth (orally) are useful for neuropathic pain. The most commonly used one is mexiletine (Mexitil), whose original use was to correct rhythm abnormalities in the heart, but tocainide (Tonocarel) and flecanide (Tambocor) are also available.

## ORAL LOCAL ANESTHETICS

| DRUG NAME | MANUFACTURER | GENERIC NAME |
|---|---|---|
| Mexitil | Boehringer Ingelheim | mexiletine |
| Tambocor | 3M Pharmaceuticals | flecainide |
| Tonocard | AstraZeneca | tocainide |

## *Anticonvulsants*

Anticonvulsants, originally prescribed in the treatment of seizure disorders, are now finding even greater use in alleviating chronic neuropathic pain. Carbamazepine (Tegretol), clonazepam (Klonopin), valproate (Depakote), and phenytoin (Dilantin) have been used for some time for pain, including headache pain. Tegretol and Dilantin interact with many other drugs, a drawback in pain management. Currently, the anticonvulsant most widely used for pain is gabapentin (Neurontin). This drug has no known drug–drug interactions, so it can be used in combination with opioids and other medications. Two important studies demonstrated the analgesic efficacy of gabapentin in the treatment of diabetic neuropathy[12] and shingles pain.[13] The findings of these two studies resulted in FDA approval of gabapentin for post-herpetic neuralgia (PHN or shingles pain). Gabapentin is also widely used for other types of neuropathic pain, such as CRPS (reflex sympathetic dystrophy), phantom limb pain, HIV-related sensory neuropathy, trigeminal neuralgia, multiple sclerosis pain, migraine headache prevention, and pain associated with spinal cord injury. *The Medical Letter on Drugs and Therapeutics*) reported in April 2004 in an article titled "On Drugs and Therapeutics," that among Medicaid recipients in Florida receiving gabapentin, 71 percent of the prescriptions were for chronic pain, and only 8 percent were for FDA-approved indications (seizures and post-herpetic neuralgia).

To be effective for chronic pain, gabapentin should be prescribed in much higher doses than for seizure disorders, up to 3,600 mg per day. Unless you've been prescribed at least 1,800 mg per day, you haven't had an adequate trial. Because gabapentin is sedative, you will be started on a very low dose and titrated upward over a few weeks. Most people become tolerant to the sedative effect of gabapentin and are eventually able to take the large doses required for pain relief.

Newer anticonvulsants that are being tried for chronic pain include topiramate (Topamax), tiagabine (Gabatril), and lamotrigine (Lamictal). Topiramate is especially useful for prevention of migraine headaches. Unlike other anticonvulsants, it tends to cause weight loss rather than gain and may be the drug of choice for obese patients suffering from migraine headaches. When given to migraine patients for six months, topiramate prescribed at either 100 or 200 mg per day was very effective in preventing migraines.[14] During the first month of treatment, the drug significantly reduced the number of migraine episodes in comparison with another group of patients who did not receive the drug. Topiramate continued to be effective throughout the treatment period.

In a study of patients with diabetic neuropathy, topiramate at a mean daily dose of $161 \pm 78$ mg gave significantly greater pain relief and better sleep than did a placebo.[15] The patients on topiramate also lost several pounds, compared with no change in the control group. This recent study gives hope that Topamax will be useful in various types of neuropathic pain.

An even newer relative of gabapentin is pregabalin (Lyrica), which is expected to be available in the United States in the summer of 2004. It was recently tried for eight weeks in patients who still had pain at least three months following healing of a herpes zoster rash (PHN).[16] In those patients who received the active drug rather than placebo, pain was significantly relieved one day after treatment was begun, and for the duration of the study. Their sleep improved, their overall functioning was better, and the side effects were tolerable. Pregabalin seems like an effective drug in the treatment of PHN, and will undoubtedly be tried for other types of neuropathic pain.

## ANTICONVULSANTS

| Drug Name | Manufacturer | Generic Name |
| --- | --- | --- |
| Dilantin | Parke-Davis | phenytoin |
| Gabitril | Cephalon | tiagabine |
| Klonopin | Roche Laboratories | clonazepam |
| Lamictal | GlaxoSmithKline | lamotrigine |
| Lyrica | Pfizer | pregabalin |
| Neurontin | Parke-Davis | gabapentin |
| Tegretol | Novartis | carbamazepine |
| Topamax | Ortho-McNeil | topiramate |

NEUROLEPTICS. Neuroleptics are drugs traditionally used for schizophrenia and other psychotic illnesses. Two new drugs in this class, however, olanzapine (Zyprexa) and risperidone (Risperdal), have shown some efficacy in treating chronic pain.

## NEUROLEPTICS

| DRUG NAME | MANUFACTURER | GENERIC NAME |
| --- | --- | --- |
| Risperdal | Janssen | risperidone |
| Zyprexa | Lilly | olanzapine |

TOPICAL ANALGESICS. As we saw in chapter 2, in response to tissue injury, peripheral nerve fibers transmit noxious signals to the spinal cord, where they are processed and either magnified or suppressed, and then sent upward to the brain. Topical agents intercept the peripheral signals, decreasing the input to the spinal cord. They are particularly effective in cases of peripheral nerve damage or tissue inflammation due to injury.

Topical analgesics and transdermal preparations have different mechanisms of actions although both are absorbed through the skin. The drug in transdermal patches, such as fentanyl (Duragesic), testosterone (Androderm), and clonidine (Catapres-TTS), gets into the bloodstream and works systemically. In other words, the body treats the drug the same as if it came in through the mouth or by injection. In contrast, topical analgesics, also called "targeted peripheral analgesics," work only at the site of application and do not produce a significant concentration of the drug in the bloodstream even if they are used repeatedly. As a result, they have very few side effects and very little interaction with other drugs. In other words, they are very safe.

Lidocaine is a local anesthetic that may be familiar to you if you've had dental work or a laceration sutured. Lidocaine gel comes in a toothpastelike tube and is useful for various painful skin lesions. In a suspension, it can be swished in the mouth for relief of mouth ulcers. These uses are basically for acute pain. But lidocaine also comes in large patches (Lidoderm) that are applied to intact skin, where they adhere. The instructions are to leave the patch on for 12 hours out of every 24, but a report on patients who left each patch on for 24 hours three days in a row showed that it was safe and well tolerated).[17] Lidocaine patches are FDA-approved only for the relief of pain associated with post-herpetic neuralgia (PHN, or shingles), but in fact they are used for all kinds of surface pain, where they block pain-related nerve impulses going to the spinal cord. For example, a *group* of 16 patients with myofascial pain was treated with Lidoderm patches for

28 days. Half the patients had significant improvement in their pain, activity level, ability to walk and work, and sleep.[18]

Lidoderm patches don't actually cause numbing of the skin (anesthesia) because they don't sufficiently penetrate the epidermis, but they do relieve pain. The manufacturer recommends applying up to three patches at a time. They can also be cut into smaller pieces. It may take a week or two of using the patches to get the maximum pain-relieving effect.

## TRANSDERMAL MEDICATIONS

| DRUG NAME | MANUFACTURER | GENERIC NAME |
| --- | --- | --- |
| Androderm | Watson | testosterone |
| Catapres-TTS | Boehringer Ingelheim | clonidine |
| Duragesic | Janssen | fentanyl |

## TOPICAL ANALGESICS

| DRUG NAME | MANUFACTURER | GENERIC NAME |
| --- | --- | --- |
| Lidoderm | Endo Labs | lidocaine |
| EMLA cream | Astra-Zeneca | prilocain + lidocaine |
| capsaicin | several | capsaicin |

EMLA CREAM. An older topical anesthetic cream, often used in children, is EMLA cream, a mixture of two local anesthetics, prilocaine and lidocaine. It is very effective in numbing the skin for shallow skin procedures. However, the cream must be applied at least one hour in advance of the procedure.

CAPSAICIN. Capsaicin, the pungent ingredient in hot chili peppers, is useful for alleviating surface pain. Capsaicin causes the release of substance P, a pain-producing transmitter, from afferent nerve cells. Repeated application of capsaicin cream causes the depletion of substance P from the cells, and thus pain relief after several days of consistent use. Capsaicin cream has been available for some years in several strengths, and is applied four to six times a day to intact skin over painful areas. Its primary use has been in relieving PHN. One drawback is that severe burning pain often occurs the first few times the drug is applied to the skin.

Capsaicin may also be effective for nonspecific back pain. Applied in the form of a plaster for three weeks in patients with back pain, this medication relieved the pain significantly better than did placebo plasters.[19]

A new way to use capsaicin has been tried in patients with PHN. First, a topical anesthetic was applied to the painful area to numb it. Next, a high-concentration capsaicin patch was applied for one hour to the same area of skin. Because of the prior application of a local anesthetic, the 44 patients treated did not experience the expected pain resulting from such a high dose of capsaicin. On the contrary, they had a significant decrease in pain that lasted up to four weeks.[20]

TOPICAL NSAIDS. Topical NSAIDs are not yet available commercially, but a study that compared the efficacy of 1,200 mg per day of oral ibuprofen with a 5 percent gel of topical ibuprofen6 found the two treatments to provide equivalent pain relief in patients with acute soft-tissue injuries.[21] Topical NSAIDs are likely to be better tolerated than the pills. Anti-inflammatory drugs, including ibuprofen, flurbiprofen, diclofenac, and naproxen, have been prepared in topical formulations and have been shown to be effective in relieving various types of soft-tissue pain such as sprained ankle, muscle strain, and soft-tissue injuries.[22]

MENTHOL. Menthol is a common ingredient in many over-the-counter analgesic preparations because of its cooling, soothing effect. A recent study showed that menthol may exert part of its pain-relieving effect through the activation of kappa-opioid receptors, which are the same receptors that interact with opioid drugs.[23] As old-timers have claimed for years, menthol appears to have a biological pain-relieving effect.

NMDA ANTAGONISTS. In chapter 2 you saw that N-methyl-D-aspartate (NMDA) receptors in the spinal cord worsen neuropathic pain and facilitate the development of tolerance to the pain-relieving effects of prescribed and endogenous opioids. NMDA-receptor antagonists can therefore be expected to alleviate neuropathic pain and to prevent or reverse opioid tolerance. Several drugs already in use are in fact NMDA antagonists. One of these is the D-isomer of methadone. Methadone is a synthetic opioid that consists of two mirror-image configurations (called isomers) of the same molecule. The L-isomer provides the most pain relief, but the D-isomer is an NMDA antagonist. Some evidence suggests that methadone (compared with other opioids) is particularly effective in neuropathic pain, and at least part of the reason may be its D-isomer.

Dextromethorphan is probably familiar to you as a component of some medicine (such as Robitussin-DM cough syrup). Dextromethorphan, a cough suppressor, is actually the D-isomer of levorphanol, a long-acting opioid. Some studies suggest that dextromethorphan, when added to morphine and other opioids, can potentiate (increase) their pain-relieving effects and decrease the likelihood of tolerance.

Ketamine, traditionally used as an intravenous anesthetic during surgery, has also been tried in the treatment of several types of neuropathic pain. A review of the efficacy of ketamine gave mixed results, with some evidence for pain relief in fibromyalgia, phantom limb pain, and PHN. The authors of the review concluded that in cases when standard analgesic options have been unsuccessful, it's worth trying ketamine as a "third-line" option.[24] Unfortunately, ketamine has significant side effects, including vivid dreams, high blood pressure, nausea, and muscle twitching, and not much is known about its long-term effects.

MUSCLE RELAXERS AND SLEEPING PILLS. At some point, your doctor has probably prescribed a muscle relaxant for pain, stiffness, or muscle spasm. Common drugs in this class are cyclobenzaprine (Flexeril), carisoprodol (Soma), methocarbamol (Robaxin), orphenadrine (Norflex), chlorzoxazone (Parafon Forte), metaxolone (Skelaxin), and diazepam (Valium). You may have noticed that all these drugs tend to relax your brain as well as your muscles; in other words, they are sedative. It's unclear whether they actually relax muscles, but they do relieve muscle pain, and they are often used in combination with analgesics.

Although many people swear by the muscle relaxants they use, published studies give a more mixed picture. For example, 77 patients who visited an emergency room (ER) for acute back strain were treated with ibuprofen; half of them also received cyclobenzaprine (Flexeril) in the ER and a prescription for home use. At 3, 24, and 48 hours, there was no difference in pain relief between the two groups. Of course, the body's response to acute pain in the first two days may differ from its response to ongoing back pain, so this study might not be the last word on muscle relaxants and chronic pain.[25] Muscle relaxants do not selectively relax tight muscles; rather, their effect is likely due to a generalized sedative effect on the brain.

For severe muscle spasms, which may be found in some people with diseases such as multiple sclerosis, some back injuries, or after a stroke, baclofen

(Lioresal) and tizanidine (Zanaflex) are useful. Tizanadine is approved for treatment of increased muscle tone associated with spasticity, but has no direct effect on skeletal muscle.

## MUSCLE RELAXERS AND SLEEPING PILLS

| Drug Name | Manufacturer | Generic Name |
|---|---|---|
| Ambien | Sanofi-Sythelabo | zolpidem |
| Ativan | Wyeth Pharmaceuticals | lorazepam |
| Dalmane | ICN Pharmaceutical | flurazepam |
| Flexeril | McNeil Consumer | cyclobenzaprine |
| Lioresal | Sun Pharma | baclofen |
| Norflex | 3M | orphenadrine |
| Parafon Forte DSC | McNeil Consumer | chlorzoxazone |
| Restoril | Geneva and Mylan | temazepam |
| Robaxin | Baxter Anesthesia | methocarbamol |
| Skelaxin | Monarch | metaxalone |
| Soma | Medpointe | carisoprodol |
| Sonata | Monarch | zaleplon |
| Valium | Roche Products | diazepam |
| Zanaflex | Elan | tizanidine |

Both muscle relaxers and sleeping medications seem to work via the same mechanism—sedation. Benzodiazepines have been used for many years to relieve muscle spasm, anxiety, and insomnia. Because they stay in the body for many hours (that is, they have a long half-life), the benzodiazepines temazepam (Restoril), flurazepam (Dalmane), and lorazepam (Ativan), have helped people stay asleep. Because they take effect in 45 to 60 minutes, they are not that effective at helping people fall asleep. Temazepam's long half-life (10 hours) means you may experience sleepiness into the following day. Benzodiazepines tend to lose their efficacy after several weeks, so you may need to take a break from your sleeping pill for a while until you are once again able to benefit from them.

Two newer drugs with shorter half-lives can help you fall asleep. Zolpidem (Ambien) has a quicker onset of action—about 15 minutes—and a half-life of about three hours. It will help you fall asleep, and to stay asleep for about six hours. Zaleplon (Sonata) also takes effect within 15 minutes or so, but its duration of action is even shorter than that of zolpidem, so it won't help you stay asleep for long. On the other hand, you can take a second dose of zaleplon if you awaken in the middle of the night.

Your sleep cycle depends in part upon production of the sleep-inducing chemical melatonin by the pineal gland in the brain. Melatonin has been synthesized and is sold as a sleep-promoting agent, but its efficacy hasn't been proven in controlled trials.

## A Cocktail of Medications May Help

Most chronic pain patients are treated with more than one medication for their pain. It makes biological sense to combine medications with different mechanisms of action, such as an anti-inflammatory, muscle relaxant, adjuvant medication, and opioid. The combination of different drugs is sometimes additive, but sometimes two drugs are even synergistic, meaning that their combined effect is greater than just the sum of the two drugs.

Here, for example, is what happened in a study of mice given ibuprofen and hydrocodone (an opioid [narcotic] analgesic) alone or in combination. The mice were positioned so that their tail lay on a metal grid that was heated. The investigators timed how many seconds it took for the mice to move their tail off the heated grid; the more painful the grid, the quicker they will remove their tails. Mice given hydrocodone experienced some pain relief, so that they were slower to move their tails away than were mice given no hydrocodone. Ibuprofen alone made no difference whatsoever. But in the mice who were given both drugs, the hydrocodone was seven times more effective than hydrocodone alone in relieving pain! Clearly, there was a strong synergistic effect between the opioid and the anti-inflammatory in their ability to relieve pain, which supports the common practice of prescribing both of these painkillers together to patients with pain.[26]

## Additional Medications for Specific Diseases

Let's discuss additional medications for three of the most common chronic pain syndromes I see in my practice: fibromyalgia, headaches, and osteoarthritis. Again, this discussion will not be comprehensive, but will focus on recent research.

## Fibromyalgia

The less that is known about a disease, the more various medications are likely to be touted as effective. Fads are common in such diseases; newspapers, magazines, and support groups on the Web frequently report on some wonderful new remedy. A patient should be discerning as to what medications are tried, and it's always a good idea to ask your physician about any possible side effects, or drug-to-drug interactions, before trying some new treatment.

Fibromyalgia (FM) pain is a condition for which there are no well-established effective treatments. Poor sleep is considered a possible causative factor. FM patients complain that poor sleep worsens their symptoms, and an improved sleep pattern is a major goal for most FM patients. Many FM patients have alpha brain waves (normally associated with awake states) during the night. A new drug that is currently FDA-approved only for narcolepsy is undergoing trials in FM patients with alpha-brainwave problems. Thus far, in small trials, gamma-hydroxybutyrate (now called sodium oxybate [trade name Xyrem]) improved both sleep pattern and pain in such patients as well as decreased their fatigue.[27,28] The use of this drug for fibromyalgia, however, is still very much in the experimental stage.

## Headaches

Several groups of drugs, taken regularly, can decrease the frequency of headaches. These include beta-blockers such as propranolol (Inderal) and timolol (Blockadren), tricyclic antidepressants such as amitriptyline (Elavil) and nortriptyline (Pamelor), and anticonvulsants such as divalproex (Depakote). People who have more than two or three headaches per month can benefit from taking these preventive medications on a regular basis. Once migraine headaches begin, most cases can be effectively treated with triptans, such as sumitriptan (Imitrex), zolmitriptan (Zomig), naratriptan (Amerge), rizatriptan (Maxalt), eletriptan (Relpax), and frovatriptan (Frova). Triptans are most effective when taken early in an attack, when the pain is still mild. For patients who need very rapid action, Imitrex is available in an injection. If nausea makes it unrealistic for you to take a pill, you can choose from a nasal spray formulation of

Imitrex or Zomig, or a tablet that dissolves quickly on the tongue without water (available with Zomig and Maxalt). Whichever triptan you try first, you have a 60- to 70-percent chance of it working. If it doesn't, however, the good news is that you have a high likelihood of obtaining benefit from one of the other triptans. Don't give up on this class of drugs just because one or two of them haven't worked.

Some patients use simple analgesics such as aspirin, acetaminophen, caffeine, and NSAIDs daily for chronic headaches. Frequent use of such drugs can cause rebound headaches, which are usually treated with the same drugs, and a vicious circle results. Other medications can help break the cycle, and sometimes a brief hospitalization is required.

About 18 percent of women suffer from migraine headaches; 60 percent of them report an exacerbation of headaches around the time of menstruation, and about 10 percent of women have exclusively menstrual migraines. The cause may be falling estrogen levels around the time of menstruation. For this reason, a useful preventive treatment for menstrual migraines is a transdermal estradiol patch applied three days before the onset of menstruation and continued for six days.[29]

Some physicians have found bedtime melatonin to be useful in preventing migraine headaches that awaken patients from sleep.[30] One aspirin a day can also reduce the incidence of migraines, especially migraines with aura.[31]

Another common type of headache is chronic daily headache, which is defined as the presence of a headache at least 15 days per month. Most cases of chronic daily headaches are believed to be caused by overuse of pain medications, especially barbiturates (such as butalbital [Fiorinal], ergotamines, triptans, benzodiazepines [such as Valium or Xanax]) and some analgesics.[32] About 80 percent of patients with chronic daily headaches improve by at least 50 percent just by successfully getting rid of their analgesics. Unfortunately, it's difficult to get people to do this, since the initial effect will be an increase in headaches.

If you have such headaches, you must be prepared to be uncomfortable for a few weeks in order to get long-term headache improvement. Fortunately, several medications can help make the process a little more bearable. The general principle is to taper the medications that are most likely to cause rebound and to substitute short-term medications that are less likely to cause rebound. Metoclopramide (Reglan) and hydroxyzine

(Vistaril), are not likely to cause rebound. Sleep disorders can be treated with a tricyclic antidepressant. A decreasing regimen of steroids, such as prednisone, given over several days, can also help. In one study, the anticonvulsant Neurontin, in doses of up to 2,400 mg per day, significantly increased the proportion of headache-free days in patients with chronic daily headache.[33]

## Osteoarthritis

Many people take a combination of over-the-counter glucosamine and chondroitin sulfate for osteoarthritis. What is the actual evidence of their efficacy? A recent comprehensive review of clinical trials in patients with knee osteoarthritis concluded that glucosamine at a dose of at least 1,500 mg per day is effective in reducing pain, improving function, and slowing down the degenerative changes in bone cartilage of the knee. Chondroitin sulfate also significantly reduced pain and improved function. Both substances are also very safe.[34]

It's now clear that glucosamine and chondroitin sulfate are effective treatments for osteoarthritis of the knee. Trials have shown that at a dose of at least 1,500 mg per day, glucosamine is about as effective as NSAIDs in improving pain and function. A really exciting finding is that it may also slow down the bone changes of osteoarthritis that can be seen on X-rays.[35,36]

To complete our tour of current and future medications for chronic pain, in the next two chapters we'll conclude with a detailed description of opioids (narcotics), their usefulness, their side effects, and why both doctors and patients are often reluctant to use them in treating chronic pain.

# 5

# OPIOIDS

## *What They Are and When They Are Useful*

*After years of being a computer programmer, I took on a project that required me to be on the computer keyboard about 12 hours a day. I suddenly started to experience severe pain in my hands whenever I typed. I tried rest and various alternative methods to input information into my computer, such as foot pedals and a voice recognition system, but nothing worked well enough. After a few months I had to quit my job. By this point, I was on very close terms with pain, but I hoped that eventually I would heal with enough rest and separation from the causes of my injury. Unfortunately, things didn't get better after this. In fact, the problem got worse, and soon spread to my shoulders, neck, and back. Eventually, I was diagnosed with acquired dystonia as well as repetitive stress injury.*

*I could not tolerate any pressure on my hands for more than a few seconds. A bit too much lifting, holding, or squeezing would give me days of pain. I could not hold or carry objects. I arranged elaborate schemes to move objects from one place to another, to open or close doors, and to open jars and bottles. I couldn't type five keystrokes without pain . . . . Eventually I even had to shorten my signature—writing my full signature caused pain. It was difficult to keep track of anything because I couldn't write or type. I could not drive, which drastically affected my social life, and made it hard for me to get to my physical therapy and doctor appointments.*

The pain spread to my shoulders and neck. I could not look at anything very long without a lot of pain unless it was exactly at eye level or slightly above. Even then, I could not look at anything close for very long. I could not read more than a page or two before the pain stopped me. I could not watch television more than 15 or 20 minutes. Movies were better because they were far away, but I had to sit exactly in the center—one seat off and my neck was in serious pain from the slight twisting. I could not lie down for very long, nor could I sit for very long. I often felt horribly depressed and just wanted to crawl into bed. It was hard to talk on the phone— headsets made my neck hurt, and holding the phone made my hands hurt. The straw that broke the camel's back, however, was not being able to read. Instead, I sat around bored and agitated, with absolutely nothing to do that wouldn't cause pain, and contemplated suicide.

I was finally referred to a chronic pain doctor, who put me on multiple medications including muscle relaxers, sleeping pills, and huge doses of Neurontin, which gave me some relief. He was willing to try any type of medication, except opioids (narcotics). Once he prescribed a few Vicodin (hydrocodone) for when I was desperate, but that was it. At age 29 I was on Social Security Disability, basically confined to home, and my life seemed to be over. My parents, who were worried about my depression, finally persuaded me to move back to my home city.

In my home state, where the doctors seemed less frightened of opioids than in Silicon Valley, I began seeing a doctor who started me on a trial of sustained-release morphine, which truly worked wonders, and had many fewer side effects than I possibly could have imagined given the potency of the medication. Suddenly I was able to drive again! I could also write without problems, and even type a few keystrokes! My doctor increased my dose until I was fairly comfortable. Now, I can type a fair amount—sometimes up to two to three hours a day! Other things, like reading, are easier. I've been on the same dose of morphine for a couple of years now and am much more functional. I am now attending art classes at the local university and can do the work required, which includes writing, drawing, and sculpting. I used to play the piano, and after years of avoiding the piano keyboard I have recently begun playing for a few minutes a day. I'm hoping to strengthen my hands so I can get back to the music I loved. I have a life again.

—WALTER, A 32-YEAR-OLD
FORMER COMPUTER PROGRAMMER

THROUGHOUT HISTORY, THE MOST EFFECTIVE PAIN-RELIEVING medications have been various forms of morphine. Generations of soldiers have been treated with morphine on the battlefield. But more than any other class of drugs, opioids (relatives of morphine) elicit strong opinions from physicians and the public, some strongly favoring their use, others considering them drugs to be avoided at all costs. Part of the problem is that most people, including some doctors, know very little about these drugs. Many draw conclusions and make decisions about opioids based on myths and misunderstandings. In this chapter, my goal is to describe these drugs to you, explain their appropriate use, and identify the controversies surrounding their prescription. In chapter 6, I will address the tremendous confusion about opioids and addiction, and will introduce you to the perspectives of professional organizations and regulatory agencies regarding the medical use of these drugs.

## What Are Opioids?

Morphine, the original drug of this class, is a purified form of opium, a chemical that is found in opium poppies. Derivatives of morphine are called opiates, and synthetic chemicals that behave like morphine in their ability to bind to opiate receptors in the body, relieve pain, and have other morphinelike properties are called opioids. The term opioids is also used to refer to all drugs with morphinelike properties.

Opioids are effective pain relievers for all types of pain, including neuropathic pain, which was until recently believed to be resistant to this class of analgesics. Higher doses of opioids may be needed to treat neuropathic pain than to treat other types of pain.[1] Nonetheless, this class of pain medications is definitely useful for neuropathic pain. For example, a randomized trial of controlled-release oxycodone in patients with post-herpetic neuralgia (PHN, or shingles) found that oxycodone, in an average dose of 45 mg per day, was effective in alleviating the steady pain, paroxysms of sudden spontaneous pain, and allodynia (pain sensations arising from usually nonpainful stimuli such as an item of clothing touching the skin).[2]

Morphine's analgesic effect takes place in several sites in the brain and spinal cord, including the midbrain and dorsal horn. It also acts on the limbic system, which is known to play a major role in both pain and pleasure. It's not surprising then that some people become addicted to opioids. The ability of morphine to produce analgesia (pain relief) varies greatly from person to person. This has also been found in animal studies, where different strains of lab animals have markedly different sensitivities to various opioids. According to Dr. Ronald Melzack, a psychologist who made extensive studies of the way pain signals travel through the body, "An important message emerging from studies of such variation is that the need for a high dose is not necessarily a sign of addiction."[3] The various opioids do not differ significantly in their ability to relieve pain, although some are more potent than others (meaning that smaller doses are required for the same effect). They all have the same basic side effects, although some opioids are more constipating, sedating, or nauseating in some people than are others. If a patient has difficulty tolerating a particular opioid, it may be worthwhile trying a different one.

Opioids relieve pain by binding to receptors that are antinociceptive; that is, they counteract pain signals. The three most important classes of opioid receptors are mu, kappa, and delta. Opioids bind predominantly to the mu receptor. Opioid receptors are found in the central nervous system (brain and spinal cord) and the gastrointestinal tract. They are also present, though to a lesser extent, in the peripheral tissues.

Like many other drugs, various opioids are available in more than one form: injectable, oral (pills and lozenges), transdermal (skin patches), rectal suppositories, and sprays. Because chronic 24/7 pain is best treated by long-acting drugs, several opioids that are inherently short-acting are available in sustained-release forms that permit a steady level in the bloodstream over many hours.

## The Drugs

MORPHINE. Morphine, the original opioid, was first extracted from poppy seeds in 1806 and has been used ever since. Morphine is broken down in the liver. Injected drugs act faster than do pills because when a drug is injected, it bypasses the liver and goes straight into the bloodstream. Not surprisingly then, it takes less morphine—about one-third the dose—to relieve pain when the drug is injected than when it is taken orally. This is why people are often given injections rather than pills for acute pain. For chronic pain, however, there is no benefit to injecting morphine, or any other pain reliever, rather than taking it by mouth.

After processing in the liver, morphine metabolites (breakdown products) are excreted in the urine. About half the morphine is converted to morphine-3-glucuronide (M3G) and another 10 percent to morphine-6-glucuronide (M6G). Both of these metabolites accumulate in the body and, with chronic use, are found in much greater concentrations in the blood than is the morphine itself. M6G is also a painkiller and, in fact, may be an even stronger analgesic than morphine. M3G has no analgesic activity and can cause hyperalgesia (increased pain sensitivity) and allodynia (pain perception from normally nonpainful stimuli). In high concentrations, it can also cause confusion, muscle tremors (myoclonus), and seizures.[4] Paradoxically, M3G can also cause increased pain.[5] Patients on high-dose morphine who experience these side effects will probably do better if switched to a different opioid. Patients whose kidney functioning is impaired should avoid using morphine for chronic pain, because both M3G and M6G are significantly increased in their blood and can lead to toxicity.

Morphine is available in several different formulations. In addition to immediate-release pills, the drug is marketed in several sustained-release formulations. MSContin and generic versions of it last 8 to 12 hours. Kadian and Avinza are marketed as once-a-day formulations, but Kadian often requires twice-a-day dosing. Avinza actually lasts 24 hours, and has the added feature that part of it is released quickly for a rapid response, and the rest during the remaining 24 hours.

CODEINE. Codeine, in combination with acetaminophen, is one of the most widely used opioids prescribed for pain relief. Unfortunately, at more than minimal doses, codeine causes more side effects, such as nausea and constipation, than do other opioids. Also, in order for codeine to provide pain relief, it must be converted to morphine. This occurs in the liver, by means of the enzyme CYP 2D6. In the United States, about 7 to 10 percent of Whites and 3 percent of Blacks lack this enzyme, with the result that these people will not obtain effective pain relief with codeine, even at high doses. Additionally, the activity of the enzyme CYP 2D6 is inhibited by several commonly used medications, including fluoxetine (Prozac), paroxetine (Paxil), cimetidine (Tagamet), and propoxyphene (Darvon), meaning that codeine might be less effective for you if you are also on these medications. Although codeine provides pain relief for most people who use it for acute pain, it is not a good choice for chronic pain because of its short duration of action, high incidence of constipation and nausea, and lack of efficacy in people lacking the enzyme needed to activate it.

HYDROCODONE. Hydrocodone is the main active ingredient in several widely used pain medications such as Vicodin, Lortab, and Norco. It is somewhat less potent than oxycodone.

OXYCODONE. Oxycodone, a potent synthetic opioid, is about 1.5 times as potent as the same dose of morphine given by mouth. A single dose provides pain relief for about four hours. Unlike morphine, the metabolites of oxycodone do not have any activity, either for pain relief or for irritation of the central nervous system. This, of course, is an advantage of oxycodone over morphine. An extended-release formulation of oxycodone (OxyContin) provides pain relief for up to 12 hours. The tablet is formulated to release some of its contents within 30 to 60 minutes, providing fast pain relief, and the rest gradually over 12 hours. You may have read articles or seen TV programs stating that OxyContin is particularly dangerous because it has a high-abuse potential. The truth is that all sustained-release pills can be misused and abused. This does not take away from the efficacy of sustained-release medications for relief of 24/7 pain.

HYDROMORPHONE. This derivative of hydrocodone is about five times as powerful as morphine. It is available in injections but also as a pill. Currently, only a short-acting formulation is available (Dilaudid), which is useful in breakthrough pain, but a long-acting controlled-release version is now in clinical trials.

FENTANYL. Fentanyl is a potent synthetic opioid, about 80 times as strong as morphine. It has been used as an intravenous injection for many years for surgical procedures, but is also available in a transdermal delivery system. Embedded in a patch (Duragesic patch) that releases the drug into the skin over three days (two in some people), it is very useful in the treatment of chronic pain. When applying the patch, it's important to press it against your skin for a full minute with the palm of your hand.

The warmth of your hand helps the adhesive bind to your skin. You should also know that heat increases the delivery of the drug through your skin; for this reason, sitting in a hot tub while you're wearing the patch is not a good idea. After the fentanyl diffuses through your skin, it is stored in the subcutaneous fat (fat layer under the skin). People who are very thin may have trouble absorbing the medication. If you are not well padded, it's best to apply the patch to the abdomen or buttocks, areas in which thin people have some fat. When the first patch is applied it takes almost a whole day for the full effect, and when the patch is removed, its effects continue for several hours.

When used for chronic pain, transdermal fentanyl was shown in a recent study to be significantly less constipating than sustained-release oxy-codone or morphine.[6] Fentanyl is also available as a raspberry-flavored lozenge on a stick—in other words, a lollipop—that delivers fentanyl through the mucosa (lining) of the mouth, as well as through the gastrointestinal tract when it is swallowed. Oral transmucosal fentanyl citrate (OTFC, or Actiq) is very effective for breakthrough pain. A quarter of the fentanyl is quickly absorbed through the oral mucosa into circulation, while the rest is swallowed and is more slowly absorbed through the gastrointestinal tract. It has a very rapid onset of action—about 5 to 10 minutes—and the peak blood level is reached in only 20 to 25 minutes. It is particularly effective for rapid-onset intense pain, such as in migraine headaches; the use of OTFC can prevent an ER visit for an injection. Transmucosal fentanyl is also very useful for office procedures—such as a skin biopsy, suturing, sigmoidoscopy, or splinting a fracture—where short-duration pain is anticipated. The biggest drawback to using fentanyl lollipops is their cost, currently about $18 for a single 800-mcg lozenge and about $13 for the 400-mcg dose.

Although OTFC is useful for many kinds of breakthrough pain, it is FDA-approved only for cancer pain. A study of its long-term safety and efficacy in cancer patients at home found that it was safe, gave excellent pain relief, and most patients did not require increased dosing over several months of treatment.[7]

OXYMORPHONE. An extended-release form of the potent opioid oxymorphone is now undergoing clinical trials and may soon be available as another option in the treatment of chronic pain.

LEVORPHANOL. This synthetic opioid, related to the cough-medicine ingredient dextromethorphan, has a longer duration of action than morphine. It is not used much but is a very effective analgesic.

METHADONE. You may have heard of this synthetic opioid, which has been used for many years in the treatment of narcotic addiction, as a means of preventing withdrawal and diminishing craving. Many addicts have been able to lead normal lives while taking methadone for years without any adverse effects. Methadone has a long serum half-life—up to three days—so that one dose a day suffices to prevent withdrawal symptoms. For pain relief, however, most people require three or four doses per day, which is a disadvantage. This is counterbalanced, however, by the very low cost of methadone compared with other sustained-release opioids. The long half-life of the drug means that dosage increases must be done slowly, only once every few days. Otherwise, the drug can accumulate in the system and result in an overdose.

Methadone is a combination of two mirror-image forms (isomers), called d-methadone and l-methadone. The pain-relieving effect of methadone comes mostly from the l-form, but d-methadone is an NMDA-receptor antagonist, and therefore stimulates the body's own pain-relieving cascade. Because of this effect, methadone may be particularly effective in neuropathic pain.

Methadone is metabolized extensively in the liver, where several other drugs can either slow down or speed up the process. Taking methadone along with these other drugs will result in higher or lower methadone blood levels than in a patient who is taking only methadone. For example, a patient, who is also taking the anticonvulsant Tegretol may need twice the dose of methadone to get the same pain relief as someone not on Tegretol. Once again, if your doctor is trying to decide which opioid is best for you, it's important that you tell him about every other medication you're taking.

Another problem with methadone is that switching to methadone from another drug is not straightforward. If your doctor wants to change your pain medication from morphine to oxycodone, the usual conversion ratio of 1.5 to 1 means that if you've been taking 30 mg of morphine, an equivalent (equianalgesic) dose of oxycodone will be about 20 mg. If you've been taking 120 mg of morphine, you'll probably do well on 80 mg of oxycodone. But unlike the consistent conversion ratios between most other opioids, the ratio of methadone to other drugs is variable. For example, a patient on a relatively low dose of morphine, say 60 mg per day, will require perhaps 10 to 20 mg of methadone per day to get the same pain relief, a ratio of 6 to 1 or 3 to 1. But for a patient on 600 mg per day of morphine, an equianalgesic dose of methadone may be 50 mg of methadone, a ratio of 12 to 1. This makes it hard to convert patients from other opioids to methadone.

Finally, among those on methadone for chronic pain or addiction maintenance, a report was published on a few people who were on moderate to high doses of methadone (80 to 1,000 mg per day) and who developed a potentially fatal rhythm disorder of the heart, called *torsades de pointes*.[8,9] Although such a risk is small, some doctors now obtain an electrocardiogram in patients who are on very high doses of methadone to be sure that their electrical conduction is normal.

Methadone is an effective, inexpensive painkiller that has been appropriately getting more use in the past few years, but these difficulties mean it must be prescribed with caution, by knowledgeable physicians.

MEPERIDINE (DEMEROL). Sickle cell anemia is an inherited disease that causes red blood cells to be deformed so that they can clog small blood vessels in the bones and other tissues, causing painful oxygen deprivation in these tissues. "Sickle cell crises," especially frequent in African-Americans in their teens and twenties, cause severe pain in the back, chest, abdomen, arms, legs, and head. They usually require hospitalization for pain relief. When I was in training 25 years ago, the standard treatment for such patients was intravenous fluids and repeated intravenous injections of the opioid meperidine (Demerol) for pain relief. Meperidine is still used in some emergency rooms for treatment of severe headaches and by some surgeons for postoperative pain.

Some years ago, I gave a talk on pain management at a hospital that frequently admitted patients with sickle cell crises. The physicians there told me that doctors used to believe that seizures were a symptom of sickle cell crisis. We now know that the cause of those patients' convulsions wasn't their disease, but their pain treatment: meperidine.

Meperidine is a synthetic opioid that is converted in the body to normeperidine, a metabolite with a 15- to 20-hour half-life that accumulates in the body with repeated dosing and can cause irritability, tremors, muscle twitching (myoclonus), and seizures. This is likely to happen even more quickly in people who are dehydrated or whose kidney function is impaired. Because of this problem, the American Pain Society recommends limiting the dose of meperidine to 600 mg per day for only two days. For patients more than 60 years old, the limit is 400 mg per day.[10] Another problem with meperidine is that, unlike other opioids, its toxicity is not reversed when the antagonist naloxone (Narcan) is administered.

PROPOXYPHENE (DARVON). This weak synthetic opioid, once a very popular medication for mild to moderate pain, is gradually disappearing from use. It is no more effective than aspirin or acetaminophen and, like meperidine, has a toxic metabolite (norpropoxyphene) that can cause irritability, muscle twitching, and seizures. It has no advantages over other pain medications.

## OPIOIDS

| DRUG NAME | MANUFACTURER | GENERIC NAME |
|-----------|--------------|--------------|
| Actiq | Cephalon | oral transmucosal fentanyl citrate (OTFC) |
| Avinza | Ligand | morphine sulfate |
| Darvon | AAI Pharma | propoxyphene |
| Demerol | Sanofi-Synthelabo | meperidine |
| Dilaudid | Abbott | hydromorphone |
| Kadian | Alpharma Branded | morphine sulfate |
| levorphanol | several | levorphanol |
| Lortab | UCB Pharma | hydrocodone and acetaminophen |
| Methadose | Mallinckrodt | methadone |
| MS Contin | Purdue Frederick | morphine sulfate |
| Norco | Watson | hydrocodone and acetaminophen |
| Numorphan | Endo Labs | oxymorphone |
| OxyContin | Purdue Frederick | oxycodone |
| Vicodin | Abbott | hydrocodone and acetaminophen |
| codeine | several | codeine |

## *Partial Agonists and Agonists/Antagonists*

Joan was a 32-year-old woman who had frequent, severe migraine headaches. Her neurologist had tried prescribing multiple medications for prevention of her headaches, but nothing seemed to work. When a migraine developed, she didn't respond to sumatriptan (Imitrex), the only triptan available 10 years ago. Finally, her neurologist put her on butorphanol (Stadol) nasal spray. A couple of sprays of this opioid gave her relief at times, but she still ended up in the emergency room once or twice a week. When she came to see me, I prescribed methadone for her, which she began taking three times a day every day. On this regimen, her headaches were controlled and she no longer needed to spend time in the emergency room.

One evening I got a call from Joan's husband, who sounded desperate. He said Joan was shaky, had abdominal cramps and diarrhea, felt anxious and frightened, and didn't know what was happening. A few more questions and I found out that Joan had developed a migraine that evening, had found an old bottle of Stadol nasal spray in the bathroom cabinet, and had sprayed two sprays into her nostril. What Joan was experiencing was acute withdrawal from methadone precipitated by the antagonist action of butorphanol. This is not dangerous, but can be very uncomfortable and frightening. Not knowing that Joan still had some of this medication remaining, I hadn't specifically warned her of the risks of combining its use with a pure opioid agonist (the methadone she was taking regularly).

As stated earlier in this chapter, opioids bind to three classes of receptors: mu, kappa, and delta. Opioids interact with these receptors in various ways, leading to the following three classifications:

- **Full opioid agonist**, also called a pure mu agonist, is an agent that binds to the mu opioid receptor and stimulates a physiologic response—analgesia.
- **Partial agonist** binds to only part of the mu receptors, so that it provides less pain relief. Partial agonists have a ceiling effect, above which they do not produce any more pain relief.
- **Mixed agonist-antagonist** produces analgesia by binding to the kappa receptor. It also binds to the mu receptor, but it does not produce analgesia; instead, it either just takes up space, preventing a full agonist from having any pain-relieving effect at this site, or it actually has the opposite effect. When a mixed agonist-antagonist is administered together with an agonist, the antagonist effect at the mu receptor can cause an acute withdrawal syndrome.

Buprenorphine (Buprenex, Suboxone), which is a partial agonist, and the agonist-antagonists nalbuphine (Nubain), butorphanol (Stadol) and pentazocine (Talwin, Talacen) can cause opioid withdrawal when given to patients who have already taken opioid agonists. Unlike pure opioid agonists, partial agonists such as buprenorphine and agonist-antagonists such as butorphanol (Stadol) have a maximum dose above which they are not more effective and, in fact, may be less effective than at lower doses. This limits their use to treating moderate but not severe pain. In a sublingual form, buprenorphine is finding increased use in detoxification for narcotic addicts, but its use in chronic pain is limited.

Pentazocine (Talwin) is hardly used anymore. Its pain-relieving effects result primarily from its interaction with the opioid kappa receptor, where it can cause unpleasant psychiatric effects. These effects are increasingly likely in long-term use of this drug, so such use is not recommended for chronic pain.

## How Effective Are Opioids for Chronic Non-cancer Pain?

The experience of pain management physicians is that long-term opioid treatment for chronic pain is effective and safe. Randomized double-blind studies (in which neither doctor nor patient knows what medication the patient is taking) are difficult to do, so that rigorous published studies are rare. However, several observational studies have reported outcomes of the use of opioids for chronic pain and have supported their efficacy.

One of the earliest studies looked retrospectively (after the fact) at 38 patients who'd been treated with various opioids for long periods of time (19 for more than 4 years) for non-cancer pain of various types. Most patients reported adequate pain relief, and only two patients had management problems. Both of them had a history of prior drug abuse.[11] In a study of 100 patients treated with various sustained-release opioids for non-cancer pain, 51 percent reported good pain relief, 28 percent partial pain relief. All the patients who had a reduction in pain also reported improved function. Among the patients treated with morphine, the average dose was 255 mg per day. The majority of patients continued on stable doses of their opioid medication, indicating that tolerance to the pain-relieving effects of the drug did not develop.[12]

In another study, more than 500 patients with various types of chronic non-cancer pain were begun on transdermal fentanyl patches (Duragesic) and were followed for a median of 10 months. Patients who had a history of opioid abuse were excluded from the study. Pain was significantly improved within two days, and the quality of life within a month. Ninety percent of patients who obtained significant pain relief continued to have pain relief throughout the study. The dose required for pain relief, which averaged 37.6 mcg per hour, did not change significantly during the first 8 months. A few patients (25) who were followed for 4 years had a gradually increasing dose requirement, which averaged 67.3 mcg per hour after 48 months. Some of this increase may have been due to progression of their pain syndrome. Patients with neuropathic pain, for whom opioids were formerly believed to be ineffective, did as well as patients with nociceptive pain.[13]

In a small study conducted for 32 weeks, 36 chronic back pain patients received either a combination of sustained-release morphine regularly twice a day and oxycodone (as needed for breakthrough pain) or naproxen. The opioid group had significantly less pain and less emotional distress than the group receiving naproxen. At the end of the study, all but one of the 25 patients on opioids were successfully tapered off the drugs without difficulty.[14]

In another trial of an opioid to treat osteoarthritis pain, controlled-release oxycodone at an average dose of 40 mg per day, was superior to no oxycodone in reducing pain, and improving mood, sleep, and enjoyment of life. Fifty-eight patients completed 6 months of treatment, 41 completed 12 months, and 15 patients had 18 months of treatment. During long-term treatment, the mean dose remained stable and pain intensity was stable.[15] This study supports the view that chronic opioid treatment is safe and effective, and patients are unlikely to become tolerant to the pain-relieving effect of the drug.

It used to be thought that opioids were ineffective for chronic neuropathic pain, such as peripheral diabetic neuropathy or post-herpetic neuralgia (PHN, or shingles). However, that is not the case. Some patients may require higher doses of opioids for neuropathic pain than for musculoskeletal pain, but it's definitely worth trying opioid treatment for any type of pain. For example, a randomized controlled trial comparing methadone to an antidepressant for treating shingles pain showed that both treatments were effective.[16]

## *Which Opioid Is Best for Me?*

Opioids are a lot more similar to one another than they are different. They all have the same general effects and similar side effects. Some opioids are more potent than others, meaning you need a lower dose to get the same effect. For example, hydromorphone is about five times as potent as morphine; oxycodone is about 1.5 times as strong as morphine. However, when given in equivalent doses, these drugs are equally effective in alleviating pain. Thirty mg of morphine, for example, is likely to be as effective as 20 mg of oxycodone. In some situations, a fentanyl patch might be a better choice than a pill—for example, people who've taken too many pain pills in the past or in those who have difficulty swallowing. Also, with people who require a lot of nursing care, it might be simpler for a caregiver to apply a patch once every 3 days than to give a pill twice a day. Another reason to choose one opioid over another is that morphine is more likely to cause itching than does oxycodone or fentanyl. If morphine makes you itch, your doctor will probably switch you to a different opioid.

A literature review of the comparative efficacy and safety of long-acting opioids in the management of chronic non-cancer pain looked at 16 randomized (the preferred type of study) and eight observational studies and concluded that there was not enough evidence to prove that various long-acting opioids differ in efficacy or safety.[17] Remember, though, that people differ genetically and in other ways in their sensitivity to various opioids. For an individual patient, one opioid may be more effective or cause fewer side effects than another. The authors also concluded that there is fair evidence that short-acting oxycodone and long-acting oxycodone are equally effective for pain control. However, the long-acting formulations have other advantages—there is no concern about the toxicity of interaction with aspirin or acetaminophen, the long duration assures better sleep, and there is less clock-watching while waiting for the time to take the next pill.

As stated before, all opioids have the same basic mechanism of action—they relieve pain by binding to opioid receptors. All opioids have the same kinds of side effects, the most important ones being sedation, nausea and vomiting, and constipation. However, there are significant individual differences in the way people respond to various opioid drugs. For example, at a given level of pain relief with a particular opioid, one person may have very little constipation, but another person may have to stop the treatment because her constipation is so severe. The same is true of the degree of pain relief. One patient may get excellent relief with morphine, whereas another—who has the same type of pain problem—may continue to have severe pain despite getting huge doses of the same drug. In one report, a cancer patient got no relief from morphine, no matter how high the dose, but became very comfortable when she was switched to hydromorphone (Dilaudid). Another patient, with chronic back pain, did much better with methadone than morphine.[18]

The differences in response may be due to many factors, such as the type and intensity of pain, the patient's expectations, and psychological factors such as depression or anxiety. Additionally, genetic factors may be extremely important. This has been shown experimentally in lab animals. In mice, for example, one strain may be 100 times more sensitive to morphine than another strain, and these differences can be related to specific genetic differences in the opiate receptors of the different mouse strains. The same is true for sensitivity to other opioids.

The take-home message is that if a patient's chronic pain is resistant to high doses of one opioid, the next step is to try a different opioid, and yet another if needed. Don't decide that opioids are useless for the particular pain problem until several have been tried, each in large doses.

## Long-Versus Short-acting Opioids for Sustained Pain

Even if you have round-the-clock pain, your doctor may have prescribed a regimen of a short-acting painkiller such as Vicodin (hydrocodone plus acetaminophen) or Percocet (oxycodone plus acetaminophen) to be taken several times a day as needed. Visualize what such a schedule does to the concentration of say, oxycodone, in your blood stream. When you take a dose, the drug's level in your blood rapidly increases, providing you with pain relief and, for some people, a slight buzz or else a brief cloudiness or sedation. Within a few hours, the blood levels drop, leading to a recurrence of the pain. As blood levels go up and down like a roller coaster, the pain relief and side effects often do the same.

In contrast, a sustained-release form of the same drug will give much smoother blood levels, and therefore more effective pain relief with fewer side effects. In addition, because you don't have to get up in the middle of the night to take another pain pill, your sleep is likely to improve. Several opioids are available in sustained-release forms. Ironically, methadone, which is the only opioid of the bunch that truly has a long half-life in the body, does not provide sustained pain relief and must be taken three or four times a day for pain. (On the other hand, because of the long half-life, one dose per day will effectively prevent withdrawal, which is why methadone clinics that treat heroin addicts supply them with methadone only once a day).

In chapter 2 we spoke about central sensitization and neuronal plasticity. To review, repeated stimulation by ongoing signals from nociceptive neurons (caused by ongoing pain) sensitizes neurons in the dorsal horn of the spinal cord, which can cause such permanent changes in the spinal cord and brain that a given signal produces more pain (hyperalgesia). The way to prevent this undesirable outcome is to avoid repeated pain signals. Long-acting opioids, which provide consistent levels of pain relief for many hours, are more effective than short-acting opioids at preventing pain. It takes a reduced amount of drugs to prevent the recurrence of pain than to treat recurring pain.

This was shown in a study that compared immediate-release versus sustained-release oxycodone given after outpatient knee surgery done under general anesthesia. Patients who regularly received long-acting oxycodone (20 mg of OxyContin every 12 hours) experienced less pain and used less pain medicine during the first 3 days than did patients treated "as needed" with immediate-release oxycodone. In addition, the OxyContin group had less sedation, better sleep, and less postoperative vomiting.[19] In another study, immediate-release and controlled-release oxycodone were equally effective, but the ER (extended release) formulation required only twice-a-day dosing.[20] The same conclusions were reached in a study comparing sustained-release oxycodone (OxyContin) with short-acting oxycodone/acetaminophen (Percocet) in patients with osteoarthritis.[21]

## Chronic Pain and Breakthrough Pain

Although the severity of pain may vary from day to day in people with chronic pain, many people experience transient increases in their baseline pain level. Some of these episodes, called breakthrough pain, are predictable, occurring with increased activity or assuming certain positions. People experience increased pain when they first awaken, or before they start moving around in the morning or after sitting still for a while. Others have breakthrough pain at the end of the dosing interval of their regularly scheduled pain medications. Yet other episodes of breakthrough pain are unpredictable—it's unclear what brings them on.

Because breakthrough pain is common in patients with chronic pain, patients being treated with long-acting opioids often need a second prescription for an opioid with rapid onset and short half-life. This second prescription, which may be for Vicodin, Percocet, or immediate-release morphine or oxycodone, is available for those times during the day when you experience temporary increased pain. If you find yourself taking many doses daily of your breakthrough pain medication, your doctor will probably choose to increase your baseline dose of long-acting opioid. Breakthrough pain medications are meant for transiently increased pain, not as part of your regular pain regimen.

## What Do I Do for Breakthrough Pain?

There are several options for breakthrough pain. All have a quick onset and relatively short duration: The oral medications relieve pain within 30 to 60 minutes, and their effect lasts from 3 to 6 hours. The most commonly used are the long-available combinations of hydrocodone and acetaminophen (Vicodin, Lorcet, Norco, etc.) and oxycodone and acetaminophen (Percocet). Hydrocodone is also available in combination with aspirin (Lortab), as is oxycodone (Percodan). Oxycodone and morphine are available in immediate-release form without either aspirin or acetaminophen, and these preparations are useful if the amount of breakthrough pain you need exceeds the daily safe allowance of aspirin or acetaminophen in the pills.

Another alternative is to use the rapid-acting oral transmucosal fentanyl citrate (OTFC) lollipops [Actiq]. In a study of migraine patients, 28 used their usual medications for migraine attacks and at-home OTFC for severe episodes. All but two obtained significant pain relief and were able to avoid an emergency room visit. During a 1 year period, these patients used fentanyl lozenges for an average of seven migraine attacks.

In another study of 20 migraine patients who used OTFC for severe episodes, the number of emergency room visits decreased from 2.8 visits per month before beginning the medication to 0.3 visits per month when using the lozenges. Only four patients had any ER visits during this period. Migraine patients reported that their pain significantly decreased within 15 minutes of using Actiq, and they continued to improve over the next 2 hours.[22]

## *Is There a Maximum Safe Dose of Opioids?*

When it comes to prescribing drugs for high blood pressure, the standard approach is to increase the dose of antihypertensive until the blood pressure is normal, and/or to add another antihypertensive and increase the dose of that drug upward until the goal blood pressure is reached. Similarly, in prescribing for depression, the dose of antidepressant is increased until the depression resolves. The same is true in prescribing for diabetes, seizure disorders, and most other conditions. Yet when it comes to opioids, many physicians fear prescribing more than an arbitrary number of pills or more than a certain number of milligrams of morphine or other opioid. This really makes no sense. Opioids are just another class of medications, and their dose should be increased until there is adequate pain control with a minimum of side effects.

Opioids are actually a very safe class of drugs. Unlike acetaminophen or aspirin and other NSAIDs, there is no upper limit beyond which pure opioid agonists are unsafe or will damage the body. For patients who don't obtain adequate pain relief with low doses of opioids, physicians' reluctance to prescribe high doses is not based on safety issues, but usually is caused by their fears of regulatory scrutiny.

For a pure opioid, the appropriate dose is the one that relieves a patient's pain throughout the dosing interval without causing significant side effects. Most patients require doses of less than 250 mg of morphine (or equivalent) per day, but patients with severe cancer or non-cancer pain may require up to 1 to 2 grams of morphine per day. Some cancer patients need huge doses, up to 5 grams *per hour* of intravenous morphine (which is three times as potent as morphine pills). The textbook of the American Society of Addiction Medicine states:

Opioids may be used safely and effectively at even massive doses (such as several hundred mg of IV morphine per hour) in individuals who have gradually increasing exposure to these analgesics over a prolonged period of time.[23]

Some of the variability in the dose that is needed to relieve pain is caused by the nature of the pain problem or extent of the disease. But some is due to genetic differences between people in their response to different opioids. Some people are very resistant to one opioid, but respond well to another.[24] Research in both animals and humans has shown that one reason is genetic differences. For example, a mouse study found that one strain of mice is more resistant to heroin than to morphine. The reason is a genetic difference in their opioid receptors.[25] In humans, the best-known genetic case of varying responses to pain medications is with codeine, which, in order to relieve pain, must be converted to morphine. As I mentioned earlier in this chapter, people who lack the gene for the liver enzyme required to convert codeine to morphine will not get pain relief even from high doses of codeine. Another liver enzyme, CYP 3A4, is required for the metabolism of the opioid analgesic alfentanil, which is used intravenously during surgery. Differences in the activity of this enzyme may explain why there is a large variation in the amount of this drug that different patients require for anesthesia.[26]

The lesson from these studies is that if you need a very high dose of the drug you are taking, it's possible you are resistant to that particular opioid. You might get better pain relief from a different opioid.

## Will I Need to Keep Increasing the Dose to Get Pain Relief?

TOLERANCE AND PSEUDOTOLERANCE. The need for an increasing dose to get the same effect is called tolerance. Tolerance to the analgesic effects of opioids is rare.[27] Until recently, high doses of opioids were used primarily to treat terminally ill cancer patients. In such patients, it's been known for more than 25 years that even long-term use of opioids does not result in tolerance or addiction. The experience of chronic pain specialists is that once an effective dose of pain medication is given, the dose often stays the same for a long time.[28] When cancer patients require increased doses of opioids, it's usually because their disease is progressing, not because they have developed tolerance to the pain-relieving effect of their drug.

The same is true of most non-cancer patients. Once the dose required for pain relief is established, it usually remains the same unless the underlying disease progresses. This has been shown in many studies.[29,30,31] Dr. Daniel Brookoff, associate director of the Comprehensive Pain Institute at the Methodist Hospital of Memphis, Tennessee, says, "The clinical implications are clear but under-appreciated: Inadequately treated pain is a much more important cause of opioid tolerance than the use of opioids themselves."[32]

In a recent study, 71 patients with back pain completed 1 year of treatment with a sustained-release form of morphine called Avinza. Their average starting dose was 184 mg per day, increasing to 217 mg per day over 6 months, and remaining stable from months 7 to 12. After the first month, their pain level did not change.[33] These doses are considered quite high by some physicians, but this study shows that after an initial increase in pain, which was most likely due to increased activity, the dose remained stable for many months and there were no untoward adverse effects.

Concerning tolerance, a consensus statement issued in 1996 by the American Academy of Pain Medicine and the American Pain Society states:

> Tolerance or decreasing pain relief with the same dosage [of opioid] over time has not proven to be a prevalent limitation to long-term opioid use. Experience with treating cancer pain has shown that what initially appears to be tolerance is usually progression of the disease. Furthermore, for most opioids, there does not appear to be an arbitrary upper dosage limit, as was previously thought.[34]

Dr. Russell Portenoy, a highly respected specialist in treating chronic pain, wrote:

> A large body of clinical experience indicates that tolerance to analgesic effects is rarely the driving force for declining analgesic effect. Opioid doses typically stabilize during long-term

administration, and when analgesic effects decline, a worsening physical lesion or changing psychological status is usually apparent. Contrary to conventional thinking, the development of analgesic tolerance appears to be a rare cause of failure of long-term opioid therapy.[35]

Recent studies suggest that some people who take high doses of opioids eventually develop an increased sensitivity to pain, needing ever-increasing doses. Although this phenomenon is unusual, these people develop a true tolerance to the pain-relieving effects of opioids.[36,37] The NMDA receptor may be involved in this, and NMDA receptor antagonist drugs such as methadone and ketamine might help reverse the process. In people taking morphine, it's possible that the increased pain is due to the accumulation of the metabolite morphine-3-glucuronide (M3G), but this does not explain increased pain in patients receiving other opioids. More research in this area is needed before any firm conclusions can be drawn.

Hyperalgesia, or increased sensitivity to noxious (painful) stimuli, is a well-recognized symptom of opioid withdrawal in opioid-tolerant people. People in withdrawal from opioids often complain of abdominal and muscle pain. A person who's been taking opioids for an extended period of time and suddenly stops is likely to experience more pain from a painful stimulus than someone who isn't in withdrawal. Animal studies have shown that hyperalgesia is more intense (increased pain) when the doses of opioids have been intermittent and that its development can be prevented by NMDA antagonism.[38]

In patients on opioid maintenance for the treatment of pain, hyperalgesia can be detected even in the presence of opioids, especially high-dose opioids given intravenously or intrathecally (into the spinal canal).[39,40] In other words, they've developed some resistance to opioids. It appears that opioid administration not only provides analgesia but concurrently sets into motion certain anti-analgesic or hyperalgesic processes, which serve to counteract or oppose the analgesic effects.[41] In other words, tolerance develops to the pain-relieving effect of the drug. We don't yet know if this also happens when treating chronic pain with long-acting opioids. Fortunately, what we do know is that when chronic pain patients are treated with sustained-release opioids in the form of pills or patches, tolerance is uncommon. When it does occur, tolerance can be managed by increasing the dose of opioid and/or adding an NMDA antagonist.

## The Need for More Pain Relief

Consider the following scenario, played out over and over again in doctors' offices:

> Gerald A, age 43, is referred to Dr. Z for treatment of chronic back pain. Mr. A relates to Dr. Z how his first herniated disk happened at age 35 and was operated on. A year later, his back pain recurred and he had a second operation, and 3 years later a third. Now, although he continues to have debilitating back pain, his neurosurgeon has told him surgery cannot help him. Mr. A has found that if he spends most of his time reclining on a sofa he can tolerate the pain, which he rates at 3 to 4 out of a maximum of 10. But when he sits for a long time, walks around, or lifts anything, the pain increases to an unbearable 8 to 9 out of 10. He doesn't work, he's given up his sports activities, and he doesn't leave his home unless necessary.
>
> Dr. Z prescribes 20 mg of sustained-release oxycodone twice a day for Mr. A, and a week later, Mr. A reports that his pain is now averaging only 2 out of 10. But 2 weeks later, the pain is back up to an average of 7 out of 10 during the day, and he would like to increase his dose. Has Mr. A developed tolerance to the pain-relieving effects of oxycodone?

In the prior section I explained that tolerance to the pain-relieving effects of opioids is uncommon. Once a chronic pain patient is stabilized on a dose of pain medication, it tends to stay the same, or nearly so, for a long time. So why did Mr. A need a higher dose of oxycodone? The answer in most cases is the patient's level of activity. The two goals of treating chronic pain are: (1) diminished pain and (2) improved function. In Mr. A's case, it turned out that after starting to take oxycodone, he had less pain, and he increased his activity level. He was helping his wife with the housework and had gone out with her to a restaurant for the first time in months. He was walking his dog for a few minutes each day. The increased physical activities resulted in increased pain. In order for Mr. A to average 3 to 4 out of 10 *while active*, he will need additional oxycodone. In the continuing scenario:

> Dr. Z increases Mr. A's dose of sustained-release oxycodone to 40 mg twice a day and encourages him to be physically active. On this regimen Mr. A resumes physical therapy to strengthen his back muscles, reports better sleep, and becomes better able to enjoy his life.

This is, of course, a description of a positive outcome, which doesn't always happen. But the point is that the outcome of being treated with opioids for chronic pain should be judged by the quality of the person's life, not by the dose of medication they require. Mr. A's case is an example of what has been called *pseudotolerance*,[42] a need for increased opioid medication for pain, which *looks like* tolerance, but is in fact caused by other factors. One is increased activity. Another cause, which may happen after months or years on the medication, is worsening of the underlying condition. This is, of course, extremely common in the treatment of cancer pain, but is sometimes found in non-cancer pain as well.

## What about Side Effects?

One of the biggest fears both doctors and patients have about opioids is that they have serious side effects or can damage the body. The reality is, however, that when opioids are used as prescribed, they are very safe drugs. First, let's discuss the most common and expected side effects: sedation, nausea, constipation, and sexual dysfunction. Fortunately, most people who are prescribed opioids quickly develop a tolerance to the sedative and nauseating effects of these drugs. Constipation, on the other hand, is a persistent symptom.

## Sedation

It's very common to feel sleepy or "drugged" when you first start taking an opioid, or when your dose is increased, but your body rapidly becomes resistant to this effect, which usually is gone within 3 to 7 days.[43] When patients are extremely sedated by opioids, they may experience a slow down in their breathing. This is termed *respiratory depression*. The American Academy of Pain Medicine/American Pain Society Consensus Statement on the Use of Opioids for the Treatment of Chronic Pain states:

> It is now accepted by practitioners of the specialty of pain medicine that respiratory depression induced by opioids tends to be a short-lived phenomenon, generally occurs only in the opioid-naïve patient [someone who hasn't taken opioids before and now is given a large dose], and is antagonized by pain. Therefore, withholding the appropriate use of opioids from a patient who is experiencing pain on the basis of respiratory concerns is unwarranted.[44]

In those cases in which the person continues to feel drugged or sleepy or not entirely clearheaded, the addition of psychostimulants—arousal drugs—such as a methylphenidate (Ritalin, Concerta) or amphetamine (Dexedrine, Adderall) can help the patient feel normal.[45] According to *The Medical Letter on Drugs and Therapeutics*, a highly respected newsletter that evaluates drugs, "Opioid-induced sedation can be ameliorated by giving small doses of dextroamphetamine [Dexedrine] or methylphenidate [Ritalin] in the morning and early afternoon."[46] Because both of these drugs are Schedule II "controlled substances" and there are special laws regarding prescribing them, physicians who are fearful of prescribing controlled substances are less likely to provide these medications. Nonetheless, most patients who take them to counteract opioid-induced sedation find them very helpful.

A new drug called modafinil (Provigil), although officially approved by the FDA only for daytime sleepiness due to narcolepsy, obstructive sleep apnea, and shift work sleep disorder, is increasingly being used to counteract the sedative effects of opioids. One dose of this well-tolerated medication in the morning increases the wakefulness of people whose opioids keep them sleepy.

Other drugs have also been tested in small numbers of patients and were found to be helpful. One of these is donepezil (Aricept), a drug that is approved for patients with early Alzheimer's disease, to slow the progression of their dementia. In a small trial, 5 mg of donepezil lessened sedation and fatigue in patients who reported sedation with the use of opioids for ongoing cancer pain.[47]

## Is It Safe for Me to Drive a Car if I'm Taking an Opioid for Chronic Pain?

The answer to this question depends upon the patient and the circumstances. It usually takes 3 to 7 days for the body to overcome sedation produced by opioids. When you first start taking the medication, or when you first increase the dose, I recommend not driving. After you're on the same dose for a few days and feel normal rather than sedated or foggy, then you can drive, even if you've just taken a dose of your pain medication.

Support for this view comes from many studies. For example, 144 patients with low back pain were administered two neuropsychological tests of psychomotor functioning before being prescribed opioids in a recent study. The tests determined their ability to concentrate (a type of mental activity or cognitive functioning) and to perform timed hand to eye coordination tasks (a type of fine motor skill). Ninety and 180 days after beginning regular use of transdermal fentanyl (Duragesic patch) up to 100 mcg per hour (average, 43 mcg per hour), and/or Percocet (oxycodone with acetaminophen) up to 12 per day (average 36 mg per day), they took the same tests again. The surprising result was that the test scores significantly *improved* while the patients were taking opioids for pain, which suggested that their ability to think or react was not impaired.[48] The explanation for the improved test scores is most likely as follows: Because pain can adversely affect your brain's functioning, pain relief has the potential to improve thinking. The results suggest that long-term opioid treatment does not result in fine motor or cognitive impairments and may improve cognitive functioning.

Dr. R.N. Jamison, the lead author of this study, said, "It might be a good idea for departments of transportation and other groups to reexamine their safety guidelines on how much opioids can be tolerated when using heavy equipment and driving."[49] In another study of 21 patients who were using Duragesic patches for at least 2 weeks at doses of 25 to 400 mcg per hour (median dose 50 mcg per hour), these patients performed as well as controls on a series of computerized tests that measured a variety of driving-related tasks.[50]

Another group of researchers recently reviewed 48 publications about the effect of opioids on driving skills. Most studies showed no impairment of psychomotor activities in patients maintained on opioids, no impairment when patients were tested on driving simulators, and no increased incidence of motor vehicle violations or accidents. In addition, they found strong consistent evidence in multiple studies for no impairment of psychomotor abilities immediately after being given doses of opioids.[51] An earlier study reviewed the epidemiological evidence regarding any association between opioid use and drunk driving and between opioid use and motor vehicle accidents. There was no association between opioid use and either drunk driving or car accidents.[52] The authors of the latter study concluded, "The results of this systematic review support the contention that patients taking opioids may be allowed to drive."

On several occasions, chronic pain patients have reported a high level of pain but have added, "But that's probably because I didn't take my pain medicine this morning because I had to drive here." They acknowledge that they don't *feel* sedated right after taking a painkiller, but they just want to be extra sure that their driving won't be impaired. Studies like the ones just described can reassure such patients that, unless they actually feel fuzzy or sedated, it's safe to take a dose of opioid and then drive.

A statement by Dr. Russell Portenoy written 8 years ago is still just as valid. He wrote, "Long-term opioid use is usually compatible with normal functioning and, in clinical practice, instructions to limit driving or other activities are not given unless overt impairment is observed."[53]

In its latest guidelines for the treatment of persistent pain in older persons, the American Geriatric Society has this to say about driving while taking opioids: "It is advisable to allow several days at the maintenance analgesic dose before advising the patient to resume driving."[54]

## Nausea

Nausea is another common side effect of opioids, occurring initially in most users. Fortunately, tolerance rapidly develops. If you are one of those people who almost vomits just from looking at an opioid pill, isn't your only option. A better one is to begin with a very small dose of the drug, for example one-quarter of a Vicodin or Percocet tablet, and increase by small increments after two or three doses. The smallest doses are unlikely to provide much pain relief, but they will quickly help your body tolerate the drug without nausea. For those people who still have residual nausea, very effective drugs are available. Older medications such as Compazine are usually effective. Nausea that results from delayed stomach emptying can be treated with metoclopramide (Reglan) or cisapride (Propulsid). For severe nausea, some new drugs were developed originally to combat the nausea of cancer chemotherapy, but are useful for nausea of other causes. These include ondansetron (Zofran) and granisetron (Kytril). Their biggest drawback is their high cost.

## Constipation

Constipation is the passage of fewer than three bowel movements per week, or having to strain at stool or having hard stools much of the time. Some people's normal pattern may be only one or two stools a week, which is fine as long as they don't have painful hard stools and as long as this isn't a recent change in their bowel habits. Constipation tends to increase with age, and is more likely in people whose diet is low in roughage, who don't drink enough fluids, who are physically inactive, or who take certain drugs, including opioids. Opioids bind to mu receptors in the gut, where they suppress peristalsis, the rhythmic movement of food through the digestive tract. Intestinal contents move more slowly through the gut, giving the body more time to remove water from them. The result is less frequent, harder stools.

Unlike nausea and sedation, which tend to diminish with continued opioid use, constipation persists. The higher the dose you are on, the more likely you are to have constipation. This is why if your doctor prescribes opioids for chronic pain, she or he is likely to suggest an ongoing bowel program for you. This program starts with increasing your fluid intake, fiber in the diet, and exercise. But this approach is often not enough. Most people who are prescribed opioids for chronic pain are advised to take a stool softener such as docusate (Colace) and a bowel stimulant such as senna (Senokot-S) on a daily basis to prevent problems.

Stool softeners increase water absorption in the stool (that is, if you are drinking enough fluids), while stimulant laxatives stimulate peristalsis, the movement of stool through the intestinal tract. Two tablets of Colace and two of Senokot-S daily are a good preventive regimen for many people. If you are not sure about this, consider the alternative—waiting until you are so blocked up that you need an enema or even manual dis-impaction!

If, despite these medications, you still become constipated, other types of laxatives can come to the rescue. One commonly used agent is lactulose syrup (Enulose), a sugar that attracts large quantities of water into the intestine. It may take a couple of days to work, and may cause bloating, cramping, and gas production, but it is very effective. Another powerful laxative that works the same way is polyethylene glycol (Miralax powder), which is preferred by some people because it is taste-less, in contrast to the very sweet taste of lactulose.

A drug that is used primarily for constipation-predominant irritable bowel syndrome (IBS) is finding new use for other types of constipation. Tegaserod (Zelnorm) is a drug that stimulates motility. Taken twice a day, it significantly relieved constipation within a day or two in 40 percent of more than 1,200 patients.[55] Zelnorm is now being tested for constipa-tion caused by opioids.

## Sexual Dysfunction

Many men who are treated with opioids for chronic pain experience sexual difficulties. Physicians and patients used to believe that the most likely reason was that pain and depression decreased sexual performance and desire. But it's now recognized that the chronic use of opioids can significantly lower serum testosterone in men, which in turn decreases sexual interest and potency. In premenopausal women, serum estrogen levels are also significantly low. In one study, serum luteinizing hormone (LH) and follicle-stimulating hormone (FSH) were low to low-normal in both men and women on opioid therapy.[56]

The effect of opioids on sex hormone levels is much more common than previously recognized. For example, a recent study reported on 20 men with cancer-related chronic pain, who were disease-free for at least 1 year and had been taking at least 200 mg of morphine per day (or equivalent dose of another opioid) for at least 1 year.[57] Their median serum testosterone level was 140 ng/dl, which is well below the normal range of 241 to 827 ng/dl. Their median levels of FSH and LH, which are produced by the pituitary glad in the brain, were also below normal. If opioids lowered testosterone levels in the testes, the pituitary gland would have responded with increased levels of FSH and LH. The finding that these two hormones were not elevated, and in fact were below normal, shows that opioids affect sex-hormone production at the brain level. The men in this study also reported markedly decreased sexual desire.

If you are experiencing this problem, ask your physician to order a test of your total and free serum testosterone levels. If your levels are low, various testosterone preparations are available for replacement. Testosterone is not usually given as pills, because they can cause inflammation of the liver (hepatitis) as well as liver tumors.

Injections of testosterone cyprionate (Depo-Testosterone) or testosterone enanthate (Delatestryl; Testro-L.A), given every 2 to 4 weeks, have been in use for many years. They are relatively inexpensive and may be the only treatment your insurance company will pay for. Their drawback, aside from the discomfort of repeated deep injection, is that the blood levels of injected testosterone gyrate from peak to trough—above normal a few hours after the injection, then gradually decreasing to below normal by the time the next shot is given. Your mood and sexual interest are likely to yo-yo along with the shots.

Testosterone replacement is now available as a gel that is applied daily to the shoulder or chest (Androgel, Testim), or as a transdermal patch applied daily to the skin. The Androderm patch is applied to the upper arm, thigh, back, or abdomen, while the Testoderm patch is placed on the scrotum. Another possibility is a buccal tablet (Striant), which is placed inside the upper lip where it adheres to the gum. A new tablet is applied twice a day. The gel, patch, and buccal tablet all provide steady blood levels of testosterone.

## Other Side Effects Related to Opioid Use

Other side effects include:
- **itching**, which tends to be more common with morphine. This can be dealt with by substituting one of the synthetic opioids

such as oxycodone or methadone. If the itching is mild, an antihistamine may give sufficient relief.

- **difficulty initiating urination (urinary retention)**. This occurs infrequently, usually in older people. This effect is usually transient.
- **central nervous system (CNS) effects**. Some patients who are on prolonged high-dose opioids, especially people whose renal function is decreased, can develop some neurological problems. These can include confusion, hallucinations or delirium, seizures, severe sedation, and increased pain. This type of toxicity is uncommon.
- **osteoporosis**, which is a decrease in bone density that may increase the risk of fractures. One of the actions of the hormone testosterone is to maintain good bone density. It is probable that opioid-related osteoporosis is in most part due to a prolonged testosterone deficiency (see "sexual dysfunction" on page 97), but there is also some evidence that opioids may directly interfere with bone formation.[58]
- **immunosuppression**. Studies in laboratory animals have shown that prolonged use of opioids can suppress the immune system, as can abrupt withdrawal of opioids. People whose immune system isn't functioning well have poor resistance against infection, and their wounds heal slowly. It is not yet known how important these effects are in humans with chronic pain.

## Will Taking Opioids Prevent Me from Feeling Pain from Other Causes?

On a recent routine visit for follow-up of her chronic pelvic pain due to interstitial cystitis, a patient sported a new cast on her arm. A week earlier she had tripped on a rock and fallen, fracturing her wrist. She related her experience in the emergency room:

*My wrist was killing me, but after reading in my chart that I was on 90 mg per day of sustained-release morphine, the emergency room doctor wouldn't give me any more pain medicine. He said that the large amount I was already taking should take care of the pain. But it didn't. I was miserable for the first couple of days.*

Unfortunately, this case is not unusual. Being on a regular regimen of an opioid, even in high doses, does not make you immune to feeling pain. Many physicians don't realize this. If you should break a bone, undergo surgery, or have appendicitis, you will still hurt, and you will need additional pain medication, at least as much as someone else who's not taking opioids on a regular basis. If you need surgery, you should discuss this in advance with your surgeon to be sure she or he understands this.

## Opioids in Combination with Other Drugs

As you've learned throughout this book, most patients who are being treated with opioids for chronic pain are also taking several other drugs. Combining drugs is based on the principle that pain medications that have different mechanisms of action can give added benefit when combined. Moreover, adding a drug such as ibuprofen (Motrin, an anti-inflammatory drug [NSAID]) or gabapentin (Neurontin, an anticonvulsant) can result in a reduced need for an opioid. Indeed, both doctors and patients have found this to be true. A recent study using laboratory animals confirmed this. When their tails were placed under a heat lamp, mice who were injected with hydrocodone (an opioid) tolerated the heat significantly longer than control mice before they flicked their tails away. Mice given ibuprofen got no benefit when compared with controls. But when the same dose of ibuprofen was administered to mice along with hydrocodone, the efficacy of the hydrocodone was markedly enhanced: Only one-sixth of the dose of hydrocodone gave them the same relief as when only hydrocodone was used.[59]

## Why Are Doctors Reluctant to Prescribe Opioids for Chronic Pain?

You may have read in national magazines or seen on TV stories about the dangers of opioids and how likely they are to be abused or to cause addiction. These stories reflect a great deal of misunderstanding about opioids. As you have seen in this chapter, when used as prescribed for the relief of chronic pain, opioids are safe, effective, and have a low risk of addiction. Most patients do not need to keep increasing their dose. Unfortunately, physicians as well as lay people often lack education about these drugs. They confuse addiction and physical dependence, believe that tolerance to the pain relieving effect of opioids is the norm (not true!), and that they are not safe in large doses. Physicians obviously need more education about these drugs.

In addition, physicians are afraid of legal consequences for prescribing opioids. You have undoubtedly heard reports about doctors losing their medical licenses or even going to jail for prescribing opioids. Some of these doctors were indeed breaking the law by "selling" prescriptions or trading prescriptions for sex, but others are well-meaning professionals who are victims of overzealous government pursuit. Your doctor has heard these stories, too, and may consider the risks of prescribing opioids to be overly high. In California, where physicians until recently were required to fill out special government forms when prescribing drugs such as morphine, oxycodone, and fentanyl, the fear is so great that about half of all health care providers choose not even to obtain those forms. In other words, they choose not to prescribe opioids at all, even for terminally ill patients with cancer!

Fortunately, these fears are mostly unfounded. In recent years, regulatory agencies and professional associations have issued position papers that favor the legitimate prescribing of opioids for chronic pain. On Oct. 23, 2001, the U.S. Drug Enforcement Administration (DEA; the agency that licenses doctors to dispense opioids and that pursues and arrests people who abuse or sell drugs) joined 21 of the nation's leading pain and health organizations to call for a balanced policy governing prescription pain medications such as OxyContin. DEA administrator Asa Hutchinson said:

> Both health care professionals and law enforcement and regulatory personnel share a responsibility for ensuring that prescription pain medications are available to the patients who need them, and for preventing these drugs from becoming a source of harm and abuse. We don't want to cause patients who have legitimate needs for those medications to be discouraged or afraid to use them. And we don't want to restrict doctors and pharmacists from providing these medications when appropriate. At the same time, we must all take reasonable steps to ensure that these powerful medications don't end up in the wrong hands and lead to abuse.

We want a balanced approach that addresses the abuse problem without keeping patients from getting the care they need and deserve.[60]

At the same meeting, Russell Portenoy, M.D., chairman of Pain Medicine and Palliative Care at Beth Israel Medical Center in New York City, said:

"The repeated accounts of misuse have skewed people's perceptions about drugs like OxyContin. The reality is that the vast majority of people who are given these medications by doctors will not become addicted. Unfortunately, some doctors may now be frightened to prescribe these medications because of fear of addiction and the new social stigma."

The DEA and health groups called for a renewed focus on educating health professionals, law enforcement, and the public about the appropriate use of opioid pain medications in order to promote both responsible prescribing practices and limit instances of abuse and diversion.

Drug addiction is common throughout the world. The fear of drug addiction is a major barrier to prescribing opioids. In the next chapter we will discuss the nature of addiction, its relationship to the medical use of opioids, and what happens in cases where people have both an addiction problem and a chronic pain problem.

# 6

# ADDICTION OR PHYSICAL DEPENDENCY?

## *The Truth Behind the Terms*

*My doctor was treating me for months with sustained-release oxycodone for my arthritis pain. I read an article that said oxycodone is bad for you, so I decided to stop it. A few hours later I got so sick! I hurt all over, I had diarrhea, I couldn't sleep, and I was nauseated. I felt like I had a terrible case of the flu, so I called my doctor. He told me it wasn't the flu, it was withdrawal symptoms from the oxycodone. Well, it's a good thing I stopped those pills. My doctor had turned me into a drug addict!*

—ARTHRITIS PATIENT INTERVIEWED ON TV

YOU MAY KNOW SOMEONE WHO WAS PRESCRIBED high doses of a corticosteroid such as prednisone for lupus, shingles, or some other disease. When it was time to stop the medication, the prescribing physician most likely didn't simply tell the patient to stop it. Instead, the doctor instructed the patient to taper the medication, gradually decreasing the dose over days or weeks. The reason for this is that suddenly stopping drugs such as prednisone results in specific adverse effects on the body. Corticosteroids are a class of drugs that produce *physical dependence*, meaning that abrupt discontinuation after the body has become accustomed to the presence of this drug results in *withdrawal symptoms.* Physical dependence is a form of physiologic adaptation to the continuous presence of certain drugs in the body.

Opioids are another class of drugs that produce physical dependence. People who have been on more than small doses for more than a few days or weeks may develop some of the following flu-like symptoms if they stop suddenly: restlessness, tearing of the eyes, runny nose, yawning, profuse perspiration, goose bumps, chills, and muscle aches. Other withdrawal symptoms from opioids are sleeplessness, nausea, loss of appetite, vomiting, diarrhea, and increased blood pressure or heart rate.

The person who experiences withdrawal symptoms from suddenly ceasing to take opioids is no more a drug addict (that is, someone who is psychologically dependent) than is the patient who gets very sick after suddenly stopping prednisone. In both cases the person has become physically dependent on the drug, which is not at all the same thing as being addicted. In fact, physical dependence in pain patients is not a sign of psychological dependence or addiction.

Moreover, most people who have been physically dependent on prescribed opioids are able to withdraw from them easily when pain is resolved, and they do not return to nontherapeutic use if the medications are tapered down.

The dose of opioids at which withdrawal occurs is variable. Some people experience symptoms when they stop after weeks of taking fairly low doses, whereas others do not, even with large doses. In one report, patients who had been taking less than 60 mg per day of OxyContin for some weeks did not experience withdrawal symptoms when they stopped, whereas a couple of patients did have symptoms after stopping 60 or 70 mg per day.[1] It's best to assume that if you stop any opioid suddenly, you'll have some symptoms. If you want or need to stop the medication, you should discuss with your doctor how to taper down the dosage.

## The Nature of Addiction

In the past, there was a great deal of confusion between addiction and physical dependence, made worse by the fact that the Diagnostic and Statistical Manual of Mental Disorders (DSM IV)—the "bible" of psychiatric disorders—refers to drug addiction as drug dependence.[2] Addiction was thought to result from the hijacking of the brain by a drug: Take the drug enough times, and you will inevitably become addicted. After you have become physically dependent, it was believed that you would be driven to continue taking the drug in order to prevent withdrawal symptoms. This, of course, did not explain the behavior of drug addicts who resumed using heroin or alcohol even after being detoxed, that is, long past when they would have experienced any withdrawal symptoms. Nor did this theory explain why some drugs such as marijuana, cocaine, and amphetamines, which do not have a specific set of withdrawal symptoms, can still be highly addictive.

We now know that addiction is not driven primarily by attempts to prevent withdrawal. Instead, all drugs that can produce addiction are capable of producing rewards, that is, pleasurable feelings, in the brain.[3] The pleasurable feelings result from increases in the neurotransmitter dopamine in the limbic system, including the nucleus accumbens and the ventral tegmental area. Addiction is thought to occur in vulnerable individuals when repeatedly rewarding drug use triggers a biologic change in the brain such that the person develops a strong drive to use the drug. This results in preoccupation with use, cravings, impaired control over use, or continued use despite harm. The vulnerability to addiction results from a combination of genetic factors, childhood and adult experiences, environmental factors, and drug availability.

Although people who are addicted to a drug are still officially called "drug dependent," the term "dependence" no longer reflects current understanding of the scientific basis of addiction. So what are the chief signs of addiction? According to the DSM-IV, when a person's relationship with a drug has the following three elements, he or she is an addict:

- **Loss of control**, also called compulsive use. One example is the person who stops at the bar after work, intending to have a couple of beers then go home for dinner—only to show up at home at 10 P.M. after having a dozen drinks.
- **Continuation despite experiencing significant adverse consequences**. This might be the person who continues to drink alcohol despite being warned by her doctor that her blood pressure is too high and her heart is damaged, or despite being arrested for drunk driving, or even after losing a job because of too many absences caused by hangovers.
- **Preoccupation or obsession with obtaining or using the**

**drug**. An example would be the person who devotes a lot of time and energy to purchasing drugs on the street, or who, instead of concentrating on his work, spends time at work thinking about that evening's opportunity to party.

The take-home message about addiction is that it is a psychological, not a physical, phenomenon. People can be physically dependent on a drug without being addicted. They can be addicted to a drug without being physically dependent. And, in some cases, they might be both physically dependent and addicted. Next time you hear someone talking about addiction, stop and clarify for yourself whether they are in fact describing addiction or physical dependence, or a combination of the two.

## Pseudoaddiction

Carl, age 36, had lost his knee and lower right leg in a motorcycle accident at age 25. Since then, he'd had severe phantom limb pain in his right leg. His previous physician, Dr. Jones, who'd been prescribing 90 Percocet a month to Carl, dropped him as a patient when he found out that Carl had been getting pain medications from a second physician. As Carl explained to his new physician, Dr. Smith:

> *I told Dr. Jones that three Percocet a day wasn't enough. I'd get some relief for about 4 hours with each dose, but I still had 12 hours a day when I was miserable. I'd take all the pills while I was working, so I could do my job, but I couldn't sleep at night because of the pain, and I was still hurting some during the day. Dr. Jones said he wouldn't prescribe any more than 90 pills a month, so in desperation I went to another doctor and didn't tell him about Dr. Jones. With the two prescriptions, I was able to take eight Percocet a day, which gave me good relief. When Dr. Jones found out, he said I was clearly just a drug-seeker, and he dropped me. If I had enough pain relief, I'd never go to another doctor; I knew it was wrong, but I couldn't think of another way out.*

Dr. Smith decided to give Carl the benefit of the doubt. She prescribed the dose of oxycodone that Carl said was effective, but in a sustained-release preparation, and gave Carl 16 pills (two per day), enough for 8 days. A week later he was back, comfortable, and with two pills left in the bottle. He stayed on that dose for the next 2 years, without any further problems.

After reading the list of three types of behaviors that signify addiction, you might have realized that some chronic pain patients indeed look like addicts. Carl, for example, took more pills than prescribed, which might suggest loss of control. He risked adverse consequences (and indeed, he experienced one—getting dropped by his doctor) to get his pills. And he surely spent a lot of time figuring out how to get enough. Yet Carl was clearly not an addict; he was an undertreated pain patient.

"Doctor shopping," or getting pain medications from more than one physician, is a red flag for drug abuse or addiction—but does not necessarily mean that the patient is a drug addict. It can be a sign of undertreated pain. The same is true of aggressive demands for more pain medication, or obvious exaggeration of pain behavior in an attempt to convince the doctor that the pain is severe. This pattern of behavior has been termed *pseudoaddiction*, and it is now recognized to be caused by undermedication of pain.[4]

If your chronic pain is being undertreated, it's possible that your physician may be uncomfortable with prescribing more than small doses of opioids. Have a discussion with him about this issue. Consider asking for a referral to a pain-management specialist to evaluate your needs. If you can't come to some consensus with your physician, you would be better served by considering changing physicians rather than engaging in doctor shopping, asking friends for pain pills, or taking more pain pills than prescribed. Pseudoaddiction behaviors can have serious consequences, and are also likely to end up in your medical record, which will make it harder for you to win the trust of your next physician.

## The Use and Abuse of Opioids

All opioids can be abused. The short-acting drugs are the most popular among addicts, because their rapid effect means more euphoria. However, addicts have learned how to defeat the slow-release mechanism of the long-acting drugs so as to make these preparations produce a "high" as well. Even the fentanyl patches, from which it's harder to extract the active ingredient than it is from pills, have been abused. But physicians are prescribing more opioids than ever before. What has happened to the likelihood of abuse during this time?

In 2000, a report appeared that compared the number of opioid prescriptions written by U.S. physicians in 1990 and 1996 with the number of cases of opioid abuse reported in those same years by U.S. hospitals.[5] Between 1990 and 1996, the use of most opioids increased significantly— for example, doctors prescribed 59 percent more morphine, 23 percent more oxycodone, 19 percent more hydromorphone, and 1,168 percent more fentanyl (Duragesic patches, which contain fentanyl, first became available in 1991). Also between 1990 and 1996, the number of patients abusing morphine increased by only 3 percent, whereas abuse of other opioids decreased by 15 percent to 59 percent. These results strongly suggest that increased medical use of opioids to treat pain is not accompanied by increases in abuse of opioids.

Unfortunately, in the years since this report, things have changed. Illicit use of prescription opioids has increased disproportionately more than legal use, and the prevalence of prescription opioid abuse is now similar to that of heroin or cocaine abuse.[6] This is worrisome but expected. The appropriate solution, of course, is not to decrease the prescribing of opioids to legitimate pain patients, but rather to reformulate prescription opioids to make it harder to abuse them. This goal is currently being actively pursued by several pharmaceutical companies (see chapter 16).

## The Opinion of Professional Organizations and Regulatory Agencies about Opioids for Chronic Non-cancer Pain

Many physicians hesitate to prescribe opioids for the treatment of chronic non-cancer pain because they are unfamiliar with recent positions about such treatment that have been expressed in recent years by professional organizations and regulatory agencies. The following are examples of the opinions of some of these organizations.

THE AMERICAN SOCIETY OF ADDICTION MEDICINE. The American Society of Addiction Medicine, the major professional organization for addiction medicine physicians, wrote in its position paper on opioids and pain, "Physical dependency on opioids is an expected occurrence in all individuals in the presence of continuous use of opioids .... It does not, in and of itself, imply addiction."[7]

Regarding the concern of physicians that they might get into trouble if they are ever duped by a drug-abusing patient, this policy statement also states:

> Despite appropriate medical practice, physicians who prescribe opioids for pain may occasionally be misled by skillful patients who wish to obtain medications for purposes other than pain treatment ....The physician who is never duped by such patients may be denying appropriate relief to patients with significant pain all too often .... Physicians who are practicing medicine in good faith and who use reasonable medical judgment regarding the prescription of opioids for the treatment of pain should not be held responsible for the willful and deceptive behavior of patients who successfully obtain opioids for nonmedical purposes.

AMERICAN ACADEMY OF PAIN MEDICINE, AMERICAN PAIN SOCIETY, AND AMERICAN SOCIETY OF ADDICTION MEDICINE. In 2001, three major U.S. professional organizations for pain and addiction medicine published a consensus statement in which they stated that the lack of uniform definitions of the concepts of physical dependence, addiction, and tolerance "contribute to a misunderstanding of the nature of addiction and the risk of addiction, especially in situations in which opioids are used ... to manage pain. Confusion regarding the treatment of pain results in unnecessary suffering, economic burdens to society, and inappropriate adverse actions against patients and professionals."

After defining these terms (see the *Glossary* for their definitions) the consensus statement continues:

> Most specialists in pain medicine and addiction medicine agree that patients treated with prolonged opioid therapy usually do develop physical dependence and sometimes develop tolerance, but do not usually develop addictive disorders.
>
> An individual's behaviors that may suggest addiction sometimes are simply a reflection of unrelieved pain or other problems

unrelated to addiction . . . .Patients with unrelieved pain may become focused on obtaining medications, may "clock watch," and may otherwise seem inappropriately "drug seeking." Even such behaviors as illicit drug use and deception can occur in the patient's efforts to obtain relief. Pseudoaddiction can be distinguished from true addiction in that the behaviors resolve when pain is effectively treated.[8]

In 2003, several of the authors of this consensus statement published a paper on definitions related to the medical use of opioids. They stated:

A patient who is prescribed opioids that control his or her pain is able to use them according to an agreed upon schedule, does not routinely request early refills, has stable or improving function, reports reasonably stable pain control, and is willing to consider additional treatment approaches is not likely to be addicted to the medications.[9]

FEDERATION OF STATE MEDICAL BOARDS OF THE UNITED STATES, INC. The Federation of State Medical Boards of the United States, Inc., is an association of the medical licensing boards of the majority of states in the United States. Their members share information and formulate guidelines that are subsequently adopted by the various individual state medical licensing boards. In 1998, this organization adopted a set of model guidelines for the use of controlled substances (such as opioids) for the treatment of pain. The document included a set of definitions, such as "Pseudoaddiction: Pattern of drug-seeking behavior of pain patients who are receiving inadequate pain management that can be mistaken for addiction," and guidelines for evaluating the use of controlled substances in patients with pain. They also stated:

The Board recognizes that controlled substances, including opioid analgesics, may be essential to the treatment of acute pain due to trauma or surgery and chronic pain, whether due to cancer or non-cancer origins . . . . Physicians should recognize that tolerance and physical dependence are normal consequences of sustained use of opioid analgesics and are not synonymous with addiction.[10]

In 2004, a panel of experts in pain management and addiction medicine recommended revised guidelines to the Federation, which include a statement encouraging each state medical licensing board to consider the undertreatment of pain as much of a violation of the standard of care as other kinds of prescribing violations.

AMERICAN PAIN FOUNDATION. On their Web site, the American Pain Foundation, which is an information, advocacy, and support organization concerning pain issues, wrote:

> Doctors and pharmacists need to be diligent in taking security measures to keep opioid medications out of illegal and improper hands. Regulators and law enforcement officers should be tough in combating the illegal diversion of opioids into street traffic, but they should do it in a balanced way that doesn't discourage the safe and legal use of opioid medications for pain care. And the news media should always balance news about opioids with information about their value to people with severe chronic pain.[11]

## State Laws

In a federal system such as we have in the United States, both state and federal governments can make laws in any particular area. However, you may not have realized that state laws can be stricter but cannot be more lenient than federal laws. A current example of the tensions that this dichotomy can produce involves the medical use of marijuana. Several states (including California and Arizona) have passed laws permitting physicians to prescribe marijuana for medical purposes. However, the federal government does not permit this. Consequently, physicians in Arizona and California who prescribe medical marijuana risk prosecution under federal law.

The laws in different states also differ with regard to opioid prescriptions. Until recently, several states (including New York and California) regulated the prescribing of Schedule II drugs (drugs regulated by the Drug Enforcement Administration [DEA]) such as morphine and oxycodone by mandating the use of special prescription pads for these drugs. The pads had three copies, one of which went to the state government where, theoretically, physicians' prescribing practices were closely monitored. As a result, physicians in these states were fearful of prescribing Schedule II drugs.

Recently, however, most states eliminated the triplicate prescription forms. California, the last holdout, will switch in 2005 from triplicates to counterfeit-resistant forms. This change will undoubtedly result in an increased willingness of physicians to legitimately prescribe strong opioids for patients with chronic pain.

## Dealing with Disapproval from Family and Friends

Getting effective pain treatment from your doctor is sometimes not the end of your difficulties. According to Walter, the 32-year-old former computer programmer quoted at the beginning of chapter 5, whose life was greatly improved after he began treatment with opioids for his work-related injury:

> *Because I'm on high doses of opioids, my father is convinced that I'm a drug addict, despite the fact that I've never abused drugs. Nothing anyone says to him can convince him that opioids can be a legitimate treatment for chronic pain. He thinks that all of my problems are due to the pills I'm taking, and that the fact that I won't stop means I care more for my drugs than for him. We've become completely estranged because of his attitude.*

This same attitude was voiced by several of my own patients. Kay, who used to be very athletic and now is limited by severe back pain, said:

> *Everyone's reaction when I tell them I'm on those [opioid] meds is that I shouldn't depend so much on the medication. They ask, isn't there anything else you can do? It bothers me that they say that, as if they don't believe me that I'm trying, or they don't trust me. They say, "You're not strong enough . . . It's all mental . . . . You're just addicted, it's not for the pain." They just don't understand. I wish they'd stop telling me to get off the medication.*

Wilma, who has painful reflex sympathetic dystrophy of the arm, and does *not* have any history of drug misuse, said:

*My two sisters and my son thought I was faking the pain just to get the pain medication. My older sister told my mother the doctor was giving me methadone because I was a heroin addict. I didn't even know she'd done this until after my mother was dead!*

It's painful to get this type of reaction from people you care about. In some cases you can educate them by giving them this book, or asking your doctor for information to give them, or by bringing them with you to your doctor's appointment to hear her explanation. The last suggestion is particularly advisable if the disapproving person is your spouse, parent, or adult child. It's important to get your family's support for your treatment. It's advisable for physicians to encourage patients to bring family members to the office so that they can ask the doctor questions and see firsthand that their relative is indeed using a recommended medication.

When asked how her family could best help her, one woman said:

*The best way people can help me is to understand that what I'm doing [taking opioids] is not bad for me, it's necessary in order to get through each day. I don't take them to get high. I want people to be able to know how much pain I have.*

If your friends or family members are unwilling to reconsider their position, you may simply have to agree to disagree. Repeatedly arguing with them or trying to convince them is unlikely to succeed; it will only make you feel worse. Sometimes, the best way of convincing them is to demonstrate to them, over time, that because of the medications you take you are able to do more and have a more active and enjoyable life.

## Treating Pain in People with an Addiction History

The prevalence of addiction in the American population is about 10 percent, meaning that one in 10 people has a current or previous addiction problem. This means that many people have both an addiction problem and a chronic pain condition. Prescribing opioids for current addicts is a difficult situation, often requiring the involvement of an addiction medicine specialist. But people who are in recovery from chemical dependency, even for many years, are often discriminated against when it comes to chronic pain management. Physicians are reluctant to treat them with opioids, fearing they will relapse.

The actual risk of addiction from prescribed medications is not known. Several studies published many years ago that involved large populations of burn patients and headache patients found a very, very low risk of addiction in these patients.[12] But these studies did not identify pre-existing addicts, did not clearly define addiction, and were carried out for only a short time. What is clear is that people with an addiction history—but who may not have used alcohol or drugs for many years—are at an increased risk of relapse if their chronic pain is *not* adequately treated. They are at risk of reaching for the bottle or getting some drugs on the street in order to numb their pain. Medical treatment is clearly a better choice.

In an important study, 20 chronic pain patients who had a known history of substance abuse were treated for a year with opioids. All but three of the patients were not working and were on long-term disability. Eleven patients did not abuse their prescription medication, and they were compared with nine who did.[13]

The characteristics of the 11 patients who took their medications only as prescribed were:
- a history of alcohol abuse alone rather than other drugs.
- if there was a history of abuse of several drugs, it had stopped years before.
- active involvement in Alcoholics Anonymous or other recovery program.
- a stable family and support system.

The patients who abused their pain medications were usually detected by their physicians within 3 months. They were more likely to seek pain medications from multiple physicians, to report lost or stolen medications, to make frequent calls to the clinic, and to keep increasing their dose.

Clearly, a history of drug abuse, including alcoholism, requires caution before a decision is made to prescribe opioids for chronic pain. This study suggests, however, that with attention to various risk factors and behaviors, patients can be selected who will benefit from opioid treatment for their chronic pain without relapsing to addiction or abusing their drugs.

Nonetheless, patients with concomitant pain and current substance abuse disorders need treatment for both, even though the treatment may be both time- and labor-intensive. One pain clinic that had a multidisciplinary substance abuse treatment program reported on a group of 44 dually diagnosed patients (that is, those who had both pain and chemical dependence [66 percent were addicted to opioids]).[14] They were put through a 10-week outpatient addiction program while being treated for their chronic pain. The patients showed significant improvements in pain, emotional distress, medication reduction, and coping style. Half the patients were off all opioids at a 12-month follow-up; the others had been transitioned to therapeutic doses of long-acting opioids and were doing well.

What about the legal status of prescribing opioids for persons with an addiction history? The U.S. Code of Federal Regulations for prescribing a Schedule II controlled substance clearly states (section 21CFR, 1306.7) that a controlled substance can be prescribed for the treatment of pain in any patient, including those with a history of abuse or addiction.

The Federation of State Medical Boards, in their Model Guidelines,[15] does not rule out prescribing opioids for patients at risk for addiction. They have stated:

> If the patient is determined to be at high risk for medication abuse or have a history of substance abuse, the physician may employ the use of a written agreement between physician and patient outlining patient responsibilities, including:
> - urine/serum medication levels screening when requested.
> - number and frequency of all prescription refills.
> - reasons for which drug therapy may be discontinued (i.e., violation of agreement).

The management of pain in patients with a history of substance abuse or with a comorbid psychiatric disorder may require extra care, monitoring, documentation, and consultation with or referral to an expert in the management of such patients.

## Opioids and Alcoholics Anonymous

Recovering alcoholics who are on opioids for chronic pain have reported negative reactions from their AA friends:

*They don't call me anymore. I can't go to as many meetings as I used to,
probably because I'm on pain meds. My sponsor fortunately has stuck by
my side. But my AA friends are now avoiding me. I'm very disappointed;
maybe I expected too much of them. My outside friends, on the other
hand, have been very supportive.*

—SAMANTHA, 51, SOBER FOR 15 YEARS IN AA

*The people at AA said, "Don't take pain pills." It made me think I'm
not trying hard enough, and that's not true. I felt I had to choose between
AA and pain relief, so I stopped going to AA.*

—DORIS, 56, SOBER FOR 16 YEARS IN AA

*After giving up drugs and alcohol I worked as a drug and alcohol coun-
selor for 30 years. I wish I'd have gotten help sooner for my back pain, but
I was afraid to go to the doctor because I didn't want him to say no, and
I didn't want to get re-addicted. I still go to AA daily, but I don't discuss
my [opioid] medications there because they don't want you to take
anything, even for depression, much less pain meds.*

—TAMARA, 58, IN RECOVERY FOR 32 YEARS

If you are a former alcoholic or drug addict now working a 12-step
recovery program, you may be interested in knowing what the AA
literature has to say about taking prescribed medications. In their
pamphlet, *The AA Member—Medications and Other Drugs*, they write:

Remember that as a recovering alcoholic your automatic response
will be to turn to chemical relief for uncomfortable feelings and to
take more than the usual, prescribed amount. Look for nonchemical
solutions for the aches and discomforts of everyday living . . . .
Because of the difficulties that many alcoholics have with drugs,
some members have taken the position that no one in AA should
take any medication. While this position has undoubtedly
prevented relapses for some, it has meant disaster for others . . . .
Just as it is wrong to enable or support any alcoholic to become
re-addicted to any drug, it's equally wrong to deprive any alcoholic of medication which can alleviate or control other disabling
physical and/or emotional problems.[16]

Nonetheless, if you are taking various prescribed medications such as opioids, antidepressants, or muscle relaxants, you might find resistance from some AA members. But their resistance stems from their personal experience and prejudices and does not represent AA as a whole. Rather than giving up your AA involvement, I suggest you find a sponsor who understands—or who has an open mind and is willing to be educated—and find AA friends who can support you in your course of action.

As to what you can do to minimize your own risk of relapse, you must intensify your recovery activities, and monitor yourself carefully for any relapse-prone behaviors. Sometimes enlisting the help of others can also help safeguard your sobriety. Here is what Steve, a 40-year-old former drug addict related after a year of treatment with opioids for chronic back pain:

> *All my life I've been chasing pleasure. It got me in a lot of trouble. Eventually I quit the drugs I'd been using in my youth, but soon I discovered cocaine. I loved it! I used to use my back pain as an excuse to drink or get drugs. I'd go from intense pain to extreme euphoria.*
>
> *Getting pain relief with long-acting opioids has really stabilized my life. The doctor and I agreed that my wife would dispense the pills to me, just to be sure I'm not tempted to overdo it. My agreement with the doctor includes that my wife will call her if I hassle my wife at all about the medications. That takes the heat off my wife. In the past it's been hard for me to have balance in my life. That's why I like this program, the strict structure regarding my opioid medications. I have no desire to do drugs. Transcendental meditation has really helped me. I get up each morning and give thanks. I've found other ways to make people happy, especially with my music. I have new creative ideas every day. Subtle changes are now exciting to me.*

In my own practice I have had many patients who had a history of drug dependence but were able to take opioids for chronic pain without any tendency to relapse to their addiction.

## Are Opioids Really Safe?

Unless you don't watch TV and don't read newspapers, you have undoubtedly seen and read frightening reports about the painkilling drugs we've discussed in this chapter. You may have heard, for example, that OxyContin is "the new heroin" in its ability to hook people and that people have overdosed on it. You may have read about people selling their prescribed opioids. You may have seen interviews with entertainers and commentators who blame treatment for pain for getting them addicted to opioids. On a TV program, *Sixty Minutes*, an osteoarthritis patient acknowledged that OxyContin had effectively relieved her chronic pain, but then she related that she stopped it because she'd heard how dangerous it was. She went on to report that she experienced very unpleasant withdrawal symptoms after stopping the opioid. She concluded that OxyContin had turned her into an addict and, accordingly, she was planning to sue its manufacturer.

You might wonder whether it's too risky for you to take these drugs for your chronic pain problem. Here are some things to consider. First, having read the beginning of this chapter, you undoubtedly recognize that the osteoarthritis patient on the *Sixty Minutes* program was confusing addiction and physical dependence. Yes, she had become physically dependent, as shown by the withdrawal symptoms she experienced after stopping her painkiller. But no, there is no evidence that she was addicted. Her mistake was to stop her medication suddenly. Any patient who decides to stop taking an opioid for chronic pain should first discuss it with her prescribing physician. The doctor may be able to alleviate your concerns about continuing to take the drug. If you both agree that cessation is a good idea, then the way to do it is to taper the dose, which will prevent withdrawal symptoms.

Second, blaming your prescribed pain medication for your addiction problem is a popular strategy for those who don't want to take responsibility for their behavior. People who become truly addicted to prescribed pain medications are usually people who had previous addiction problems or other vulnerabilities. It is very unlikely that someone without a prior addiction history will become addicted just by taking pain medications. Also, *all* pain medications have the potential to be misused, and addicts have figured out ingenious ways to defeat the safeguards in any painkiller.

It is certainly true that opioids can be abused. In addition, almost every medication has risks, therefore you and your doctor must weigh the risks and benefits of taking opioids with the risks and benefits of other drugs. For example, a headline in the *New York Times* on Sept. 21,

2002, read: "FDA panel calls for stronger warnings on aspirin and related painkillers."[17] The article reported: "The committee said certain groups of patients, including the elderly, should be warned that they risk stomach bleeding or kidney failure by taking anti-inflammatory drugs (NSAIDs), [even when] taking the drugs as directed.… On Thursday, the panel voted overwhelmingly to recommend stronger warnings for acetaminophen, which is the main ingredient in Tylenol. The FDA says thousands of consumers take unintentional overdoses of acetaminophen, resulting in 100 deaths from liver failure each year."

The lesson from the *New York Times* article is that the medications that have been touted as safer alternatives to opioids have their own risks, which are significant. Don't rule out opioids on the basis of adverse reports in the media; discuss all the options with your physician.

# 7

# GETTING INSIDE
# YOUR SKIN

## *Invasive Procedures*

O RAL MEDICATIONS, EXERCISES, AND REST ARE
therapies that are called "noninvasive." Sometimes doctors will
recommend what are called "invasive procedures" to alleviate
pain. These include injections and operations. Operations will be
described in chapter 8. With injections and other devices, medications
can be delivered to parts of the body that are not otherwise accessible,
such as specific nerves, joints, ligaments, tendons, and areas around the
spine. Injections and other devices can deliver corticosteroids, local
anesthetics, and other substances, to relieve muscle spasm, painful joints,
tender points, and trigger points.

### *Injections for Chronic Low Back Pain*

Chapter 1 listed some of the causes of chronic back pain. Often the specific cause of the back pain is impossible to find or there may be several
sources of the pain; therefore there are many treatments for back pain.
Among them are various types of injections. To understand these, you
need to know a little about the structure of the back.

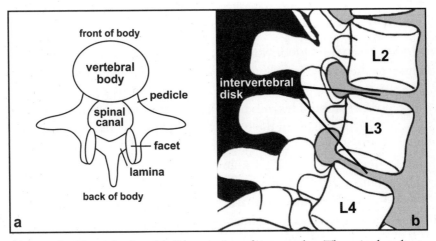

**Figure 3.** *Normal spine. (a) Cross-section of one vertebra. The spinal cord goes through the spinal canal. (b) Lateral view of the lumbar spine.*

## The Structure of the Back

The vertebrae are cylindrical bones with flat surfaces on the top and on the bottom. The vertebrae of the spine form a continuous column from the neck to the sacrum, and support the body in its upright posture. Each vertebra is cushioned from its neighboring bone by a soft and spongy "disk" (see Figure 3). A common source of back pain is degeneration of these intervertebral disks; this process can deform the spine, and the damaged disk material can press against the adjacent nerves and cause pain that can radiate down the arms and/or legs.

An important function of the vertebrae is to protect the spinal cord, the delicate highway of nerves that send signals up and down the periphery to and from the brain. The spinal cord is protected by surrounding bone and also by several membranes that separate it from the surrounding ligaments. The spinal cord is surrounded by fluid, the cerebrospinal fluid (CSF), which flows around the brain and spinal cord. The membranes surrounding the brain and spinal cord prevent this fluid from escaping into the rest of the body.

## Types of Injections for Low Back Pain

Most people with chronic low back pain have had some type of injection into the back. The following is a list of injections of different types of painkillers and the locations where they are injected.

- Corticosteroids and local anesthetics can be injected into specific joints on the back of the bony spine (facet joints).
- A local anesthetic is sometimes injected into the ligaments, tender points, trigger points, acupuncture points, or within the intervertebral disks.
- A local anesthetic can also be injected near a nerve to block its ability to send pain signals (nerve block).
- Medications can be injected or delivered directly into the spinal canal in order to relieve pain at the spinal cord. This is described below.

## Epidural and Intrathecal Injections

A solution of local anesthetic, usually along with a corticosteroid, can be injected into the space just outside the dura, which is the outermost membrane of the spinal cord. This is called the *epidural space*. The drugs will diffuse (spread out) and affect nerves and other tissues. The anesthetic can numb nerves directly as they leave the spinal cord. The steroid can un-pinch nerves that are being compressed by swollen ligaments or other tissues, because the steroid can decrease the swelling of these tissues and thereby give the nerves more room.

How effective are back injections? A review of 21 randomized trials of injections for chronic back pain concluded that the efficacy of injections is uncertain.[1] However, the reviewers added that because the studies did tend toward positive results with only minor side effects, "…there is currently no justification for abandoning injection therapy for patients with low back pain." Therefore, if spinal injections have helped you, then by all means continue them.

## Intraspinal Pump

Another option for treating severe back pain is an intraspinal pump, a device that delivers a constant level of pain medication directly into the intrathecal space, which is the space right near the spinal cord that contains the cerebrospinal fluid (CSF). With a minor surgical procedure, a catheter (thin plastic tube) can be inserted and left in the intrathecal space of the spinal canal, attached to an external pump that pumps the pain medication into the body at a predetermined rate. The drugs used are often some combination of an opioid, the alpha-agonist clonidine, a local anesthetic, and a muscle relaxant. The advantage of this method of pain control is that the medication is being delivered directly to the area of pain rather than having to travel throughout the body, and therefore the patient will require much smaller doses of medication. Side effects such as nausea, sedation, and constipation are also minimized. For this reason, intrathecal medication delivery is particularly useful in patients who need exceedingly high doses of pain medication. Another benefit is that because the drugs can flow up and down the spinal canal, wide areas of pain can be treated. The disadvantages of an intraspinal pump are the need for an operation, the risk of infection or bleeding, and the need to refill the pump at regular intervals (such as every month).

Intraspinal pumps are usually used for somatic pain rather than for neuropathic pain. The reason is that with neuropathic pain, very high doses of opioids are often required, and gradually increasing doses may be necessary.

## Spinal Cord Stimulators

In chapter 9 you will learn about transcutaneous nerve stimulation (TENS), a means of relieving pain by applying electrical current through pads applied to the outside of the skin. This approach is based on the gate theory, which relies on the observation that when nerves are stimulated in one way (such as with an electric current), they do not respond to other types of stimulation (such as pain stimuli). Because pain signals travel more slowly than other types of signals, the other stimuli will override the pain signals.

Spinal cord stimulators (SCS) are also devices that deliver pulses of electricity to the spinal cord. They can be considered a more aggressive form of TENS, useful for patients who don't respond well enough to TENS. The electrodes of the device are permanently implanted near the spinal cord. The procedure is either done through the skin (percutaneously) or by an open surgical procedure. The leads are then connected to an implanted radio frequency (RF) controlled receiver or to an implanted pulse generator (IPG) that supplies power to the electrodes. When nonpainful electric pulses from the spinal cord stimulator flood the nerves, they decrease the pain felt by the person. Because the system is self-contained, patients can resume doing all their daily activities, including bathing and swimming.

Spinal cord stimulators are particularly useful in alleviating neuropathic pain, which is a burning pain from damaged nerves. This includes phantom limb pain, peripheral vascular disease, reflex sympathetic dystrophy, multiple sclerosis, arachnoiditis, injuries to the brachial plexus in the arm, and pain after failed back surgery.

The results with SCS have been mixed. Appropriate patients must be carefully chosen. If the disease of reflex sympathetic dystrophy (RSD), also called complex regional pain syndrome (CRPS), is treated early, the results are better than if it is treated late. If particular nerves can be identified as the cause of the person's neuropathic pain, it's possible to target those nerve roots and implant the electrodes so as to send electrical pulses to those specific nerves, thereby decreasing the pain.[2]

The advantage of an SCS over an intraspinal pump is that there is no need for medication refills and no risk of medication side effects. A disadvantage is that it is useful primarily for peripheral pain (such as in the arms or legs), but less effective for central pain (pain originating in the spinal cord). It is also not usually effective for pelvic pain. Another disadvantage is its cost, currently in the range of $40,000 to $60,000. However, years of expensive pain medication can also add up to many thousands of dollars. A recent review article compared the costs of implanting a spinal cord stimulator with the costs of noninvasive ongoing treatments for pain.[3] The conclusion was that whatever medical problem led to the chronic pain, the costs of implanting the stimulator were consistently offset by a decrease in post-implant health care costs. It is cost effective to use a spinal cord stimuator.

## Injecting Trigger Points and Tender Points

Trigger points are tender areas located in tight bands of muscle, tendons, or ligaments. Trigger points produce a pain that is deep and aching, and muscles with trigger points are weak. When a trigger point is palpated, the muscle will twitch and the person will experience pain directly over the area and also in a particular pattern in other areas (referred pain). Trigger points can be found in any skeletal muscle, but are often found in the neck and shoulders. They may be part of tension headache, temporomandibular joint (TMJ) pain, and low back pain. Myofascial pain syndrome is also a common muscle disorder caused by trigger points.

Tender points are also in muscles and cause pain when compressed, but unlike trigger points, tender points do not cause referred pain; the pain is only located directly at the affected spot. Tender points, unlike trigger points, usually occur symmetrically: Both sides of the body are equally affected. They are often associated with a total body increase in pain sensitivity. Fibromyalgia is the best known example of a disorder with tender points.

Steroid injections combined with a local anesthetic directly into a trigger point can eliminate the pain, although the relief is usually temporary. There is usually soreness right after the injection, followed by relief. Stretching the affected muscle right after injection improves the effectiveness of the injection. The patient is asked to actively move each injected muscle through its full of range of motion three times. Chapter 9 will describe an alternative treatment for trigger points, termed *spray and stretch*: The affected muscle is sprayed with a coolant such as ethyl chloride, which provides local anesthesia, and the muscle is then passively stretched. This is done several times. Steroid injections are also widely used in treating the tender points of fibromyalgia.

## Knee Osteoarthritis: Intra-articular Injections

STEROIDS. The most common material injected into a joint (intra-articular injection) is corticosteroids (such as methylprednisolone [Solu-Medrol]). Steroids can reduce pain and inflammation in patients with osteoarthritis, so they are particularly useful for an acutely inflamed or "flared" joint. The mechanism of action of steroids is not clearly understood, but they clearly provide pain relief. In the past, there was concern that repeated injections into the knee joint might cause destruction of the cartilage, but a recent well-designed study showed that they are, in fact, safe.4 A patient can feel secure and comfortable continuing to get such injections.

HYALURONIC ACID. You may have seen advertisements on TV for a new treatment for knee osteoarthritis—injections of hyaluronic acid. This substance, naturally present in the synovial fluid of the knee joint, forms a lubricant that allows smooth motion of the knee joint. The synovial fluid in patients with knee osteoarthritis is less viscous (thinner) than the normal joint fluid. It was thought that injecting normal hyaluronic acid into the knee might alleviate pain by improving the quality of the joint fluid.

In 1997, the FDA approved injections of hyaluronic acid (Hyalgan, Synvisc) into the knee joint. Several studies have shown that intra-articular injection of hyaluronic acid in people with osteoarthritis of the knee relieves joint pain and improves functioning, and that this effect lasts for months. Some people experience pain reduction for up to one year after such an injection. A review, however, pointed out that similar results are seen with placebo injections, and that it is still uncertain whether hyaluronic acid injections actually have any benefit.[5] A recent meta-analysis of hyaluronic acid injections for knee osteoarthritis evaluated the efficacy of once-weekly injections into the knee joint for at least three injections. The researchers found the results of various studies to be variable, and concluded that intra-articular hyaluronic acid has only a small benefit when compared with an intra-articular placebo. The data do not support the efficacy of such injections. Injection of the most viscous types of hyaluronic acid may be more effective than thinner preparations, but the results were not consistent enough to make any recommendations.[6] A reasonable conclusion from this study is that hyaluronic acid injections are an expensive treatment whose value is still uncertain.

Recently, a randomized, blinded study compared the efficacy of intra-articular injections of a steroid (betamethasone) and hyaluronic acid in 100 patients with knee osteoarthritis. Half the patients received a single steroid injection, the other half three weekly injections of hyaluronic acid. There was a modest improvement in pain and function in both groups, but no significant differences between them at 3 or 6 months later.[7]

BOTULINUM TOXIN. Botulism is a potentially fatal type of food poisoning in which a toxin produced by the bacterium *Clostridium botulinum* paralyzes the muscles and can cause breathing to stop. The toxin, however, has now found some positive uses. You have undoubtedly heard of injecting botulinum toxin (Botox) to erase facial wrinkles. You may not be aware that it is also useful in relieving muscle spasm that causes chronic pain. One example is the use of Botox injections to relieve the painful muscle spasms of a patient's hand after a stroke.

A recent report described its use in a condition termed *piriformis syndrome*, which consists of pain in a buttock (but not the back) that radiates down the leg. Standard therapy of this condition consists of analgesics, steroid injections, and physical therapy. Four patients with piriformis syndrome received this treatment. Four others instead received injections of botulinum toxin A into the piriformis muscle. Three of the patients who received the injections had complete pain relief within 10 days, and all four were able to return to unrestricted physical activity, but only one of the four patients who received the standard treatment was able to return to unrestricted physical activity.[8]

Botox may turn out to be very useful in other painful muscle syndromes such as the painful muscle spasms of multiple sclerosis (MS). Five MS patients who had experienced many severe episodes of muscle spasm daily were injected with botulinum toxin in the hyperactive muscles. The muscle spasticity was relieved in all the patients for about 3 months.[9]

Botulinum toxin has also been used successfully in treating chronic headaches. Up to 30 injections are given at multiple sites in the face, neck, and scalp. Most patients notice improvement in their headaches within 3 to 7 days after injection, and the relief lasts 3 to 5 months. The procedure is repeated every 3 to 4 months, and the benefit often increases with subsequent injections. It sounds unpleasant and the cost is high, but for people who haven't benefited from other treatments, this may be worth a try.

Another use for botulinum toxin is for upper back pain. When 25 patients with such pain received a single treatment of Botox into the mid-belly of the affected muscles (up to four injections per treatment) and then received physical therapy, they reported significant decreases in upper back pain by the fourth week, with maximal improvement by the eighth week.[10]

## Procedures to Destroy Nerves

One way to relieve pain is to interrupt the transmission of pain signals from the periphery or through the spinal cord. This can be done surgically, chemically, or with heat.

In patients with painful abdominal or pelvic cancer, alcohol or phenol can be injected into the celiac and hypogastric plexuses, areas where nerves are concentrated. The caustic chemicals will inactivate the nerves and decrease pain. This procedure, however, hasn't shown a lot of benefit in non-cancer pain.

A heated (radiofrequency) probe can be positioned to destroy specific peripheral nerves and provide pain relief in conditions such as facet joint arthropathy (a type of back pain) and trigeminal neuralgia. When this procedure was used on half of a group of patients who had low back pain at a single painful vertebral level, the treated group had significantly less pain than a control group who received only injections of lidocaine, a local anesthetic, in the area of the nerve.[11] This is yet another treatment option for persistent low back pain.

Destroying sympathetic nerves has long been a procedure to relieve the pain of complex regional pain syndrome (CRPS, formerly called reflex sympathetic dystrophy [RSD]). Seven patients who had sympathetic nerves severed surgically in the mid-back all experienced a reduced amount of pain after surgery and an improved quality of life.[12]

# 8

# DEALING WITH PAIN DURING SURGERY

## When to Use Pre-emptive Pain Relief

*From the earliest days of medicine, surgeons have tried all manner of primitive techniques to ease their patients' pain. The Egyptians, for example, used diluted narcotics. Other surgeons made their patients drunk with brandy and then tied them to wooden benches that served as operating tables. In Europe, some surgeons choked their patients unconscious before operating. Still others applied pressure to a nerve or artery to make an area "fall asleep." In the sixteenth century, the French surgeon (and barber) Ambroise Pare . . . put a wooden bowl over the head of a patient and pounded a hammer against it to knock him unconscious.*

*In the days before anesthesia, a surgeon's reputation was determined by the swiftness of his scalpel. By the nineteenth century, Dr. Robert Liston was amputating legs at University College in London in less than thirty seconds. Liston . . . was considered the finest and swiftest surgeon of his day.[1]*

—L.K. ALTMAN, *WHO GOES FIRST*

FOR MANY PEOPLE WHO HAVE CHRONIC PAIN, SURGERY is an important means of obtaining relief. This chapter will describe surgical treatments for specific chronic pain syndromes. But there is another connection between surgery and pain: All types of operations involve pain. Beginning with the first use of ether during an operation in the mid-nineteenth century, advances in painless surgery quickly followed. Ether, chloroform, and nitrous oxide, the earliest anesthetics, have been replaced by safer, better drugs with fewer side effects. Today an entire medical specialty, anesthesia, is devoted to making surgical procedures as safe and painless as possible. Although we may experience pain postoperatively, we all expect to be pain-free during the operation.

## Avoiding Pain During Surgery

For some types of operations, your doctor may give you a choice between two kinds of anesthesia—general or regional. With either type, you will not experience pain; the key difference is whether you will be asleep or awake. Under general anesthesia, you are unconscious, unable to move, unaware of your surroundings, and you will not remember what happened during the operation. With regional or local anesthesia, you are awake and more or less aware of what is being done to you, although the anesthetized part will be numb. You will be able to move some parts of your body, and you will remember what happened. I say "more or less aware" because today there are so many anesthesia options that patients often get a combination of drugs. For example, a patient who undergoes hand surgery for arthritis might get a nerve block near the axilla (armpit) that deadens the arm. But, in addition, she might also get an injection of a drug that will heavily sedate her. As a result, the patient will be conscious but not really aware of what's happening.

No matter what type of anesthesia, an anethesiologist will be present to continuously monitor the patient's vital signs—heart rate, respiration, temperature, and oxygen saturation (how well the lungs are absorbing oxygen).

### GENERAL ANESTHESIA

Of the earliest general anesthetics, all of which are gases—diethyl ether, chloroform, and nitrous oxide—the first two are no longer used because there are safer agents with fewer side effects. Ether, for example, is flammable and can cause explosions. Nitrous oxide (laughing gas) is still widely used today, despite its propensity to cause postoperative nausea and vomiting. When used alone, nitrous oxide is not potent enough to be a complete general anesthetic. However, it can be used alone for sedation, or combined with one of the other inhaled anesthetics or injected liquid anesthetics for general anesthesia.

The inhalational anesthetics (gases) that are widely used today, primarily sevoflurane, desflurane, and isoflurane, are potent, nonflammable, and minimally metabolized. The last characteristic means that, unlike halothane, a popular gas that was metabolized (processed) in the liver and caused its damage with repeated use, today's anesthetic gases are safe for the liver. Anesthetic gases are quickly absorbed through the lungs and travel via the blood vessels to the brain, where they act.

Most adults are first anesthetized with liquid intravenous anesthetics. Once they are asleep they may receive an anesthetic gas. Liquid anesthetic drugs are injected directly into the bloodstream, through which they rapidly reach the brain. Examples of injected drugs are barbiturates, propofol, ketamine, and etomidate, as well as larger doses of opioids (such as morphine) and benzodiazepines (Valium-like drugs such as Versed [midazolam]). Propofol has antinausea properties, so it is particularly effective if a patient has a tendency to become nauseated and vomit after surgery. In lower doses, propofol is also used for sedation during regional anesthesia. A commonly used injected barbiturate anesthetic is sodium thiopental (Pentothal). This drug is fat-soluble and acts very quickly. If you receive sodium thiopental and then you are asked to count backward from 100 after the drug is injected, you probably won't remember counting past 95. In addition, some injected anesthetics are used in low doses for sedation. A small dose of an opioid or a benzodiazepine can significantly decrease anxiety. These drugs are used in these doses either as a premedication prior to general anesthesia or as "twilight sleep" for sedation when used in conjunction with local or regional anesthesia.

## REGIONAL ANESTHESIA

Regional anesthesia, as the name suggests, numbs a region of the body rather than the entire body via a local anesthetic. When large sections of the body, such as an entire leg or the abdomen, need to be anesthetized, the anesthetic is injected into the subarachnoid space of the spine (spinal anesthesia) or in the epidural space (epidural anesthesia), causing loss of sensation in the lower part of the body. Spinal and epidural anesthesia are widely used on women during childbirth. For spinals and epidurals, opioids such as morphine or fentanyl can be injected along with the local anesthetic.

For arm or hand surgery, the local anesthetic is injected into the brachial plexus, a large nerve bundle in the axilla (armpit). Depending on the site of the surgical procedure, the area around other nerves is also injected. The resulting numb area may be as small as one finger. When used as part of combination anesthesia, a regional block assures that the patient will experience no pain during the operation. If a long-acting local anesthetic such as bupivacaine (Marcaine) is used, the body part will remain numb for several hours after the end of the procedure. This can be a definite advantage compared with experiencing immediate postoperative pain.

## Minimizing Postsurgical Pain

As the previous section described, pain during an operation can be totally prevented. Pain *after* an operation is a different story. Many procedures typically result in a significant amount of pain for hours, days, or weeks after the procedure. Several approaches have been developed to decrease postoperative pain. Depending on the expected amount and duration of the pain, and how soon after surgery you are able to eat or at least take oral medications, you may receive one or a combination of the following pain relievers.

### PAIN PILLS OR INJECTIONS GIVEN AS NEEDED
The doctor's order specifies the minimum number of hours between doses, such as "every 4 to 6 hours as needed." With this approach, the patient has to ring for the nurse whenever the pain level rises. If the nurse is busy, he may have to wait. If it's too soon for the next dose, the patient has to suffer. If he asks for pain medication more often than the nurse is comfortable with, she may label him a "drug seeker" and treat him with less respect. This is the way postoperative pain medications were given for many years.

### PAIN PILLS OR INJECTIONS GIVEN ON A TIMED BASIS
The doctor's order specifies how often the medication is to be given, such as every 4 to 6 hours, with the proviso to "hold if asleep or sedated." Instead of the patient having to ask for the medication, he automatically

gets it unless he declines it or is asleep or seems too sleepy. (The reason for the caution if the patient isn't alert is that opioids are sedative in people who aren't used to taking them, so that the physician is concerned about knocking the patient out with too much medication.) To prevent possibly undertreating the pain, the physician might add an order that additional medication can be given "every 4 to 6 hours as needed" or a similar regimen. Both the "as needed" and the timed approaches require the nurse to be involved with every dose, which is a hassle for an already-busy nurse.

## PATIENT-CONTROLLED ANALGESIA

When significant postoperative pain is to be expected, this modern pain management approach is definitely the way to go. Patient-controlled analgesia (PCA) begins with a computerized pump with a reservoir containing a solution of morphine or fentanyl, or other opioid, sometimes along with other medications (such as a local anesthetic). Tubing from the pump to a vein (intravenous PCA) or the epidural space of the spinal canal (epidural PCA) delivers the medication to the patient. The pump is programmed to deliver a constant flow of medication, termed the *basal rate*. The basal rate is set at the level that the anesthesiologist believes will give adequate pain relief most of the time. In addition, the patient is given a button, attached by a cable to the pump, which she can press to get additional bursts of the pain medication. In order to prevent excessive dosing, the pump is programmed to respond to the button's signal only after an interval (called the *lockout period*), say 10 minutes, has passed since the previous signal. The pump keeps a record of exactly how much and when medication has been dispensed. The basal rate and lockout period can be adjusted by the physician depending on the patient's needs. The benefits of the PCA pump are:
  • better pain control.
  • no need for the patient to wait more than a brief time for a dose.
  • no need for frequent visits by the nurse.

Depending on the circumstances, the PCA pump may be used for one to several days. When the pain level decreases, and the patient can take medications orally, the pump is removed and the patient is then prescribed pain pills as needed.

## Pre-emptive Analgesia

Pain prevention is also an appropriate goal in the treatment of acute moderate-to-severe pain that is expected to last more than 24 hours.2 Consider the following scenarios:

1.  You go to the dentist to have a cavity filled. Knowing that drilling into a tooth is painful, the dentist first numbs the area with an injection of novocaine (Procaine) and then drills. By the time the novocaine has worn off (about 2 hours later), the drilling is long since finished. You experienced no pain during the drilling, and since drilling hurts only while it's being done, you'd have been just as happy to have the numbness go away as you were leaving the dentist's office.

2.  You smash a finger while closing your car door. The fingernail has become displaced, and the nail bed under it has a gash in it. Your bleeding finger is a mess, but it is temporarily numb, as sometimes happens with injuries. You wrap the hand in a towel and drive to the emergency room (ER), where a physician injects bupivacaine (Marcaine), a long-acting local anesthetic, near the major sensory nerve in your finger, and then sends you for an X-ray. The X-ray shows you've broken the fingertip. The ER physician sews up the laceration in your anesthetized finger, wraps it up, and sends you home. Eight hours later the Marcaine wears off, and you are surprised that there is only mild pain in the finger. (This happened to me!)

3.  You go to the hospital for a scheduled total knee replacement. During the operation, you are unconscious and experience no pain. But as soon as you awaken, you realize your knee is killing you. The nurse asks if you want some pain medicine, and quickly administers it to you. Over the next few days you require repeated doses of pain medication.

4.  You go to the hospital for a scheduled total knee replacement. During the operation, you are unconscious and experience no pain. As the surgeon is closing up your

knee, he injects Marcaine into the area. When you awaken in the recovery room, you have pain, but less than did your friend who had the same operation in the scenario number 3.

There is a difference in the way pain was managed in these scenarios. In the first case, because pain was expected only during the drilling, a short-acting local anesthetic was administered before the pain began, which got you through the entire expected duration of the pain. Once the drilling stopped, no residual pain was expected so there was no need for any further analgesia.

In scenario number 2, you were again expected to have pain during the procedure (stitching your finger), but also for some hours afterward, because of the injury, so a long-acting local anesthetic was used, which got you through the worst of the pain. These two scenarios are simple examples of *pre-emptive analgesia*, which means administering pain-relieving medications in advance of the pain. It is based on the principle that it is easier to prevent pain than to treat it. In my case (my smashed finger), it was very effective.

In the third scenario, the immediate pain of the surgical procedure was prevented by having the patient unconscious during the operation, but the expected postoperative pain was managed only by ordering pain medications to be given *after* the patient developed the pain. The patient most likely woke up in the recovery room already having a painful knee. This is the typical way that postoperative pain has been managed for generations. But things are changing!

For example, in scenario number 4, the orthopedic surgeon injected a long-acting anesthetic under the skin at the end of the procedure, not to alleviate pain during the operation, but rather for the expected postoperative pain.

In chapter 1, we made the distinction between acute pain, which serves a useful function, and chronic pain, which does not. You saw that chronic pain often results from changes in the body's nervous system that perpetuate the pain signals even in the absence of the original source of those signals. It seems that pain begets pain, and that under-treated pain can result in continuation and expansion of pain. In recent years, there has been increasing interest in learning whether predictable postoperative pain can be lessened and chronic pain prevented.

When someone undergoes surgery, the goal of preemptive analgesia is to reduce the intensity and duration of his postoperative pain, and hopefully prevent prolonged pain. Three basic ways pain can be controlled are to:

1. block it at its source—the site of injury. This is where local anesthetics act.
2. block its transmission to the brain. Spinal anesthesia and some pain medications act at this level.
3. modify the perception of pain by the brain. Various drugs, such as opioids, and nondrug modalities, such as hypnosis, work in this way.

Various drug and nondrug treatments are increasingly being tried, alone or in combination, as part of a pre-emptive analgesia plan.

## The Efficacy of Pre-emptive Analgesia

In a study of people undergoing outpatient repair of a hernia, half were given a combination of the anti-inflammatory drug rofecoxib (Vioxx), intravenous ketamine (an NMDA in chapter 4 receptor antagonist), and local anesthetic injections to the groin area before the operation, and half were not. All the patients then had the surgery under general anesthesia. During the first day after surgery, the patients who got the pre-emptive analgesia experienced only half the pain that the others did despite asking for one-third less pain medication.[3]

In another study, half of 70 patients undergoing total knee replacement received rofecoxib (Vioxx) starting on the day before the operation and continuing for 2 weeks postoperatively. Compared with the group that did not get the rofecoxib, those who did receive the painkiller needed less opioid medication during hospitalization, had less pain, vomiting, sleep disturbance, and needed a reduced amount of time in physical therapy to restore good flexion and extension to the knee.[4] Beginning treatment with an anti-inflammatory drug one day before surgery greatly benefited these patients. This is another example of the efficacy of pre-emptive analgesia in diminishing postoperative pain.

The anticonvulsant gabapentin (Neurontin), which is very useful in neuropathic pain, was compared with tramadol (Ultram) and placebo in a study of 450 patients undergoing laparoscopic cholecystectomy (gall bladder removal). The drugs were given 2 hours before the operation, which was done under general anesthesia. During the first 24 hours after surgery, the patients who had received 300 mg of gabapentin needed significantly less fentanyl (an opioid) than did those who received 100 mg of tramadol or placebo.[5]

Another class of drugs that is sometimes useful for pre-emptive analgesia is NMDA-receptor antagonists. (As seen in chapter 4, this class of drugs is particularly useful in relieving neuropathic pain.) A meta-analysis of 40 studies in which the NMDA-receptor antagonists ketamine or dextromethorphan, or else magnesium, were used to prevent postoperative pain found significant immediate and preventive analgesic benefit of dextromethorphan in two-thirds of the studies and ketamine in over half (58 percent). Magnesium had no benefit in any of the studies.[6]

Recently, researchers reviewed the multiple available animal and human studies of the efficacy of pre-emptive analgesia on acute postoperative pain.[7] Of 27 prospective, randomized, controlled trials (the most rigorous type of research trial) in humans, 12 showed that pre-emptive analgesia was effective, 10 showed no difference, and five showed it was worse than controls. The authors of this review favor giving an analgesic before surgery because it does not have a downside and might help prevent postoperative pain. If the medication is in pill form, it's best to give it 1 to 2 hours before surgery rather than on the way to the operating room, so that there is time for the medication to get into the bloodstream. They also point out that pain medicine given before or during the operation should be of sufficient duration to carry over into the early postoperative period, when pain may be at its greatest. They added: "Failure to reduce early postoperative pain significantly may diminish any potential preemptive effect during surgery." In other words, ask your surgeon or anesthesiologist to administer pain medication, which will last through the first few hours afterward, before or during the operation. I believe that this is exactly why I had such a good outcome with my smashed finger, which remained anesthetized for several hours after I left the emergency room.

## Pre-emptive Analgesia and Chronic Pain

As you read in chapter 2, pain causes the release of chemicals that mediate (induce) inflammation. Inflammation in turn can cause the development of hyperalgesia, an exaggerated pain response that may be prolonged. It makes sense, therefore, that pre-emptive analgesia might prevent hyperalgesia and chronic pain. Animal research studies on pain mechanisms have suggested that early treatment of pain might prevent peripheral and central sensitization and thereby decrease acute pain and minimize the risk of developing chronic pain.

A dramatic example of prevention of chronic pain through pre-emptive analgesia involved phantom limb pain. More than half of amputees suffer from phantom pain in the missing limb during the first year after amputation. In a group of 25 patients who underwent amputation of the leg below the knee, 11 received an epidural block in their lumbar (lower) spine before the operation began. All 25 had spinal or epidural analgesia during surgery and pain medications afterward. Six months later, all 11 patients who had received the preoperative epidural block were pain-free, whereas five of the 11 controls had phantom limb pain.[8] A brief pre-emptive analgesia procedure was indeed effective in preventing prolonged phantom limb pain.

Other studies suggest that injury-induced inflammation plays a role in the development of chronic pain. A neurotransmitter, interleukin-6, is produced at sites of trauma and travels through the bloodstream into the brain. This neurotransmitter increases production of the enzyme cyclooxygenase 2 (COX-2), which, in turn, increases levels of prostaglandins in the cerebrospinal fluid (CSF), leading to increased inflammation and hyperalgesia.[9] Anti-inflammatory drugs (NSAIDs) work at both the periphery and in the central nervous system. Doctors generally advise against taking an NSAID before surgery because such drugs can increase bleeding. However, a newer generation of NSAIDs— COX-2 inhibitors—does not affect bleeding (see chapter 4). Taking a COX-2 inhibitor such as rofecoxib (Vioxx), celecoxib (Celebrex), or valdecoxib (Bextra) before surgery not only reduces pain immediately afterward, but might also decrease the risk of developing hyperalgesia and chronic pain.

This is just a brief introduction to one of the most exciting new areas in pain management. Traditionally, physicians have focused on treating pain after it occurs. What the current research shows is that we need to pay a lot more attention to preventing pain when pain can be predicted.

## Surgical Treatments for Particular Pain Problems

This section will describe surgical treatments for the most common causes of chronic pain—arthritis and back pain.

### KNEE SURGERY FOR ARTHRITIS: TOTAL KNEE ARTHROPLASTY (TKA)

About 350,000 people in the United States undergo total knee replacement (also called arthroplasty) each year, the vast majority because of osteoarthritis. Osteoarthritis is the most common indication for total replacement of the hip and knee worldwide. In normal joints, the surfaces of the bones are covered with cartilage that allows them to glide smoothly as the joint moves. In a patient with arthritis, cartilage is damaged or lost, so that bone rubs against bone. Total joint replacement (arthroplasty) restores smooth surfaces by replacing the damaged cartilage with artificial materials. The results of knee replacements are usually excellent—about 90 percent of patients have pain relief for 10 years. Candidates for knee surgery are generally people older than 55 who've already had an adequate trial of nonoperative management, including NSAIDs, local injections, activity modification, weight reduction (if needed), and physical therapy, and who also have:

- persistent pain.
- significant restriction in their ability to function.
- significant stiffness, instability (constant giving way), and/or locking of the knee.
- X-ray evidence of knee damage.

When walking becomes too painful despite pain medications and assistive devices such as a cane or walker, it's time to consider surgery. (If you are overweight, your orthopedic surgeon will undoubtedly recommend weight loss first.) The procedure involves a 7- to 8-inch incision over the knee. The surgeon opens up the knee and cuts out the diseased joint surfaces of the tibia (shin bone) and femur (thigh bone). (See Figure 4.) The lower end of the femur is resurfaced with a metallic prosthesis held in place with a special cement, while a polyethylene-bearing surface in a metal tray is attached to the top end of the tibia by means of a peg or stem through the bone, and anchored with bone cement. The underside of the patella (kneecap) is often removed, and may be replaced by a polyethylene button.

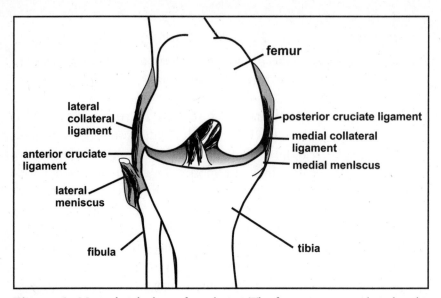

**Figure 4.** *Normal right knee, frontal view. The femur is connected to the tibia and fibula by various ligaments, and the joint is cushioned by the medial and lateral menisci and other cartilage.*

Total knee replacement is major surgery, and anyone considering this type of surgery should know that sometimes there are complications. The most common complication is loosening of the prosthesis. Others are stiffness of the knee and infection. Infected artificial knees may have to be removed, and surgery repeated after a course of antibiotics.

During your 3- to 5-day hospital stay, and for weeks afterward, you will be expected to participate in physical therapy—in a swimming pool and on land—to restore mobility and strength to the knee joint and surrounding muscles. Having your knee replaced requires a real commitment on your part to the rehabilitation process. You also need to know that artificial joints don't last forever, and they fail more quickly when more demand is put on them. Exercise is helpful, but with an artificial joint the exercise should be moderate rather than extreme.

### Evidence Concerning Efficacy of Total Knee Replacement

What do the experts say on the role of knee replacement surgery? This question was recently addressed by a panel convened by the National

Institutes of Health. After reviewing 20 years of data, the committee found that total knee replacement is safe and cost-effective for alleviating pain and improving physical function in the vast majority of patients who do not respond to nonsurgical therapies.[10] According to the report, some 90 percent of people who undergo the surgery experience rapid reduction in pain and improvement in overall quality of life. About 1 percent of prosthetic knees loosen or otherwise fail each year, most of which require repeat surgery. This is more likely among obese, male, and relatively young patients. Excessive exercise can also hasten problems with the knee prosthesis. The success rate of repeat surgery is about 70 percent.

A patient of mine, a man 60 years of age, was a former professional tennis player who, at the time of surgery, worked full-time as a tennis coach. The years of heavy use had taken their toll on his knees, and two years before I started seeing him for pain management he underwent total replacement of both knees. Against the advice of his orthopedic surgeon, he continued his demanding work unabated, and soon developed knee pain again. I added a sustained-release opioid to his regimen of NSAIDs and advised a decrease in his activity level, but he persisted. Eventually, his new knees showed X-ray signs of wear and tear, he required increased doses of painkillers. He finally resigned himself to the inevitable and reduced his amount of activity.

## UNICOMPARTMENTAL SURGERY

For patients with osteoarthritis in only half of the knee (but not both sides), osteoarthritis in either the medial (inside) or lateral (outside) compartment, a less invasive knee replacement procedure called unicompartment "mini-knee" surgery may be an option. In this operation, only the affected half of the knee is resurfaced. Through a small incision (3 to 3.5 inches), part of the surfaces of the femur and tibia are removed and small femoral and tibial prostheses are attached. There is minimal damage to the surrounding muscles and tendons. The hospital stay is shorter (1 to 2 days) and recovery is much faster. The 10-year success rate is only slightly less than that of TKA, and, if necessary, can later be converted to TKA. After recovery from this operation, you should not return to active sports such as tennis, jogging, or basketball, or the results might be short-lived.

## UniSpacer

Another less invasive surgical procedure, approved in 2001, is the insertion of a small kidney-shaped implant called the UniSpacer between the femur and tibia on the medial (inside) half of the knee.[11] In people with early knee osteoarthritis (OA) that affects primarily the medial compartment, this procedure gives moderate improvement in pain and function. The device is inserted without removal of bone and without cement. If the patient later needs a total or unicompartmental knee replacement, the surgeon slips the UniSpacer out and then performs the knee replacement. The biggest problem with the UniSpacer is that it may eventually become dislodged. If you are interested in this procedure, you need to realize that it hasn't been around for long and that long-term results are still not in. A recent report on the results of using the UniSpacer showed disappointing results.[12]

## High-tibial Osteotomy

An older procedure that can help people with arthritis on only one side of the knee is called high-tibial osteotomy. The upper end of the tibia is cut and repositioned to reorient the loads that occur during walking and running so that the loads pass through a non-arthritic portion of the knee. This procedure allows people to return to high-impact sports.[13] However, it provides less complete pain relief and is more likely to require later surgery than TKA or a unicompartmental replacement. The use of high-tibial osteotomy is decreasing in the United States.

## Arthroscopic Knee Surgery

Arthroscopy is a minimally invasive surgical procedure that has revolutionized orthopedic knee surgery. The knee was one of the first joints in which this procedure was successfully performed. Previously any repair of the knee required the knee to be opened, which in many cases resulted in some residual disability. Arthroscopy is now used in many other joints and is very common.

A small fiberoptic telescope (arthroscope) is inserted into a joint through a small incision. Saline (salt water) is then pumped into the knee to distend it and to allow the surgeon to see the structures within it. He views the inside of the knee on a monitor, and inserts additional instruments through one to four additional small incisions to carry out the procedure. Depending on the complexity of the problem, either general or local anesthesia is used. Arthroscopy is often performed on an outpatient basis.

Knee problems that are amenable to arthroscopic treatment include:
- repair or trimming of a torn meniscus (cartilage in the knee).
- mild osteoarthritis (OA) or rheumatoid arthritis (RA).
- removal of debris (small pieces of broken cartilage) in the knee joint.
- repair of a torn or damaged anterior cruciate or posterior cruciate ligament.
- inflamed or damaged lining of the joint (synovium).
- malalignment of the kneecap (patella).

The advantages of arthroscopic surgery are that it is less traumatic to surrounding tissues, the incision is smaller, there is a reduced amount of pain and stiffness, fewer complications, and recovery is quicker than when the knee is surgically opened.

Arthroscopic lavage is a procedure in which the knee joint is irrigated with copious amounts of fluid. In the past this procedure was thought to be as effective as injections of steroids into the joint. In the future, however, the procedure of washing out the knee joint through an arthroscope might be done less often because a recent trial suggested that the results were no better than placebo in relieving pain.[14]

## HIP SURGERY FOR ARTHRITIS: TOTAL HIP ARTHROPLASTY (THA)

As with knee surgery, the most common cause for total hip replacement (THA) is osteoarthritis. As the disease worsens, pain increases, and the range of motion of the hip decreases because bone spurs limit movement of the hip joint. Conservative treatment is similar to that of knee arthritis—anti-inflammatories and other pain medications, physical therapy, injections, and the use of a cane or walker. When pain remains and mobility is significantly decreased despite nonsurgical therapies, surgery is a reasonable choice. You can expect an artificial hip to last 12 to 15 years. Recent studies suggest that THA done before severe disability sets in results in a better postoperative outcome.[15]

Total hip replacement is usually done in patients who are older than 55 and have:

• severe pain that restricts their ordinary activities.
• pain that is no longer adequately relieved by pain medications, assistive devices, and restricting activities.
• stiffness of the hip that significantly decreases its range of motion.
• X-rays that show significant abnormalities.

As with other joint replacements, a total hip prosthesis has two parts—a hemispherical socket component that fits into the pelvis (hip bone) and replaces the natural cup-shaped socket (acetabulum), and the femoral portion that replaces the head of the femur. The socket device is a metal shell containing a tough plastic liner that serves as a bearing and allows smooth movement of the joint. The femoral component is made of a metal ball (some devices have a ceramic ball) and stem that is inserted into the femur.

The operation, which is done under general anesthesia, begins with a long vertical incision, about 8 to 14 inches long, on the side of the hip. (See Figure 5.) Muscles and ligaments are separated, the head of the femur is cut off, and the acetabulum is reamed out and shaped to the exact configuration of the socket prosthesis. The two components are then inserted. In some cases, bone cement (methyl methacrylate) is used; in others, the femoral component used is made with spaces that permit natural bone eventually to grow into it and fix it permanently into place.

The most significant complications of THA are:
• thrombophlebitis (blood clots in the leg ).
• pulmonary emboli (blood clots in the lung) .
• hip joint infection.
• hip joint dislocation.
• loosening of the prosthesis.

Hip dislocation—popping out of the ball from the socket—is a significant risk in the early weeks before the muscles and tendons have healed. For this reason you will be given instructions on body and leg positions to avoid; it is very important to follow these instructions religiously. Loosening of the prosthesis is a later development, usually taking place after years of good function, and requires additional surgery.

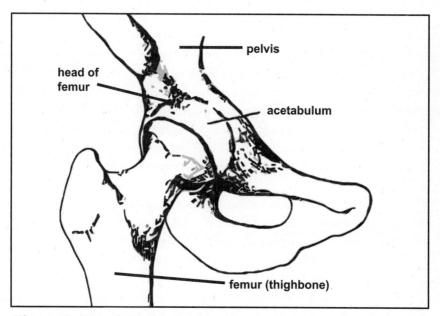

**Figure 5.** *Normal right hip, frontal view.*

Some orthopedic surgeons are now performing "mini-hip" total hip replacements, which are less traumatic to the patient and result in a shorter recovery time. Like the mini-knee procedure, these use a smaller incision.

### BACK SURGERY

The superhighway that carries nerve signals from the body up to the brain and back down to the body is the spinal cord, a delicate bundle of nerves that is essential for normal functioning of the body. To keep this bundle protected, it is surrounded by a column of peculiarly shaped bones, the vertebrae, the back portions of which form bony cylinders around the spinal cord. (See Figure 3, page 121.) Each vertebra contacts the next one at several sites, called facet joints. The 24 uppermost vertebrae are separated by fibrous cartilage pads—the intervertebral disks—which act as shock absorbers during movement and also make the spine flexible rather than rigid. Through spaces in each vertebra, a pair of spinal nerves emerge and fan out to the torso, arms, and legs.

This wonderful arrangement has several unfortunate points of vulnerability. In osteoarthritis (OA), which is an extremely common disorder of aging and overuse, abnormal bone growth gradually intrudes on the space in the spinal canal or the exit points of the nerves. The spinal nerve becomes increasingly crowded in its space and at some point may become compressed. This process is termed *spinal stenosis*, and the result is pain in the back, which often radiates to the leg. The leg pain may be accompanied by numbness and tingling. This is called *radiculopathy*, which means an abnormality of the nerve root.

The intervertebral disks are another point of vulnerability. With age, they gradually deteriorate and at some point may extrude (*herniated disk*) and bump against the adjacent exiting spinal nerve, thereby compressing it. Again, the compressed nerve may produce both back pain and radiculopathy—pain, numbness, and tingling in the leg.

As you read in earlier chapters, back pain is initially treated conservatively, with education about the back, activity modification, strengthening exercises, physical therapy, epidural corticosteroid injection, and anti-inflammatory drugs (NSAIDs) and other painkillers. In the majority of cases, no particular cause for the back pain is found (this is called "mechanical back pain") and these conservative measures are continued. Many people think that back surgery is a first-line solution to back pain. Unfortunately, unless there is a clear indication for surgery, you may have no improvement or end up even worse off than before. The most common reasons to consider back surgery are:

- progressive neurological problems, such as numbness, loss of reflexes, or bladder or bowel problems.
- sciatica, which is leg pain arising from compression of the sciatic nerve.
- instability of the joints of the spine.
- instability due to a fractured vertebra.
- presence of a tumor or infection in the spine.

## LUMBAR LAMINECTOMY
When abnormal bone growth or a herniated disk pinches one or more nerve roots in the lower (lumbar) spine, the most common operation to relieve pressure is a lumbar laminectomy. This procedure is done

through a 2- to 5-inch incision in the back. The surgeon separates the muscles overlying the spine, then removes part of the lamina, which is the bone roof of the spinal canal. This gives the surgeon access to the compressed nerve and whatever is causing the pressure—part of a herniated disk, a bone spur, or a tumor—can be removed.

After the operation, patients remain in the hospital for up to 3 days, but are immediately encouraged to walk. However, for 6 weeks, a patient should avoid excessive bending, lifting, or twisting in order to avoid pulling on the suture line before it heals. About 70 to 80 percent of patients have significant improvement in pain and function. In those who have spinal stenosis related to osteoarthritis, pain relief is usually better in the leg than in the back. Because bone growth related to the arthritis continues, the symptoms may recur after several years. Complications of surgery include the usual bleeding and infection and, rarely, damage to a nerve resulting in bladder or bowel incontinence. In 5 to 10 percent of cases, the operated joint becomes unstable as a result of bone removed during surgery. The usual solution is a fusion operation at a later date. Occasionally, a leak of the spinal fluid occurs, which results in a severe head-ache. Fortunately, this is a very temporary problem, and lying flat in bed for 24 hours usually allows the leak to seal.

## MICRODISCECTOMY (MICRODECOMPRESSION) FOR A LUMBAR HERNIATED DISK

Just as there are now "mini" procedures for repairing knee and hip problems, there is a new, smaller procedure for treatment of a lumbar herniated disk.

In a microdiscectomy, a small incision (about an inch) is made in the back, the muscles over the bony arch are moved aside, and only a small portion of the vertebral bone over the compressed nerve is removed. Once the affected nerve is seen, bone fragments and/or disk material are removed from around the nerve to relieve the pressure. As with a laminectomy, a microdiscectomy is more effective for treating leg pain (radiculopathy) than for lower back pain. Patients usually get relief from leg pain almost immediately after the procedure.

Microdiscectomy is usually performed as an outpatient procedure. Because disturbance to the structures of the back is significantly less, the risk of postoperative instability is minimal. Patients can often return to normal functioning immediately. It's advisable to undertake a program of stretching, strengthening exercises, and aerobic conditioning to help prevent a recurrence of back pain or another disk herniation.

The success rate of a microdiscectomy is about 90 to 95 percent, but some patients develop a recurrent disk herniation, most commonly within the first 3 months, but sometimes only after many years. Part of the reason for the early recurrences is that only a small portion of the disk can be visualized (seen) during the procedure. A second microdiscectomy can be done, but if the same problem recurs yet again, the patient may be advised to have a fusion operation in which all the disk material of that joint is removed and the adjacent vertebrae are fused.

## When to Wait Rather Than Have An Operation for a Herniated Disk

In general, if your leg pain due to a disk herniation is going to get better, it will do so in about 6 to 12 weeks. As long as the pain is tolerable and you can function adequately, it is usually advisable to postpone back surgery for a short period of time to see if the pain will resolve with conservative (nonsurgical) treatment alone. If it does not, then a microdiscectomy is a reasonable option to relieve pressure on the nerve root and speed the healing. Immediate surgery is necessary in cases of bowel/bladder incontinence (*Cauda equina* syndrome) or progressive neurological deficits. It may also be reasonable to consider immediate surgery if the pain is severe.

### LUMBAR SPINE FUSION

Each year, more than 150,000 people in the United States undergo fusion of the lumbar spine because their low back pain worsened with abnormal movement of certain vertebrae. The goal of this kind of surgery is to stabilize the joint and thus prevent pain. The cause of an unstable joint may be abnormal position of one vertebra relative to the next (spondylolisthesis), which can be congenital but is more often degenerative, occurring with aging. If there is spinal stenosis as well as spondylolisthesis, the patient might need both a decompressive laminectomy and fusion.

The goal of spinal fusion surgery is to stop the motion at a painful vertebral segment, which in turn should decrease pain generated from the joint. All lumbar spinal fusion surgery involves adding bone graft to an area of the spine to set up a biological response that causes the bone graft to grow between the two vertebrae to fuse them. Bone graft can be taken from the patient's hip (autograft bone) during the fusion surgery, or harvested from cadaver bone (allograft bone). Soon synthetic bone grafts will be available. Currently, a new synthetic substance, bone mor-phogenic protein (BMP), is in clinical trials. This substance helps the body create bone and may eventually replace the use of human bone grafts. Electricity can also improve bone growth and enhance bone fusion. Electrical bone stimulators, which emit a low-level electrical current, can be temporarily implanted or can be worn on the outside of the back.

Traditionally, painful movement of two adjacent vertebrae is prevented by inserting a bone graft from the hip so that the two bones will grow together and function as one unit. At present, however, a new procedure is being used more often; it is called a spinal instrumentation. This consists of inserting a perforated metallic cage in the disk space between the two vertebrae and filling it with bone-graft material so that the two vertebrae become fused. The cage restores the original height of the disk space. Additionally, the vertebrae are rendered immediately immobile by using plates or rods through which screws are placed into the adjacent vertebrae.

Although spinal fusion hastens pain relief compared with more conservative approaches, it should be used only as a last resort. Fusion may result in additional stress on the joints adjacent to the fusion site. All too often problems later develop at a level above the operated vertebra (less commonly below it), leading to yet another operation, only to be followed again by additional pain farther up the spine. This is more likely to happen if more than two disk spaces of the spine are fused, which is why two is usually considered the maximum.

## INTRADISCAL ELECTROTHERMAL ANNULOPLASTY (IDET)
A common cause of back pain is pain within the intervertebral disks. Disks are prone to wear-and-tear damage or accidental injury. The result is painful tears in the outer wall of the disk. This is probably due to irritation of small

nerves in the damaged outer wall of the disk or pressure on nerves that grow into the disk. Back pain originating within the disk is termed *discogenic pain*. The pain is not due to disk herniation, and it does not radiate down the legs.

In 1997, a new procedure was introduced, intradiscal electrothermal annuloplasty (IDET). It's based on the theory that discogenic pain can be relieved by strengthening the torn, weakened disk wall and deadening the pain nerves within. Under local anesthetic, a hollow needle is inserted into the disk. Through the needle, a thin wire is passed into the disk and then heated for several minutes up to 90 degrees Celsius (194 degrees Farenheit, almost the boiling point of water). The heated wire is kept in place for 15 minutes, during which time it shrinks the fibers that make up the disk wall, closing any tears, and also cauterizes (burns) the tiny nerve endings within the disk, making them less sensitive to pain. Several disks may be treated at one time. The preoperative pain may take several days to be relieved, and recovery from the procedure takes a few weeks. Postoperative recovery therapies include wearing a back support, getting physical therapy, and avoiding any strenuous activities.

Not everyone is a candidate for this procedure, however. To determine whether a disk is causing your pain, the physician will first order a discogram, a procedure in which the disk is injected with a contrast dye. This will cause pain to an injured disk but not in any that are healthy. If the results confirm that the pain indeed originates from inside the disk, then IDET has about a 70 percent chance of providing significant relief.

Because the procedure is so new, there are no published prospective randomized studies yet; the long-term results are also still unknown. There is some debate about how IDET really works, and not everyone gets relief. In one outcome study of IDET, 62 back pain patients were followed up for 12 to 15 months.[16] The patients had experienced pain for an average of 5 years before the procedure. At follow-up, 44 of the 62 patients (71 percent) had a reduction in pain and improved function. None had any complications or adverse events.

In a recent small retrospective study, 44 patients were interviewed a year after undergoing IDET.[17] All had had a positive discogram before the procedure. Six patients (15 percent) had lumbar surgery within a year after IDET. Of the remaining 38, 50 percent were dissatisfied with the procedure, 37 percent were satisfied, and 13 percent were undecided; 29 percent reported more pain after the procedure, 39 percent less pain, and

29 percent no change. Although IDET has been helpful for some patients, the likelihood of no benefit is significant.

## NEW SURGICAL TREATMENTS FOR OSTEOPOROSIS

Osteoporosis is thinning of the bones. All the bones of the body are involved, but because of their different structure, the vertebrae of the spine weaken to the point of fracture usually before fractures involve other bones of the body. A frequent consequence of osteoporosis is compression fractures of the vertebrae. These result in pain and in the characteristic hunched-over posture of too many older men and women. Conventional treatment of such fractures consists of analgesics, bed rest, and bracing. There are also two new surgical procedures that aim to relieve pain. One of them—*kyphoplasty*—restores the original structure of the compressed vertebrae, thereby restoring the person's height and erect posture. Both procedures are done percutaneously—through the skin.

In *vertebroplasty*, the bone cement polymethylmethacrylate (PMMA) is injected under pressure directly into the vertebral body to stabilize the fracture. It provides significant pain relief and improved function in most treated patients, but does not restore the height of the vertebral body. In kyphoplasty, the surgeon inserts an inflatable balloon into the affected vertebral body. When the balloon is blown up, it pushes the walls of the of the vertebra back to their original height. The balloon is then deflated and withdrawn, leaving a space that is then filled with PMMA. A more viscous (thicker) PMMA is used, which reduces leakage of the material from the vertebra as compared with the vertebroplasty procedure. Kyphoplasty restores an average of 97 percent of the vertebral height, versus 30 percent with vertebroplasy.[18]

It is likely that both procedures relieve pain by stiffening the vertebral body, thereby decreasing the micromotion (tiny movements) of the fractured vertebra.

## RHEUMATOID ARTHRITIS (RA)

Patients with RA are more likely than those with OA to require surgery. Some surgical procedures used in RA are soft-tissue repairs, arthroscopy, arthrodesis (fusion of joints), and total joint replacement (arthroplasty). The disadvantage of joint fusion for RA patients is that there is no longer any motion of the affected joint; the benefit is that fusion can provide ongoing pain relief and joint stability. Candidates for total joint replacement are patients who have severe joint pain or severe impairment in function and have not responded to other medical treatments. The shoulders, elbows, hands, hips, knees, and ankles can all be replaced.

# 9

# EXERCISE, PHYSICAL THERAPY, AND OTHER HANDS-ON APPROACHES

## *Do They Work?*

*Regular, moderate exercise offers a whole host of benefits to people with arthritis. Mainly, exercise reduces joint pain and stiffness, builds strong muscle around the joints, and increases flexibility and endurance. But it also helps promote overall health and fitness by giving you more energy, helping you sleep better, controlling your weight, decreasing depression, and giving you more self-esteem.*

—THE ARTHRITIS FOUNDATION

ALTHOUGH MEDICATIONS ARE A MAINSTAY for the treatment of chronic pain, they are not enough. For most musculoskeletal pain syndromes, exercise and physical therapy are important for prevention and relief of pain. Unfortunately, the belief that activity will cause pain results in physical deconditioning, which can complicate chronic pain syndromes. The reality is that in most cases, "hurt does not equal harm." When physical deconditioning is reversed with gentle and appropriate exercise, your pain levels may decrease. Graded exercise programs seek to maximize functional range of motion and correct poor posture. It's important to maintain moderate levels of physical activity, even if your pain persists, and the program should include exercises that improve flexibility, strength, and endurance.

Because a moderate exercise program should be lifelong, you need to take into account your preferences. Below are some suggestions for increasing the probability that you will continue exercising, along with comments by several of my patients about the efficacy of these strategies.

- **Make exercise a scheduled part of your day rather than hoping it will happen if you have the time**. *Take the choice out of it. If I ask myself, "Should I walk today?" or "Do I really have the time for this?", I'm likely to decide to postpone it. But if it's as much a part of my life as taking a shower or doing the dishes, then it will happen.*

- **Plan to do the physical activity at a time that will best fit your lifestyle**. *My day is full of interruptions—telephone calls, urgent demands, multitasking. There's no way I could get through my stretches plus an uninterrupted 30 minutes on my stationary cycle. So I've committed to doing it first thing in the morning, at 6 A.M. That way I can actually get a good workout.*

- **Increase your level of commitment by involving other people**. *My friend Linda and I walk our dogs every evening. It's the highlight of my dog's day, and an opportunity for Linda and me to share our day. There are times I'd rather not go, but I know I've made that commitment to Linda, and I'd feel guilty depriving my dog of his one daily opportunity to run around.*

- **Sign up for a class**. *I found an arthritis pool therapy class at my fitness center that's just at my level. Everyone else has just as severe hip or knee problems as I do, and the teacher knows what movements are good for us and which are risky. At first, it was a drag to drive to the class, but now I look forward to the workout and to getting together with the other people in the class.*

- **Hire a personal trainer**. *My trainer worked out a muscle-strengthening program for me that's tailored to my back problems. I basically don't like to exercise, but he really keeps encouraging and motivating me. The improvement in my back is why I keep coming back to the sessions!*

## Do Physical Activity and Exercise Decrease Pain?

In an interesting study done 20 years ago in Copenhagen, Denmark, some 900 people underwent a thorough back examination and physical measurements of the length and endurance of their back and leg muscles. One year later, they completed a questionnaire concerning low back pain in the preceding year. The main finding was that, in men, good isometric endurance of the back muscles seemed to prevent first-time experience of low back pain (the results for women were not as clear). Weak trunk muscles and reduced flexibility of the back were more pronounced in men who had recurring or ongoing low back pain during the follow-up year.[1] This study shows that having strong back muscles protects against developing back pain. It supports the value of exercise in maintaining good musculoskeletal health.

Whiplash injuries are another common source of chronic pain. A recent study compared two treatment approaches to this problem.[2] Ninety-seven patients who had whiplash injuries in a motor vehicle accident were randomized to either frequent active neck exercises or to initial rest, a soft collar, and gradually increased movement. The group who did active neck exercises had a significantly reduced amount of pain and a shorter time out of work. In addition, half of the actively treated group waited 2 weeks to begin treatment, while the other half started exercises by 4 days after the injury. Three years later, only the patients whose treatment began early had entirely normal range of motion of the neck. This study showed that the most effective approach is early active treatment, which can be carried out as home exercises after appropriate instruction.

## Exercise

Three studies especially illuminate the many benefits of exercise. Two used exercises that can be done without expensive equipment. A study of older adults with osteoarthritis found that exercise reduced by about 15 minutes per night the time needed to fall asleep, and increased the duration of sleep by about 45 minutes.[3] The activity included 30 to 40 minutes of home-based exercise 4 days a week, including brisk walking. In the Fitness Arthritis and Senior Trial (FAST) of older adults with knee osteoarthritis, moderate exercise including strength and endurance training improved function and reduced pain, and the results were sustained over at least 18 months.[4] The people who adhered strictly to the exercise regimen experienced a greater improvement in functioning and a greater reduction in pain. In yet another study, patients with knee or hip osteoarthritis who exercised for 12 weeks had reduced pain and disability, used less acetaminophen for pain, and made fewer doctor visits than did osteoarthritis patients who did not exercise.[5]

Aerobic exercise and weight training will not only increase your exercise tolerance, but can also decrease the chronic pain of osteoarthritis and other musculoskeletal conditions. In people with osteoarthritis, the more fit the muscles, the better the hips and knees can absorb the shocks of walking and other physical activity. The way to strengthen the muscles is by strength—or resistance—training. The Arthritis Foundation endorses weight training, and many physicians recommend it.

## Physical Therapy

Physical therapy (PT) has some overlap with a personal trainer, in that both involve a combination of stretching, aerobic exercise, and muscle-strengthening under supervision. The difference is that the physical therapist has extensive training in musculoskeletal disorders and a good understanding of the requirements and limitations involved in rehabilitating someone with chronic back pain, knee osteoarthritis, and other disorders. The therapist can evaluate your gait and posture and prescribe corrective exercises for abnormalities. Physical therapy is usually limited to the number of sessions your insurance will cover. Be sure that when you stop PT, you have a detailed home exercise program you understand and are committed to pursuing.

The physical therapist may also recommend an assistive device to help you move with less pain and more stability. For example, in osteoarthritis of the knee, using a cane in the hand opposite the side of the affected knee can reduce the load on the knee and improve its function. As part of your PT program, you might receive ultrasound, hot packs, pulsed electric current to strengthen muscles, massage, and/or a trial of a portable electrical stimulator. Some of these are discussed below.

## Transcutaneous Electrical Nerve Stimulation (TENS)

In transcutaneous electrical nerve stimulation (TENS), pulses of a low-intensity electrical current are applied to the skin. The mechanism of action is based on Melzack and Wall's gate control theory[6] (see chapter 2): If electric stimulation is applied to a peripheral site, the large-diameter nerve fibers are activated first, thus inhibiting the transmission by small nociceptive fibers. This gating effect is established at the dorsal-horn level of the spinal cord, where the transmission of pain-related impulses are inhibited. Another possible mechanism for the effect of TENS is that it somehow stimulates release of endogenous opioids. This was suggested in a study in which the opioid antagonist naloxone reversed the analgesia produced by TENS.[7] The implications of such an effect of naloxone is that the pain-relieving effect of TENS results from opioid release in the treated area.

Not all TENS treatment is the same. The electrical pulses can be short or long, and their intensity (voltage) can be high or low. Conventional TENS (also called high-frequency TENS) is administered at 50 to 120 hertz (Hz) pulses at a low intensity. Low-frequency TENS consists of longer 1 to 4 Hz pulses delivered at a high intensity. Traditionally used for back pain, TENS has also been used successfully in treating painful menstrual cramps. Studies of this use found high-frequency TENS to be more effective for pain relief than either placebo TENS or low-frequency TENS.[8,9] The implication of these findings is that if a trial of TENS doesn't give you as much relief as you'd like, before giving up on this modality altogether, talk with your physical therapist about trying other frequencies or intensities of the pulses.

## Spray and Stretch for Myofascial Pain

A person with myofascial pain syndrome experiences a deep ache that is worsened by activity. The basic problem is trigger points, areas of muscle tightening that hurt when touched. Additionally, when the trigger point is stimulated, you feel pain in areas away from the trigger point. A particular trigger point is associated with pain at the same reproducible area of the body, which may or may not be adjacent to the trigger point. The primary treatment is to release the trigger points. One way of doing this is the "spray and stretch" technique first described years ago by Dr. Janet Travell, who treated President John F. Kennedy's back pain. First, the surface of the skin over the trigger point is sprayed with a coolant spray and then the affected muscle is stretched. Massage of the trigger points can also provide relief. Other helpful treatments include ice or heat, ultrasound, TENS, acupuncture, and biofeedback. NSAIDs have shown no efficacy in relieving myofascial pain, but tricyclic antidepressants can provide some benefit.

## Traction

If you or a relative has ever gotten physical therapy for osteoarthritis of the neck, you are probably familiar with traction, an effective means of separating vertebrae and reducing the pain resulting from nerve compression. Traction is traditionally used for both neck and back pain, but it is also finding new uses. Wrist traction by means of a portable wrist traction device was recently tested in 30 patients who had mild to moderate carpal tunnel syndrome.[10] Each patient wore the device for 10 minutes once or twice a day for 8 weeks. The device placed a constant and controlled traction force across the wrist, separating and elongating the joints and soft tissues of the wrist and hand. It relieved the pressure in the carpal tunnel that caused the pain. Most patients experienced pain relief within the first 2 weeks, as well as improved sleep. In addition, nerve conduction studies showed improved functioning of the affected median nerve in most patients. (The median nerve is located in the wrist, and when it is compressed, causes carpal tunnel syndrome pain.)

This study is interesting because it shows that there are always new treatments for various chronic pain problems. As part of living with your pain, you are well-advised to keep track of new developments. Surf the Internet, ask your doctor, and talk with other people with the same problem. Be an active part of your recovery plan.

## Heat

Temperature changes have long been a staple of pain treatment. If you've suffered a sprained ankle or other acute injury, you were probably advised to put ice on it. Perhaps you were told to use ice for the first couple of days and then heat. The role of ice and heat might be confusing to you. Ice can numb pain and reduce inflammation. That's why it's often recommended as initial treatment. Heat increases the blood supply to the region and can also alleviate pain. For chronic pain, heat rather than ice will more likely reduce pain.

Heat can be delivered by means of a heating pad or by ultrasound—sound waves that can warm up body parts below the skin surface. Ultrasound is usually a part of physical therapy, whereas heating pads are usually used at home.

You have undoubtedly experienced the beneficial effect of heat, but what does the research show? A study of almost 400 patients with low back pain assigned one group to 8 hours of continuous low-level heat-wrap therapy, another to ibuprofen treatment, and a third group to a maximal dose of acetaminophen.[11] The patients treated with the heat wrap had greater pain relief than did those in the other two groups. Of course, most of us don't have the luxury of lying around for 8 hours during the day wrapped in a heating pad. But a second study enrolled 76 patients to compare the effects of an overnight heat wrap with no treatment.[12] Those who slept with the heat wrap had effective pain relief throughout the next day, with less muscle stiffness and disability and improved trunk flexibility. The benefits lasted for more than 48 hours after the treatment was completed. A cautionary note: In these studies, the temperature of the heat wrap was very carefully controlled. Sleeping on an electric heating pad can be risky, as a temperature level that feels good at first can easily be too hot for prolonged application, and can burn the skin. It's safer to sleep with an old-fashioned rubber hot-water bottle, the temperature of which gradually cools.

## *Taping for Knee Osteoarthritis*

We've already discussed the importance of exercise, physical therapy, and muscle strengthening for treating osteoarthritis (OA). Occupational therapists (OTs) can suggest canes or other assistive devices for advanced disease. Proper footwear, tailored orthoses (shoe inserts), and splints can also help. Another possibly useful approach for knee osteoarthritis is therapeutic knee taping. In a recent study, a small group of patients with knee osteoarthritis wore therapeutic tape for three weeks. Rigid strapping tape and hypoallergenic undertape were applied by physical therapists, who changed the tape weekly. Compared with patients who got no tape or had knee taping in a nontherapeutic pattern, patients whose knees were taped therapeutically had a greater reduction in pain and improved functioning.[13] It's unclear whether taping would continue to be effective and whether patients would be willing to visit a physical therapist weekly for the taping. But it's certainly an approach worth considering if what you already are doing isn't giving you enough relief.

## Back and Knee Braces

People with jobs that entail lifting sometimes routinely wear back braces on the job in an attempt to prevent back injuries. Industrial back belts are in widespread use in stores where employees lift packages. Many employers actually require workers to wear such belts. Athletes sometimes wear knee braces in the hope of avoiding knee injuries. Unfortunately, braces have not been shown to effectively reduce such injuries. For example, a large-scale prospective study of almost 14,000 employees whose jobs involved lifting found that neither frequent back belt use nor a store policy that required back belt use significantly reduced the incidence of back injury or low back pain.[14]

# 1 0

# COMPLEMENTARY AND ALTERNATIVE TREATMENTS

## A Second Health Care System

MANY PEOPLE IN THE UNITED STATES USE COMPLEMENTARY and alternative (CAM) treatments (approaches outside the usual consideration of physicians) for health problems. In 1993 telephone survey of 1,539 adults throughout the United States one in three (34 percent) reported using at least one unconventional therapy in the past year.[1] Unconventional therapies were defined as medical interventions not taught widely at U.S. medical schools or generally available to U.S. hospitals. Examples include relaxation techniques, chiropractic, massage therapy (these were the top three modalities used), acupuncture, imagery, spiritual healing, commercial weight-loss programs, lifestyle diets (for example, macrobiotics), herbal medicine, megavitamin therapy, and energy healing. The four conditions for which unconventional therapies were most frequently sought were back pain, anxiety, headaches, and chronic pain.

Most users of unconventional therapies—83 percent—also sought treatment for the same condition from a medical doctor. Interestingly, however, 72 percent of them did not inform their medical doctor that they had done so. The projected 425 million visits to providers of unconventional therapy exceeded the number of all visits to U.S. primary care physicians—388 million! It's as though a massive second health care system is quietly operating alongside the traditional one, and use of this system is increasing. This was shown in a 1997 telephone survey that found that among respondents born before 1945 ("pre-baby boomers"), three out of 10 had used some type of alternative therapy by age 33. Among baby boomers, born between 1945 and 1964, the figure was five out of 10, and among those born between 1965 and 1979 ("post-baby boomers"), a full seven out of 10 had used some alternative modality.[2] Complementary and alternative therapy is obviously increasing in popularity.

This chapter will examine the role of alternative treatments and nutritional supplements in managing chronic pain. Several of these treatments have not been extensively studied, but wherever evidence-based information is available, it will be described here. The treatments covered in this chapter are:

- massage.
- spinal manipulation.
- acupuncture.
- magnets.
- yoga.
- tai chi.
- prayer.
- diet and nutrition.
- nutritional supplements and herbal medicines.

## *Massage Therapy*

Massage therapy is probably the most popular hands-on treatment for the aching body. Four benefits of massage are:

1. Pain relief. Massage not only feels good, but it also may activate the body's pain inhibitory system, increasing the production of endorphins (the body's own opioids), and the neurotransmitters serotonin and norepinephrine.
2. Reduced muscle tension. Muscles reflexively tighten around any painful area, producing spasm. Massage loosens up knotted muscles.

3. Increased circulation. Massage can lessen swelling by pushing excess fluid into the circulatory system.
4. Improved joint mobility. By alleviating pain, massage can improve a joint's ability to move.

There is actually a whole range of massage techniques. The following descriptions were obtained from the Web site of the American Massage Therapy Association, www.amtamassage.org. You can visit their Web site to learn more about each of the following techniques.

- **Cranio-sacral massage** is a technique for finding and correcting cerebral and spinal imbalances or blockages that may cause sensory, motor, or intellectual dysfunction.
- **Deep tissue massage** releases the chronic patterns of tension in the body through slow strokes and deep finger pressure on the contracted areas, either following or going across the grain of muscles, tendons, and fascia. It is called deep tissue because it also focuses on the deeper layers of muscle tissue.
- **Swedish massage** is a system of long strokes, kneading, and friction techniques on the more superficial layers of the muscles, combined with active and passive movements of the joints.
- **Effleurage** is a stroke generally used in a Swedish massage treatment. This smooth, gliding stroke is used to relax soft tissue and is applied using both hands.
- **Petrissage** (also called **kneading**) involves squeezing, rolling, and kneading the muscles and usually follows *effleurage* during Swedish massage.
- **Friction** is the deepest of Swedish massage strokes. This stroke encompasses deep, circular movements applied to soft tissue, causing the underlying layers of tissue to rub against one another. The result causes an increase in blood flow to the massaged area.
- **Myofascial release** is a form of bodywork that is manipulative in nature and seeks to rebalance the body by releasing tension in the fascia. Long, stretching strokes are utilized to release muscular tension.
- **On-site massage** (also known as chair massage or corporate massage) is administered while the client is clothed and seated

in a specially designed chair. These chairs most often slope forward, allowing access to the large muscles of the back. On-site massage usually lasts between 15 and 30 minutes and is intended to relax and improve circulation.

- **Reflexology** is massage based around a system of points in the hands and feet thought to correspond, or "reflex," to all areas of the body.
- **Rosen method** utilizes gentle touch and verbal communication to help clients to release suppressed emotions and, subsequently, muscular tension in some instances.
- **Shiatsu and acupressure** are Asian-based systems of finger-pressure that treat special points along acupuncture "meridians" (the invisible channels of energy flow in the body).
- **Sports massage** is massage therapy focusing on muscle systems relevant to a particular sport.
- **Tapotement** is executed with cupped hands, fingers, or the edge of the hand with short, alternating taps to the client.
- **Trigger point therapy** (also known as myotherapy or neuro-muscular therapy) applies concentrated finger pressure to "trigger points" (painful, irritated areas in muscles) to break cycles of spasm and pain.

## The Efficacy of Massage Therapies

In one study, fibromyalgia patients who had a 30-minute massage twice a week for 5 weeks had significantly reduced amounts of pain and fatigue, less depression and anxiety, and improved sleep compared with patients who did not get massage.[3] A follow-up study confirmed that massage produced improved sleep.[4]

In a study of chronic tension-headache sufferers, repeated massage therapy sessions involving the neck and shoulder muscles significantly decreased the frequency of headaches by the end of the first week of treatment. Once a headache was present, however, its intensity was not ameliorated by the massage. In this study, massage therapy helped prevent but not treat tension headaches.[5]

A recent review of the evidence for the effectiveness, safety, and cost of acupuncture, massage therapy, and spinal manipulation for back pain found no apparent benefit of acupuncture. Massage, however, reduced pain more significantly than did acupuncture or muscle relaxation. Spinal manipulation was better than no therapy, but was no better than conventional therapies.[6] Alternative therapies are, at best, only modestly effective, according to Dr. Richard Saitz, who reviewed the study for *Journal Watch.*[7]

## *Spinal Manipulation*

Spinal manipulation is a widely used technique for treating low back pain. It consists of quick thrusts to bring a joint to its limit of motion. The rapid movement produces a popping sound. Two different types of specialists—chiropractors and osteopaths—perform spinal manipulation. Doctors of osteopathy (osteopaths, or D.O.s) are fully licensed physicians whose training is similar to that of medical doctors (M.D.s), with the addition of training in manual (hands-on) treatment of musculoskeletal disorders. After going to osteopathy schools, many get specialty training in the same programs as graduates of medical school and become fully trained cardiologists, oncologists, surgeons, and other specialists. Most osteopaths remain in primary care, where they provide a full range of medical care along with their skills in spinal manipulation and other hands-on techniques.

Chiropractors have a narrower focus, and are not licensed to prescribe medications or perform medical or surgical procedures. Their philosophy also differs from that of M.D.s and D.O.s. Chiropractors believe that the spine is the key to most aspects of health: When the vertebrae of the spine become misaligned (chiropractors call this "subluxated") through trauma or repetitive injury, the range of motion becomes limited and spinal nerves emerging from the spinal cord are compromised. Interruption of nerve flow can eventually lead to pain, disability, and an overall decrease in the quality of life. They believe that the removal of that interference has significant, lasting health benefits. Through the adjustment of the subluxation, the chiropractor tries to restore normal nerve expression, which leads to restored health. Some chiropractors believe that adjusting the spine can relieve many kinds of medical problems, and they attempt to treat diseases that they are not qualified to treat. This minority of chiropractors has created a mixed reputation for chiropractic in the United States, as well as some distrust by medical doctors.

The best use for spinal manipulation is for back pain and stiffness. Many patients have benefited by it and attest to its efficacy. Spinal manipulation for musculoskeletal problems is exceedingly popular. Many insurance companies now pay for chiropractic care and many patients welcome its benefits. Compared with sham treatment, spinal manipulation can significantly reduce chronic low back pain. Most studies investigating the effectiveness of spinal manipulation for chronic low back pain have reported short-term improvement in pain and/or disability. Spinal manipulation should be avoided, however, if you have a fracture, osteoporosis (bone thinness), rheumatoid arthritis, or any neck instability.

## What Does the Evidence Show About Spinal Manipulation?

In a recent meta-analysis of the results of 26 randomized controlled trials of spinal manipulation for acute and chronic back pain, the investigators reported that spinal manipulation was superior to sham therapies and to traction, bed rest, topical gel, or diathermy, but it was not superior to effective conventional treatments with analgesics and physical therapy.[8] In other words, the results of chiropractic spinal manipulation are similar to treatment with physical therapy and pain meds.

Yet another systematic review of chiropractic and massage therapy for reducing any type of pain found some "promising evidence." But convincing evidence was lacking that either chiropractic or massage are effective in reducing musculoskeletal or other pain.[9] Another group of researchers randomly assigned 321 adults who had low back pain for at least a week to the McKenzie method of physical therapy, chiropractic manipulation, or a minimal intervention consisting of provision of an educational booklet about back pain. The first two groups of patients received a maximum of nine treatments. Physical therapy and spinal manipulation were both significantly better than the booklet group in terms of pain relief and patient satisfaction. At 1 year, the booklet group was functioning somewhat less well than the other two groups. The costs of physical therapy and chiropractic were similar.[10] This study shows that chiropractic manipulation is as effective as physical therapy for low back pain. Spinal manipulation of the neck is also helpful for some patients with neck pain, but safety concerns are greater than when the low back is manipulated.

Similar conclusions about spinal manipulation for low back pain—but this time by osteopaths—was reached by researchers who compared osteopathic spinal manipulation with standard care for patients with "subacute" low back pain.[11] These patients had experienced back pain for at least 3 weeks but less than 6 months. The standard care consisted of combinations of analgesics, anti-inflammatory drugs, various types of physical therapy, and use of transcutaneous electrical nerve stimulation (TENS). After 12 weeks of treatment, patients in both groups improved, and there was no significant difference between the groups regarding pain relief or improvement of functioning. The only difference was that the spinal manipulation group used fewer medications. A weakness of the study design was that there was no control group, so it was not possible to learn how either treatment compared with no active treatment.

What can we conclude from these various studies? The natural course of acute back pain is to eventually improve no matter what treatment is applied. Both standard treatment and spinal manipulation can provide more rapid improvement, and they do it equally well. It is likely that for chronic back pain, both types of treatment are equally effective, but ongoing back pain has not been subjected to the same rigorous studies as acute back pain.

## Magnets

Each year, Americans spend about $500 million on magnets, which some believe alleviate various sources of pain. The magnets are applied to the skin in an attempt to decrease fibromyalgia, headaches, back pain, neck and shoulder pain, knee arthritis, and foot pain. Very few well-designed studies have looked at the efficacy of magnets. One of the best is a recent study in patients who had heel pain due to plantar fasciitis. They had been experiencing the typical symptoms of knifelike pain in the back of the sole, typically worse on first arising from bed. Half of a group of 101 patients were given magnetic insoles, while the remainder had similar insoles that were not magnetized. The strength of the magnets was typical of commercially available therapeutic magnets. After 8 weeks of wearing the insoles, there were no differences between the groups in the amount of pain experienced. Magnetic insoles are no more effective than regular insoles in alleviating heel pain.[12] It's probably better to focus on other ways of getting pain relief rather than magnets.

## Yoga

Yoga is an ancient Indian practice combining stretching, breathing exercises, maintaining certain postures, and meditation. Yoga therapy aims at a holistic treatment of various physical and psychological ailments, such as back problems and emotional distress. In explaining the importance to healing of an approach that includes both mental and physical involvement, Amy Weintraub, author of the 2004 book *Yoga for Depression* quotes a psychologist who treats abuse survivors: "A body-oriented treatment model speaks the language of these areas of the brain—sensation, perceptual experience, and somatic responses. Cognitive restructuring [thinking differently] is, of course, important, but the healing process must also include bodily experience."[13] Weintraub continues, "A daily yoga practice will bring your physical body and your emotional body into balance, restoring a sense of well being and energy. You will feel more energy, love yourself more, and have a happier life." The goal of yoga in the West, according to Weintraub, is to maintain emotional and physical well-being. Yoga can help diminish obsessive negative thinking, a problem that many chronic pain patients have. It can also improve depression, another common disorder found in chronic pain patients. And certainly the stretches can alleviate muscle tightness.

Regarding the safety and value of yoga specifically for people with chronic pain, Amy Weintraub writes:

> Chronic pain often goes hand in hand with depression. Those who are depressed often experience shallow, upper-chest breathing. Yoga postures and yogic breathing, called pranayama, reverse this trend. In contrast to other forms of physical exercise, in yoga, the breath is an essential part of the practice. There are breathing exercises that specifically lift the mood and energize the entire system. There are other breathing exercises that calm the central nervous system.
>
> If you are suffering from osteoarthritis of the knee or hip, be

sure that the class you are entering is a gentle beginner's class and speak to the instructor before the class. Ask her for help with props or modifications—ways to support yourself in poses that may put stress on the knee or the hip joint. You might even wish to work privately with a certified yoga teacher for a few sessions, so that you can learn ways to protect the vulnerable areas of your body when you're in a larger class. There are no specific limitations, only guidelines for practice.

1.  Always practice gentle warm-ups for the joints and the muscles, using long diaphragmatic breathing through the nostrils.

2.  Begin with yogic breathing exercises in order to expand lung capacity and increase oxygen availability.

3.  Keep your attention focused on the areas of strong sensation in your body. If there is discomfort, back off somewhat. The breath can be a great help in this. If you are consciously breathing deeply, you can be more in tune with your body's signals.

The first lesson in yoga is to pay attention to your body's signals. Yoga is not a competitive sport. In yoga practice, you are forming a healthier, more compassionate relationship with your body, not "going for the gold." As you pay attention to the breath and the sensations in your body, you begin to develop what the ancient yogis called "the seer" or witness consciousness. You cultivate an ability to be both present in the moment of sensation and to also rise above it, observing with compassion and without judgment. This developing sense of witness consciousness helps you to acknowledge the pain, be it physical or emotional, yet not succumb to it and not obsess about it. Physically, when you practice yoga, the stretch receptors send messages of relaxation to your brain. The level of cortisol, the stress hormone, drops, while the amount of prolactin and oxcytocin, the "feel-good" hormones, increases. Doing so not only can increase your ability to cope with your chronic pain, but actually help reduce it. Mentally, when you practice yoga with attention to the breath and the sensations in your body, you are developing the two pillars of yogic practice:

equanimity and self-awareness, which can help you develop a healthier relationship to your body and its limitations.

The focus on the breath and the cultivation of equanimity and self-awareness as your own inner witness grows stronger are two ways in which yoga differs from other forms of physical exercise or martial arts. The third way that yoga is different from an exercise like tai chi is that the postures work on a principle of contraction and release. As you release from a posture you have held, the areas of chronic tension in your body relax. Dr. Bessel van der Kolk believes that working with the physical state is essential in trauma recovery: "You have to work with core physiological states and then the mind will start changing." In yoga practice, as we contract and release, with attention to the breath and the sensations in the body, the physical and emotional blocks dissolve, allowing energy to move more freely through the areas of chronic pain.[14]

According to such leaders in the field of trauma recovery as Bessel van der Kolk, M.D., long-held emotions can be stored in the body as chronic tension, numbness, and pain. Many chronic pain patients have been victims of trauma. One of my patients, for example, was in an elevator when the cable broke. The elevator box fell several stories until it crashed at the bottom. The only occupant, he suffered multiple injuries to his spine. Ten years later, he was still experiencing not only chronic back pain, but psychological aftereffects.

Dr. van der Kolk, also a world-renowned expert on posttraumatic stress disorder (PTSD), is Professor of Psychiatry at Boston University Medical School, Medical Director of the Trauma Center at HRI Hospital in Brookline, Massachusetts, and coeditor with Alexander McFarlane and Lars Weisaeth of *Traumatic Stress: The Effects of Overwhelming Experience on Mind, Body, and Society* (1996). Dr. van der Kolk believes that talk therapy alone doesn't heal trauma survivors who have PTSD. Such patients dissociate themselves from the trauma experience. But when they are asked to recall the experience, they overreact, responding with hyperventilating, muscle tensing, heart pounding, crying, physical agitation, or collapse. Their entire bodies responded as if they were experiencing the trauma again. They are unable to access their trauma without becoming so physically involved that they felt re-traumatized.

No wonder they tend to remove themselves from the memories as much as possible! Dr. van der Kolk came to believe that PTSD patients needed to find some way to access their trauma, while at the same time staying physiologically quiet enough to tolerate it, so that they didn't shut down in treatment. He now recommends body therapies as the way to accomplish this.

In a recent psychiatric paper he wrote, in agreement with Ms. Weintraub:

> There are three critical steps in treating PTSD: safety, management of anxiety, and emotional processing . . . . Practical anxiety management skills may include training in deep muscle relaxation, control of breathing, and yoga . . . . The effective treatment of PTSD must involve promoting awareness rather than avoidance of internal somatic [body] states . . . . Mindfulness, awareness of one's inner experience, is necessary for a person to respond according to what is happening and is needed in the present, rather than reacting to certain somatic sensations as a return of the traumatic past.[15]

In published research studies on yoga, it is often used in combination with other alternative techniques, such as mindfulness meditation. For this reason, it is difficult to find rigorous research outcomes in which yoga was the only intervention. However, many studies in which yoga was a part of the intervention have shown how helpful it can be.

## Tai Chi

When I visited Beijing, China, a dozen years ago, as I looked out the hotel window every morning I'd see a large group of people, mostly elderly, standing in a field moving their arms and legs slowly in unison, assuming various positions repeatedly for more than an hour. They were doing tai chi, the ancient Chinese Taoist martial art that has been called "meditation in motion." That's because tai chi combines movement, holding postures, and meditation. Unlike more active aerobic exercises such as brisk walking, cycling, or swimming, tai chi is more passive, emphasizing inner strength rather than building muscles. Introduced to the United States in the 1960s, tai chi is believed to enhance balance, flexibility, posture, gait, and overall physical and mental well-being. In a recent controlled study of the efficacy of tai chi in improving the symptoms of rheumatoid arthritis, 10 patients participated in a 60-minute tai chi class twice a week for 12 weeks, while 10 others did stretching exercises. At the end of 12 weeks, half the tai chi group and none of the control group had significant improvement in their symptoms.[16] This was a small pilot study, but the results are promising.

## Acupuncture

Acupuncture, which originated in China some 2,000 years ago, is increasingly popular as an alternative treatment for pain, anxiety, weight control, and various addictions such as smoking and drugs. In acupuncture, very fine, solid needles are pushed through the skin into specific sites. These sites were mapped by Chinese practitioners long ago. Although most acupuncture consists of needling alone, in some cases, electric current is also sent through the needle, and in others, herbs are burned in a container attached to the outer end of the needle (moxibustion). Treatments involve one to 20 needles, last 20 to 30 minutes, and usually require several sessions to obtain pain relief. It is worth noting that the FDA regulates acupuncture needles as medical devices, the same as with hypodermic needles and surgical scalpels.

Traditional acupuncture is based on the concept that the continuous flow of *qi* (life energy) and *xue* (blood) is vital to health. *Qi* flows through distinct meridians or pathways that cover the body somewhat like the nerves do. Acupuncture is believed to allow *qi* to flow to areas where it is deficient and away from where it is present in excess. Acupuncture may correct imbalances of flow by stimulating specific anatomic points close to the skin.

Modern Western medicine is uncertain how acupuncture works. Reported success when using acupuncture in animals suggests that its mechanism of action is something other than placebo. There is considerable evidence that acupuncture releases opioid peptides whose actions at least partly explain its analgesic effect.[17] This is supported by the fact that the opioid-antagonist naloxone reverses the analgesic effects of acupuncture. This has been shown both in humans[18,19] and in monkeys.[20] Acupuncture has also been shown to increase the level of endogenous beta-endorphins in spinal fluid.[21]

There is positive evidence that acupuncture is effective in treating dental pain, and there is some evidence of its success in menstrual cramps, fibromyalgia, and tennis elbow. In treating myofascial pain, acupuncture appears to be as effective as anti-inflammatory drugs, with fewer side effects.[22] The National Institutes of Health (NIH) Consensus Panel concluded that acupuncture is of value for postoperative and chemotherapy nausea and vomiting and for postoperative dental pain. In a typical study, the effect of ear acupuncture on post-operative vomiting was tested in 100 women undergoing hysterectomies.[23] The patients treated with acupuncture had significantly less vomiting 12 hours after surgery.

In another study, researchers compared acupuncture to sham acupuncture in 35 people undergoing shoulder surgery.[24] They were studied for 4 months after the operation. Compared to the patients undergoing sham acupuncture, those who had real acupuncture had significantly reduced amounts of pain, used fewer pain pills, had better movement of the shoulder, and were more satisfied.

Acupuncture may be beneficial for musculoskeletal conditions such as fibromyalgia, myofascial pain, tennis elbow, and epicondylitis. The NIH Consensus Statement states that there is evidence that acupuncture is not effective for smoking cessation, however.

In a recent report, 40 patients with myofascial and trigger point pain were divided into three groups: One group was treated with acupuncture followed by active stretching exercises, one group did only the exercises, and the third group did not get either treatment. Acupuncture plus stretching was more effective than stretching alone in reducing the sensitivity of the trigger points to pressure, and more effective than no treatment in decreasing pain.[25] Another study involved two groups of cancer patients, one of whom received two courses of ear acupuncture at established points, while the other got ear acupuncture at other sites (placebo group). The treated group had significant relief of their cancer pain, whereas the placebo group did not.[26]

Following arthroscopic surgery on their shoulders, 40 patients received either real or sham acupuncture. The real acupuncture group had significantly decreased levels of pain, used fewer analgesics, had greater range of motion of the shoulder, and more patient satisfaction.[27]

Acupuncture was studied in a group of patients older than 60 years who had chronic low back pain.[28] Half received back exercises, anti-inflammatory drugs, and muscle relaxants. The other half had acupuncture with electrical stimulation for 5 weeks. The acupuncture group had greater improvement in their functioning and fewer medication-related side effects compared with the control group. The investigators concluded that acupuncture is an effective, safe adjunctive treatment for chronic low back pain in older patients.

A recent British Study supported the value of acupuncture in treating chronic headaches. Four hundred such patients (primarily with migraines) were randomized to receive either up to 12 acupuncture treatments over 3 months or their usual care. The acupuncture group experienced fewer days of headache equivalent to an average of 22 days per year. They also used significantly less medication, made significantly fewer visits to their doctor, and took significantly fewer days off work.[29]

## *Prayer*

Prayer is a common practice in the United States. A 1998 survey of over 2,000 people found that 33 percent used prayer for health concerns; 75 percent of this group prayed for good health in general, and 22 percent prayed for healing from specific medication conditions. Among those whose prayers concerned specific medical problems, two-thirds (69 percent) found prayer to be very helpful. People who prayed tended to be older, female, and better educated. The most common conditions they prayed about were depression, chronic headaches, back and/or neck pain, digestive problems, or allergies.[30] Clearly, prayer is a source of comfort to most people who use it.

What do randomized controlled trials say about prayer? First, you should be aware that some people believe it is not possible to do such studies because prayer involves a belief system different from medicine. In an attempt to avoid the subjective aspects of prayer (such as that a person who prays is likely to believe that the prayer helped, a supposition that is confirmed in the study mentioned above), several researches studied the effects of intercessory prayer. This is prayer by one person on behalf of another. A study published in 1999 randomly divided very ill patients who were admitted to a cardiac intensive care unit into two groups. The names of one group were sent to people who then prayed for them over a period of several weeks; the other group did not get prayers. The patients themselves did not know whether or not they received intercessory prayers. The results showed significantly better healing in the prayer group.[31] A similar protocol was subsequently used by researchers at the Mayo Clinic. In direct contrast to the earlier study, the Mayo study, published in 2001, found no evidence that prayer affected the health of the study subjects.[32]

What conclusion should we draw from these studies? Clearly, randomized controlled trials about the effect of prayer have given mixed results. From a perspective focused strictly on the body, it is hard to accept that prayer might aid the healing of someone who is not even aware of being prayed over. Yet, as you will see in the next chapter, "Engaging the Mind," there is increasing acceptance of the connection between the mind and the body. Many people believe in the power of prayer, for themselves and others. Healing the mind can certainly help heal the body. Prayer has no down side, and should be encouraged for those who believe in its efficacy.

## Diet and Nutrition

Did you see the 1998 film "Pleasantville," which was about two teenagers who find themselves living in a 1950s sitcom? In one scene, the traditional devoted mom served breakfast to the family and urged them to eat heartily. As the camera panned across the table laden with large plates of bacon, sausage, scrambled eggs, steak, fried potatoes, and butter-slathered toast, most people in the audience laughed. Why? Because we were groaning at all the fat and cholesterol that the family was consuming, a diet that was considered healthy in the 1950s. By 1998, the American public was obsessed with efforts to minimize the fat and cholesterol in our diets. Products advertised in large print that they contained no cholesterol or were low-fat. A high-carb, low-fat diet was considered desirable. But the pendulum is again swinging the other way: Many now consider carbohydrates to be the enemy. One man, the late Robert C. Atkins, M.D., is responsible for this revolution. Many physicians swear by the high-fat, low-carb Atkins diet as an effective way to lose weight and lower cholesterol. Currently, products are being touted as being low-carb. Even extremely unlikely products are available, such as low-carb bread and low-carb tortillas. One can only wonder at the ingredients that have replaced the carbohydrate in these products.

The low-fat versus low-carb controversy is still alive and well among health professionals. No wonder consumers are confused! The guidelines and Food Guide Pyramid recommended by the by U.S. Department of Agriculture (USDA) and supported by the Department of Health and Human Services (HHS) still emphasizes a low-fat diet based on the carbohydrates bread, cereal, rice, and pasta.[33] The guidelines and pyramid are designed to help people make healthy food choices and maintain a healthy weight. These guidelines state:

- Eat a variety of foods to get the energy, protein, vitamins, minerals, and fiber you need for good health.
- Balance the food you eat with physical activity. Maintain or improve your weight to reduce your chances of having high blood pressure, heart disease, stroke, certain cancers, and type 2 diabetes, the most common kind.
- Choose a diet with plenty of grain products, vegetables, and fruits, which provide needed vitamins, minerals, fiber, and complex carbohydrates, and can help you lower your intake of fat.
- Choose a diet low in fat, saturated fat, and cholesterol to reduce your risk of heart attack and some cancers and to help you maintain a healthy weight.
- Choose a diet moderate in sugars. A diet with lots of sugars has too many calories and too few nutrients and can contribute to tooth decay.
- Choose a diet moderate in salt and sodium to help reduce your risk of high blood pressure.
- If you drink alcoholic beverages, do so in moderation. Alcoholic beverages supply calories, but little or no nutrients. Drinking alcohol is the cause of many health problems and accidents and can lead to addiction.

The Food Guide Pyramid is a triangle divided into six parts. Each part represents one of five food groups, topped by a small triangle representing fats, oils, and sweets, which should be consumed sparingly. The area of each of the sections reflects the desired proportion of that food group in the diet. Naturally, carbohydrates are at the base, with the largest area. The five food groups and desirable portions are:

- breads: five to 11 daily servings.
- vegetables: three to five servings.
- fruits: two to four servings.
- proteins: two to three servings of meat, poultry, fish, dried beans, eggs, and nuts.
- dairy products: two to three servings of milk, yogurt, cheese, and so forth.

To get all the nutrients you need, it's important to eat foods from each group daily. The number of portions depends on how many calories you need daily, which depends on your level of activity, size, age, and sex. Sedentary women and some older adults may need only 1,600 calories, whereas teenage boys, active men, and very active women may need up to 2,800 calories per day. For most children, teenage girls, active women, and sedentary men, 2,200 calories is about right. If you need to lose weight, it might help you to know that in order to lose 1 pound, you need to reduce your calorie intake by 3,500 calories. This means that you need to eat 500 fewer calories per day than your previous intake in order to lose 1 pound per week, or 1,000 fewer calories per day to lose 2 pounds per week.

A caveat: In recent years, portion sizes in restaurants and in prepared foods have swelled. A dinner plate served in many restaurants often actually constitutes enough for two servings. Size inflation is particularly common in fast-food places. For example, one serving of meat, according to the USDA, is 3 ounces, yet a restaurant steak usually comes in 6, 8, or even 12 ounces!

## Food and Diet Recommendations for People with Chronic Pain

People with chronic pain should follow the same guidelines described above. There is no special diet that will take away the pain. Diets touted in the past for various disorders, such as arthritis, are not effective for either preventing or curing them. There are only a few specific dietary recommendations for people with some type of chronic pain.

First and foremost is the matter of weight. Obesity is a risk factor for several common diseases including diabetes, hypertension, and elevated cholesterol. It also contributes to some types of chronic pain conditions. Carrying around excess weight increases the stress on your weight-bearing joints such as the knees and hips, and makes them work harder. The added stress can accelerate the development of osteoarthritis and can increase your pain level. Being overweight can also trap you in a vicious circle: The weight makes it more painful for you to exercise, but exercise is needed to strengthen your muscles and thereby reduce the pain in the back, knees, and hips. The "solution" for too many people is to avoid physical activity, but in the long run this is no solution at all.

The real solution is to lose weight. Unfortunately, although most people know what they need to do in order to lose weight, it's hard to put those steps into action. What makes it easier is to get the support of other people. Such commercial programs as WeightWatchers don't have any magic diets. What they do provide, in addition to a typical healthy eating plan, is group support and accountability. The WeightWatchers program, for example, includes a weekly weigh-in, discussion by a leader about the challenges of weight loss and how to overcome them, and applause for those who succeed. Interestingly, these elements are also found in all the self-help programs based on Alcoholics Anonymous, programs that are very successful in helping people overcome various addictions. Accountability and group support are elements that can make the difference between success and failure in dealing with any compulsive behavior. You don't need to pay money to get this type of help. Getting together with a group of friends or family members who need to lose weight and doing it together can be equally effective. But your group needs to make a serious commitment to accountability as well as support and encouragement. Because it's hard to lose weight without doing any exercise, your group might decide to get together a couple of times a week to walk or do whatever physical activities your chronic pain problem permits.

## Specific Diseases Affected by Diet

GOUT. There are only a few conditions in which a specific diet makes a difference. Gout, a painful inflammatory joint disease, is related to elevated levels of uric acid in the blood, which accumulate in joints. Uric acid is a product of digestion of purines, found in certain foods such as meat or fish. The body's uric acid levels can rise either because the body makes too much, or because of difficulty with the kidney's ability to excrete uric acid. The most common symptom of gout is a red, swollen, extremely painful big toe, although other joints can also be affected. Higher levels of meat and seafood consumption are associated with an increased risk of gout, whereas eating more dairy products is associated with a decreased risk. A recently published study described what happened to almost 50,000 men who didn't have gout at the beginning of the study and were followed up for 12 years. During that time, 740 of them developed gout. Those who ate red meat at least twice a week increased the risk of gout by 50 percent, andthose who ate all types of seafood had an even higher risk. Interestingly, no increased risk was seen with the consumption of purine-rich vegetables, which include peas, beans, mushrooms, cauliflower, and spinach. The study found a protective effect from vegetable and dairy proteins. Eating low-fat dairy products also strongly reduced the risk of gout.[34]

It's advisable for people who've had gout attacks to avoid foods such as red meat, poultry, anchovies, herring, and scallops. Drinking a lot of fluids in order to flush out the uric acid is very advisable.

For many years, heavy alcohol consumption was believed to bring on gout attacks. Now there is scientific evidence to support that alcohol intake strongly increases the risk of gout. The actual risk is related to the type of alcoholic drink consumed, with beer being the worst.[35] Alcohol raises the levels of uric acid in the blood, so if you have any risk of gout, it's best to consume only nonalcoholic drinks.

OSTEOPOROSIS. A common cause of back pain in women is osteoporosis, the thinning of the bones that occurs with age. Men lose bone mineral more slowly, so fewer of them are affected by osteoporosis. Bone loss per se doesn't cause pain, but the weakened bone is susceptible to fractures—most commonly, vertebral fractures—that compress the spinal column, shorten height, and cause pain. In addition to any prescription medications you may be taking to prevent or treat osteoporosis, it's crucial to have enough calcium in your diet. Calcium in young people builds up bones, and in older people it slows down bone loss.

Postmenopausal women need a total of 1,500 mg of calcium per day. If you still have menstrul periods, if you are are an older woman on estrogen, or if you are a man, you will need 1,000 mg of calcium per day. Calculate how many milligrams per day you are getting from your diet; each portion of daily products gives you approximately 250 mg. Take a calcium supplement to make up the balance. Additionally, vitamin D is needed to absorb calcium. If you purchase a calcium supplement, make sure that it contains vitamin D as well.

Another important component of osteoporosis prevention is weight-bearing exercise, such as walking. You may have heard that in the early days of space travel, astronauts who spent several days in the absence of gravity returned to Earth with muscles so weak they could hardly walk. Those who were in space longer developed significant bone loss by the time they returned. These days, astronauts in space are prescribed aerobic exercises specifically designed to maintain muscle and bone mass.

INSOMNIA. People with chronic pain often have difficulty falling asleep. Tryptophan, an amino acid found in certain foods, can help you get to sleep. A bedtime snack of milk and turkey might just solve your insomnia problem. Tryptophan supplements are available, but the U.S. government has an "import alert" on their importation into the United States. In 1989, tryptophan supplements from Japan caused an epidemic of a very serious illness, eosinophilia-myalgia syndrome. The cause was originally thought to be a contaminant in one Japanese company's product, but there is still not 100 percent certainty about the cause, which is why purchasing imported tryptophan supplements may not be a good idea. The best way of ingesting tryptophan is still through foods.

CONSTIPATION. If you are taking an opioid medication for pain relief, you probably are aware that opioids produce constipation. They do this by slowing down the transit of food products through the digestive tract. Your doctor will undoubtedly recommend to you that you take a stool softener and drink plenty of liquids. In addition, you may need to counteract this slowing effect of the opioids by taking a laxative that stimulates the bowel.

Whether or not opioids are part of your medication regimen, a high-fiber diet is recommended for chronic pain sufferers. Fresh fruits and vegetables, whole-bran cereal or muffins, brown rice, and garbanzo beans are some foods high in fiber. If your current diet is low in fiber, increase it gradually—a rapid fiber increase may result in gas, cramping, bloating, or diarrhea. Your goal should be to consume at least 25 grams of fiber per day. Nutrition labels list the number of grams of dietary fiber contained in the food. Another effective daily addition to your dietary fiber is psyllium seed, found in the over-the-counter powder Metamucil. You need to drink plenty of water with psyllium. When it is stirred into juice, you should drink it right away, or else it turns into a thick gelatinous mess that is impossible to swallow.

## What About Vitamins and Minerals?

Vitamins and minerals are chemicals the body needs to function properly but cannot produce on its own. Lack of these substances can produce serious or even fatal illnesses. For example, in the sixteenth century, when maritime explorers began making lengthy trips across the oceans, a new disease, scurvy, began causing major casualties among the sailors. In 1520 while crossing the Pacific, the explorer Magellan lost more than 80 percent of his men to scurvy. The British public became aware of the disease in the 1740s after Commodore George Anson led a squadron to the Pacific to raid Spanish shipping and lost 1,300 of his 2,000 sailors to disease, mostly to scurvy. A few years later, in 1757, James Lind published *A Treatise of the Scurvy*, providing experimental proof that citrus had a rapid beneficial effect.

It's now well-known that scurvy is caused by deficiency of vitamin C, or ascorbic acid, which is found in citrus fruits. Including lemons in sailors' diets at sea abolished seafaring scurvy. Scurvy is seen now only in severely malnourished people, primarily the elderly. Vitamin C is required for the production of collagen. When the support that collagen provides to small blood vessels is inadequate, the result is bleeding in the gums, around the nails, and in the skin and muscles, general weakness, and poor tissue healing. The bleeding can result in severe anemia. Wounds don't heal, and scars from previous surgery may dehisce (open up).

Most vitamins were discovered many years ago in an effort to understand unknown diseases. For example:

- lack of vitamin A causes visual problems.
- lack of vitamin B1 (thiamine) causes a type of dementia.
- lack of vitamin B3 (niacin) causes pellagra, a disease characterized by dermatitis (severe rash), diarrhea, and dementia.
- lack of vitamin B12 causes a type of anemia.
- lack of vitamin D causes rickets (soft bones).
- lack of vitamin K causes bleeding.

The Food and Nutrition Board of the National Academy of Sciences publishes and updates the Recommended Dietary Allowances of vitamins, which is a list of the recommended minimum daily require-ments. If your diet is healthy, most people don't need to take vitamin supplements. However, on the theory that if some is good, more is better, many people take vitamin and mineral supplements. Large doses of some of these are fairly well-tolerated, but others can be toxic. In particular, fat-soluble vitamins such as A and E are stored in the body if taken in excessive doses, and can be dangerous. In contrast, excess doses of water-soluble vitamins, such as B and C, are excreted, and therefore are less toxic. It's especially important not to exceed recommended doses of the fat-soluble vitamins. Years ago, Nobel Prize winner Dr. Linus Pauling concluded that megadoses of vitamin C can prevent colds and other infections, promote wound healing after surgery, and prevent and treat cancer. These conclusions have not been validated in controlled clinical trials.

There's a great deal of ongoing research about whether particular vitamin supplements are of benefit in any diseases. Recently, much research has been focused on antioxidants. Oxidation is a metabolic process in the body that can damage tissues by modifying the structure of lipids, proteins, and nucleic acids (RNA and DNA), leading to diseases such as cancer and atherosclerosis (narrowing of blood vessels in the heart and other body parts). Four vitamins, A, C, E, and beta carotene (a form of vitamin A) are antioxidants (they prevent some oxidation). Some observational studies suggest that taking antioxidant supplements can decrease the risk of heart disease. This was not confirmed in either a recent meta-analysis of seven randomized trials (those with the best scientific validity) of vitamin E treatment or in eight different trials of beta carotene plus vitamin E.[36] Unfortunately, neither regimen showed any benefit to patients with heart disease. Additionally, a trial of vitamin A showed increased incidence of lung cancer and increased deaths in patients treated with vitamin A. Yet another trial—of beta carotene—showed more deaths in the group treated with beta carotene. High intakes of vitamin C can also lead to bloating and diarrhea.

## *Nutritional Supplements and Herbal Medicines*

Interest in nutritional supplements and herbal medicines is natural. After all, long before the pharmaceutical industry existed, people had discovered through trial and error that certain botanicals were helpful for particular ailments. These included cinchona bark for fever, purple foxglove for dropsy (severe swelling due to fluid retention), and opium poppy for pain and diarrhea. Eventually, the active ingredients of these plants were isolated: quinine for malaria, digitalis for congestive heart failure, and opium for pain. Other conventional medications derived from plants include atropine (for allergy symptoms), taxol and vincristine (anticancer drugs), ipecac (to induce vomiting), senna (a bowel stimulant), capsaicin (a pain reliever), and reserpine (an antihypertensive). So it makes sense that some plants can be effective treatments for certain medical conditions.

Many people use herbal supplements, and some can be very effective. Glucosamine and chondroitin sulfate are becoming increasingly accepted for use in osteoarthritis pain. Ginger can relieve nausea, feverfew helps headaches. Echinacea is widely used for colds.

The problem is that most dietary supplements haven't been as thoroughly researched as have conventional drugs. Of the studies that have been done, most compare the herbal remedy with placebo (no effective treatment), not with a prescription drug, so that even if some efficacy is reported, we still don't know how it compares with conventional treatments. Of the thousands of herbal medications available, only a small percentage has undergone the critical test of randomized controlled trials. To try to remedy this situation, the National Center for Complementary and Alternative Medicine (NCCAM) was established in 1998 as part of the National Institutes of Health, with the mission of sponsoring scientific research in complementary and alternative medicine (CAM). Unfortunately, its small budget has limited its ability to fund many projects, although some are now in progress.

The Natural Standard Research Collaboration, a group based at Massachusetts General Hospital, reviews the safety and efficacy of herbal medicines based on high-quality scientific studies. They also disseminate information on the interactions between drugs and herbs. Their results can be accessed online at www.naturalstandard.com. The group grades each herbal remedy from A to D with A meaning definitive evidence of benefit; B meaning high-quality evidence of some, but not definitive, benefit; C meaning less-than-rigorous studies have shown benefit, conflicting evidence of benefit, or evidence of benefit only from animal lab studies; or D meaning no benefit.

Some recent ratings[37] are:

- **Black cohosh**: *B* for hot flashes; *C* for joint pain.
- **Evening primrose oil**: *B* for relieving atopic dermatitis; *C* or *D* for Raynaud's disease and other conditions for which it is touted.
- **Saw palmetto**: *A* for benign prostatic hypertrophy.
- **Valerian**: *B* for insomnia; *C* for anxiety; *D* for sedation; avoid if you have liver disease.
- **St. John's Wort**: *B* or *C* for severe depression; *A* for mild to moderate depression; *C* for anxiety; interferes with oral contraceptives; avoid in thyroid disorders.
- **Echinacea**: *B* for treating colds; *C* for preventing colds.
- **Bilberry**: *C* for vascular and eye diseases; *D* for improving night vision.
- **Cranberry**: *B* for preventing bladder infection; *C* for treating it.
- **Wild Yam**: *C* for hot flashes.
- **Ginger**: *B* for nausea caused by chemotherapy or pregnancy; *C* for nausea after surgery and for motion sickness; *C* for rheumatoid arthritis, osteoarthritis, joint pains, and muscle pains.

Recently, a review article on herbal remedies was published in the prestigious *New England Journal of Medicine*. Four herbal preparations were discussed in detail—Gingko leaf, hawthorn leaf or flower, saw palmetto, and St. John's Wort. The results, which were not particularly encouraging, are summarized below.

- **Gingko**: Randomized controlled trials (RCTs) show superiority to placebo for dementia and some trials show a benefit for tinnitus (ringing in the ear). However, gingko can reduce blood clotting and should be avoided if you are on a blood thinner.

- **Hawthorn**: Placebo-controlled trials suggest improvement in heart function and symptoms in patients with mild heart failure.
- **Saw palmetto**: RCTs suggest improvement in urinary symptoms and flow measures in patients with benign prostatic hypertrophy.
- **St. John's Wort**: RCTs suggest superiority to placebo for short-term treatment of mild to moderate depression. However, St. John's Wort can reduce the efficacy of various conventional medications, and in combination with antidepressants that are serotonin-reuptake inhibitors (such as Prozac [fluoxetine], Zoloft [sertraline], or Paxil [paroxetine]), it can cause a troublesome central nervous system side effect called serotonin syndrome.

An herbal remedy not mentioned in these reviews is the medical use of marijuana for pain relief. Many people, experimenting on their own, have found that smoking marijuana relieves pain. Recently, in Canada, the Medical Marijuana Access Program allowed patients access to dried cannabis for medical purposes. A 2003 report from Canada describes the efficacy of smoked marijuana for relief of chronic noncancer pain in three patients. One had multiple sclerosis-related pain and muscle spasm, the second a work-related injury resulting in back and leg pain, and the third had HIV-related painful peripheral neuropathy.[38]

All had been on multiple pain medications including opioids, but within weeks after beginning to smoke marijuana daily, their pain was reduced significantly, and they were able to cut down their opioid dose by 60 percent to 100 percent. Additional medical studies of cannabinoids are sorely needed, but progress is slow because of the legal issues. Given that so many physicians are reluctant to prescribe potent pain medications that are legal, such as opioids, it's not recommended that you try any that are not; it is likely to make your physician less willing to prescribe controlled medications for your pain.

What can we conclude from this brief review of rigorous research on herbal remedies? That some of them are effective for some conditions in some people. If you have found herbal remedies to be useful in alleviating pain or other symptoms, there's no reason not to use them—unless they have interactions with prescription drugs you are taking or unless they risk causing damage to your body. That's why you need to tell your doctor about supplements that you are taking. A caution: Most physicians are not very knowledgeable about the risks and benefits of herbal supplements. They are usually not trained in anything except allopathic (traditional mainstream) medical care. It is both the difference in their training and in their belief system that is the cause of the gap in their knowledge.

If you are taking any herbal remedies on a regular basis, it's a good idea to check out their safety for yourself. The Web site www.naturalstandard.com is one place to look, although they do charge for access to their information. There are undoubtedly other, free Web sites as well.

## The Risks of Dietary Supplements

Do you believe that dietary supplements must be approved by a government agency before they can be sold to the public? Do you assume that dietary supplements are required to have warning labels of their dangers or side effects? Do you believe that the supplements' makers must have trial-based evidence for claims of safety for their product? You may be surprised to learn that none of these are true. Government regulations regarding dietary supplements are much more lax than those for drugs.

Before a new drug can receive approval from the FDA, its maker is required to present credible evidence that the drug is safe. In contrast, the law that regulates supplements, the 1994 Dietary Supplement Health and Education Act (DSHEA), allows supplements to be marketed *without* such evidence. Additionally, supplement manufacturers are not required to report adverse events to the FDA. Instead, the burden is on the FDA to prove conclusively that available supplements are hazardous. This usually happens only after multiple injuries or deaths occur. This is exactly what happened with the supplement ephedra. According to a *Consumer Reports* article, a leading ephedra manufacturer did not let the FDA know of thousands of complaints it had received over several years about ephedra (mu huang)—including heart attacks, strokes, and deaths. After the ephedra-related death in 2003 of 23-year-old Steve Bechler, a pitcher for the Baltimore Orioles, the government finally investigated and, in April 2004, outlawed the sale of ephedra–containing products.

Supplement makers do not need to conduct any safety testing before selling their product, and they don't have to put warnings on the label even if they know there are serious risks. The manufacturers are not required to test the purity of their products, so potentially dangerous contaminants may be present in the product without consumers' knowledge. One example of these is PC-SPES, a supplement formerly used for prostate cancer, which turned out to contain warfarin, a blood thinner, a drug with the potential to cause bleeding. (And it's the main ingredient of a type of rat poison!) PC-SPES also contained variable amounts of diethylstilbestrol, a compound with estrogenic activity, so many men taking it received hormonal treatment without knowing it, some in addition to the estrogen treatments they were getting from their cancer doctors.[39] Because of these findings, PC-SPES was withdrawn from sales in early 2002.

In May 2004, *Consumer Reports*, the highly respected magazine that reports on the efficacy and safety of all types of consumer products, had a lead story entitled "Dangerous Supplements," which should be required reading for everyone who takes nutritional supplements.[40] The article reported on current government regulations regarding supplements, and then listed 12 dangerous supplements currently available which the article termed "the dirty dozen," that should be avoided. (You should also recognize that dietary products often contain a combination of ingredients, so it's crucial that you read the label.) Most dangerous of the 12 is *aristolochic acid* (also known as *Aristolochia,* birthwort, snakeroot, snakeweed, sangree root, sangrel, serpentary, serpentaria, Asarum canadense, and wild ginger). It is a potent carcinogen that has caused cancer of the urinary tract, and has also caused kidney failure requiring a kidney transplant.

"Very likely hazardous" are *comfrey, androstenedione, chaparral, germander,* and *kava,* most of which are banned in other countries and have caused liver failure and death. *Bitter orange, organ and glandular extracts, lobelia, pennyroyal, skullcap,* and *yohimbe* are listed as "likely hazardous."

The following is a summary of the toxicities of 15 herbs and their drug-herb interactions.[41,42]

- **Aristocholic acid**: kidney failure; urinary tract cancer
- **Borage**: may increase seizure risk if used with anticonvulsants

- **Chinese herbal teas**: pulmonary hypertension (elevated pressure in lung arteries)
- **Echinacea**: liver toxicity if used more than 8 weeks; stimulates the immune system, so avoid if on immunosuppressants (for example, steroids or cyclosporine)
- **Ephedra**: hypertension, spasm of the coronary arteries, increased heart rate, death
- **Evening primrose oil**: may increase risk of seizures if used with anticonvulsants
- **Feverfew**: may alter blood coagulation
- **Garlic**: thyroid disorders; may affect blood coagulation
- **Ginseng**: estrogenic effects such as breast enlargement and vaginal bleeding; hypertension; may affect blood coagulation; may affect blood sugar levels in diabetics
- **Ginger**: may affect blood coagulation
- **Jimsonweed**: agitation; confusion; hallucinations
- **Kava**: has caused coma when used with alprazolam (Xanax)
- **Kelp**: goiter; increased or decreased thyroid hormone levels
- **Licorice**: hypertension; hypokalemia (low blood potassium levels)
- **Valerian**: excessive sedation if used with conventional sedatives

The lesson here is to know that just because an herb is natural doesn't mean it's safe. And just because an herb is safe when used in cooking (for example, garlic or ginger) doesn't mean it's just as safe when used in the much higher quantities and potencies that are in herbal preparations. To learn more about the safety of dietary supplements, visit the following three Web sites:

1. National Institutes of Health: ods.od.nih.gov/databases/ibids.html
2. Food & Drug Administration: www.fda.gov
3. Memorial Sloan-Kettering Cancer Center: www.mskcc.org/mskcc/html/11570.cfm

Another problem with herbal supplements is that the amount of the active ingredient they claim to contain is variable. For example, an analysis of several ginseng products, all of which supposedly had the same amount of active ingredient, varied by up to tenfold.[43] A more recent analysis of ginseng products showed up to thirtyfold differences in their active ingredients![44]

The law requires that dietary supplements not be promoted as preventing or treating a specific disease, and there must be a disclaimer provided on the label that states that the FDA has not evaluated the product. It is illegal to claim that the product affects the structure or function of the body. Next time you read the label of such a product, notice the vague language; it is likely to state only that the product "promotes health" or "maintains function."

A final risk of herbal supplements is that they may interact in adverse ways with conventional prescription drugs. A recent survey of U.S. adults taking prescription drugs found that one in six were also using at least one herbal product.[45] Some drug-botanical interactions that have been reported included excessive bleeding when gingko leaf was combined with use of aspirin, rofecoxib (Vioxx), or warfarin (Coumadin); additive digitalis-like effect when hawthorn was combined with digitalis; gastrointestinal toxic effects when garlic bulb was combined with the HIV drug ritonavir; and CNS toxicity when yohimbine bark was combined with tricyclic antidepressants.[46] It is clear that you should tell your doctor about any herbal product you are taking. Most are harmless, but occasionally adverse interactions with prescription drugs can occur.

# 11

# ENGAGING THE MIND

## *A Mind-Body Approach*

THE ENGLISH LANGUAGE IS FULL OF ALLUSIONS linking the body with the mind. The end of a relationship results in a broken heart or at least a heartache. A person who keeps bugging you to do something is a pain in the neck. An insult is like a kick in the butt. A fearful prospect feels like a knot in your stomach. An emotional burden can be a huge weight on your shoulders. As reported recently in the *Journal of the American Medical Association*,[1] many languages other than English also contain overlaps between emotional pain and physical harm.

New research on the brain supports a real—not just a metaphorical—connection between physical and emotional pain. Using functional magnetic resonance imaging (MRI) scans, scientists at the University of California at Los Angeles (UCLA) found that the emotional pain of being rejected by others activates two brain regions that also respond to physical pain.[2] Both physical and emotional pain activate a section of the brain called the anterior cingulate cortex (ACC), which is important for elaborating feelings of emotional distress and also generates signals that cause the person to act to stop the pain. When either physical pain or emotional hurt is experienced, a second section called the right ventral prefrontal cortex (RVPFC) is also activated, and helps dampen the distress signal sent by the ACC. It is not surprising, then, that such pain medications as opioids relieve both physical and emotional pain. It appears that psychological pain in humans, especially grief and intense loneliness, may share some of the same neural pathways that respond to physical pain.[3] Some antidepressants, too, can alleviate both depression and pain. Drugs that increase the levels of the neurotransmitters serotonin and norepinephrine, which affect the emotional state, can also relieve some types of chronic pain.

## Pain and Depression

Pain and depression frequently coexist. Some 30 to 60 percent of patients with depression also have chronic pain, and about two-thirds of patients with chronic pain conditions have major depression at some point in their lives.[4] Coexisting depression can make pain treatment less effective. In a study of elderly people with chronic pain, those who were also depressed reported much greater limitation in their physical functioning.[5] Conversely, pain can reduce the effectiveness of depression treatment.[6]

Depression is more prevalent among patients with chronic pain than even among patients with cancer pain.[7] Treating depression in older adults with arthritis improves not only their depression, but also decreases their pain and improves their quality of life and their ability to function.[8]

## Which Came First—Pain or Depression?

Based on a review of published studies of this issue, it appears that *in most cases chronic pain came first*, and that depression is increasingly likely with longer or more severe chronic pain. However, a history of depression may predispose people to developing chronic pain. Not surprisingly, the more severe the pain, the greater is the probability that it will be accompanied by depression, as was shown in a recent study of patients with rheumatoid arthritis.[9] A recent review of research on patients with depression and unexplained pain found that, on average, 65 percent of depressed patients have significant pain, and about 37 percent of pain patients have significant depression.[10] Depressed patients are more likely than nondepressed patients to report pain, and patients with pain are more likely than patients without pain to be depressed. Patients with pain are also less likely to have depression diagnosed and treated than patients without pain. Depression and pain often occur together, and each condition complicates the effective treatment of the other.

What makes pain and depression hard for the physician to sort out is that more than 50 percent of patients with depression complain only of physical symptoms, and at least 60 percent of those physical complaints are pain-related. This means that depressed patients are more likely to complain of various pains than of depressive symptoms. Patients with both pain and depression have poorer results if only one of the disorders is treated, and are more likely to have persistent pain than people without concomitant depression. Depressed patients with pain are less likely than nondepressed patients with pain to follow through with a prescribed rehabilitation program and are therefore more likely to relapse to chronic pain.[11] Pain is associated not only with depression, but also with anxiety. In one study, 17.8 percent of disabled workers with chronic musculoskeletal pain also had a diagnosable anxiety disorder.[12]

## Neuroanatomy: The Pain-Feelings Connection

Depression often has a biochemical basis. Many depressed people have an imbalance or a deficiency of the neurotransmitters serotonin, norepinephrine, and/or dopamine. Antidepressants that increase levels of serotonin and norepinephrine alleviate depression and also decrease pain signals.[13] In the human nervous system, pain and feelings share common pathways. The same fibers—A-delta and C fibers—transmit information about pain and emotions from the periphery to the dorsal horn of the spinal cord. There, they separate on the way to the brain: Pain and other sensation signals go up the spinothalamic tracts, whereas emotional-processing signals go up the spinoreticular pathways to the limbic areas of the brain. The limbic system is a group of structures located in the cerebrum (upper part) of the brain. It plays an important role in the expression of emotion. Patients who years ago underwent frontal lobotomy surgery became emotionally unconcerned about their pain. More recently, PET scans (which record regional blood flow in the brain) of people who were experiencing pain showed that two different areas of the brain were activated: the SI and SII (sensory component), and the ACC of the limbic system.[14] In other words, an incoming pain stimulus causes the brain to respond both with a sensation of pain and an emotion.

What the scientific research indicates is that the pain experience consists of both pain sensation and emotions. The same pathways and the same neurotransmitters (brain chemicals) are involved in both processes. If you have chronic pain, treating the body is not enough; you need to involve your mind, too.

## The Experience of Pain

The mind can be a powerful tool for coping with chronic pain. Various techniques can affect the way we perceive pain and how we interpret it. We will explore some of these techniques and will report on studies that have tested the efficacy of those techniques.

As stated before, our experience of chronic pain is not just the perception of pain. Chronic pain patients often experience a lot of emotional distress, such as anxiety and depression. They may become excessively aware of changes in body sensations, and may interpret these sensations as pain. When you feel the transitory aches and pains that everyone experiences at times, you may become anxious as you tell yourself, *Oh, no! Now I'm getting hip pain on top of all my other aching places! I thought I was getting better, but now I'm getting worse and I won't be able to do those things I was planning.*

Anxiety and depression make it harder to live with chronic pain. Anti-anxiety and antidepressant medications can help, but so can the following techniques.

## Cognitive Behavioral Therapy

The way a person thinks about his or her chronic pain problem has a great impact on how she feels. For example, rheumatoid arthritis patients who feel personal helplessness have more anxiety, depression, and functional impairment.[15] People who expect the worst, who catastrophize whatever happens to them, have a diminished ability to control their pain, whereas older adults with more effective coping strategies have a significantly lower pain level and fewer psychological disabilities.[16] Osteoarthritis patients who are able to think rationally about their pain and disability have less severe pain, better health status, and lower levels of psychological distress than do similar patients who tend to catastrophize or think irrationally about their disease.[17] Patients with post-herpetic neuralgia (shingles, PHN) who catastrophize have more depression early on and more pain at 8 weeks than do patients who don't expect the worst to happen.[18] It makes sense, then, to have a plan for changing a patient's self-defeating way of thinking and behaving.

The major goal of all behavioral strategies is to increase the patient's sense of control by decreasing the helplessness and hopelessness that are so much a part of living with chronic pain. Cognitive behavioral therapy (CBT) attempts to change a person's thinking and behavior. As the National Association of Cognitive Behavioral Therapists explains, CBT emphasizes the important role of thinking in how we feel and what we do. Cognitive behavioral therapy is based on the fact that our thoughts, rather than external things such as people and events, cause our feelings and behaviors. If we are experiencing unwanted feelings and behaviors, it is important to identify the thinking that is causing the negative feelings and behaviors and learn how to replace this negative thinking with thoughts that lead to more desirable reactions. Cognitive behavioral therapy aims to change negative thoughts and dysfunctional beliefs, attitudes, and expectations about pain, and to foster more healthy and adaptive thoughts, emotions, and behaviors. Another important component of CBT is to motivate patients to reduce their social isolation, increase their interaction with others, and engage in pleasurable activities.

Typically carried out in small group sessions of four to eight patients, CBT may also be conducted one-on-one. In therapy, clients learn to identify the common mental mistakes that people make and how to correct them. These common patterns include overgeneralization, catastrophizing, all-or-none thinking, jumping to conclusions, selective attention, and negative predictions. As a CBT client you will be asked to identify a troubling situation such as "I'm on disability because of my ongoing back pain." Next, you will be asked what you are telling yourself about the situation. This might be "I'll never work again. I'll just be a burden on my family. I'm useless." You will also be asked how you feel about the situation. "I feel depressed. I'm not worth anything anymore." Once this sequence is identified, you will be asked to consider the validity of what you're telling yourself. People often have distorted ways of thinking, such as black-and-white thinking. They tell themselves "I'll never be able to . . . I'll always feel so terrible . . ." Or they catastrophize.

"My wife won't love me anymore ... I'm a terrible burden." Or perhaps "This pain is horrible and there's nothing I can do to make it better." The therapist will keep questioning your assumptions and help you to become more realistic and to focus on the positive. The therapist will help you identify and challenge beliefs and feelings that interfere with motivation for coping efforts. The result is that you will be more motivated to make the changes that will enable you to cope more effectively.

Cognitive behavioral therapy is based on an educational model, rather than on just expressing yourself. You will be given homework assignments, and each session is structured and specific techniques and concepts are taught. Many CBT therapists include relaxation and breathing techniques in their work. The therapy is generally brief, perhaps fewer than 10 sessions. Published studies have confirmed that CBT can reduce depression and also unexplained pain.[19,20]

## *Biofeedback and Relaxation*

Biofeedback is rarely used on its own, but rather in combination with relaxation and other cognitive behavioral techniques. In biofeedback, patients' skin temperature, heart rate, and/or brain waves are monitored with instruments, and the results displayed on a screen, or given in terms of changes in colors or tones. The feedback helps people change some physical parameter over which they usually have no control, such as decreasing their heart rate, increasing the temperature of their fingertips, or inducing a particular type of brain wave seen during relaxation rather than another brain-wave type that is seen during active thinking. They may be taught how to decrease the tension in particular muscles, such as the frontalis muscle in the forehead or trapezius muscle in the neck. They receive immediate feedback letting them know how successful they were.

In response to an injury, for example to the back or knee, the surrounding muscles tighten in order to protect the injured area. They may go into spasm, which is painful. The pain sensations of the muscle spasm can cause additional muscle tightening, leading to more spasm and more pain. The primary objective of relaxation-training techniques is to relax the muscles and calm the mind. Different techniques all share (1) a repetitive focus on a word or phrase, a sound, a body sensation or muscle activity, and (2) adoption of a passive attitude toward intruding thoughts and a return to the focus of attention. The following is a list of some types of relaxation techniques, which are often used in combination.

- **Meditation** is becoming aware of current body sensations and mental activities without judging them. In some types of meditation this is facilitated by focusing on your breathing or on a word or some repetitive sound.
- **Progressive muscle relaxation** is first tensing, then relaxing a sequence of muscles.
- **Breathing techniques**: in paced respiration, breathing is deliberately slowed when the person feels anxious. In deep breathing, a deep breath is taken and held for 5 seconds, then exhaled. This process is repeated.
- **Autogenic training** helps you to imagine that your arms and legs are heavy and warm, your heart rate slow, your belly warm, your forehead cool, and your breathing slow. While doing this, you imagine a peaceful environment such as a beach or a forest.
- **Guided imagery** helps you to recall a pleasant and relaxing image and focus your attention on the sensory details, such as the light, color, sound, and texture of the situation.

Biofeedback and relaxation training can help break the cycle of spasm and pain. They can also reduce anxiety, depression, and the detective-like monitoring of the body for any additional pain or dysfunction. These techniques have found wide use in treating chronic headaches and other types of pain, as well as hypertension.

Many studies support these conclusions. For example, a 1999 study found that biofeedback and relaxation training reduced depression in chronic pain patients, as measured by improved scores on the Beck Depression Inventory, a commonly used self-assessment questionnaire for depression.[21] More recently, 25 chronic pain patients were given eight sessions of biofeedback and relaxation training and then were compared with a control group of similar patients. The treated group had significantly less anxiety and fewer physical complaints.[22] It appears that patients who learn biofeedback and relaxation training experience less anxiety and fewer somatic complaints. These techniques can empower chronic pain patients, giving them a sense of control over their stress and pain, which in turn makes the stress and pain less anxiety-provoking.

## Mindfulness Meditation

Mindfulness meditation is a relaxation technique used for relieving pain. Subjects are taught to detach themselves from the pain experience and simply observe the pain sensations without attaching meaning to them. Jon Kabat-Zinn and his partners taught this meditation technique to 90 chronic pain patients in a 10-week stress-reduction and relaxation program. Compared with another group of patients who were treated with more traditional pain-control techniques such as nerve blocks, physical therapy, and medications, patients who meditated had significant decreases in pain levels and amount of medication used, and significant increases in activity level and feelings of self-esteem.[23] Interestingly, the male patients had more mood disturbance and psychological symptoms than the females, and were less successful in improving these symptoms during meditation training than were women.

## Hypnosis

Have you ever seen—or read about—people who, under hypnosis, seem to feel no pain when stuck with a needle? When I was in China some years ago, I saw a film about the use of hypnosis for anesthesia in major surgery. In the film, the patient walked over to the operating table and lay down, and was then hypnotized. After that, with no additional anesthesia, her abdomen was opened and surgery proceeded. When she was awakened shortly after the operation ended, she appeared comfortable.

Hypnosis is a state of altered consciousness in which there is narrowed awareness, focused attentiveness, selected wakefulness, and heightened suggestibility. One form of hypnosis is a trance, or a conscious state of awareness, in which a person can be absorbed in his own thoughts and ideas so much that he may perceive and respond to those thoughts and ideas as if they were real. Dr. Steven Gurgevich, a psychologist who specializes in medical applications of hypnosis and who writes about its use in surgery and in chronic pain, stresses that all hypnosis is actually self-hypnosis. The hypnotist's role is to provide instructions and to guide the patient in shifting consciousness to become absorbed in pleasantly relaxing thoughts, ideas, images, and feelings, and to be distracted from adverse or noxious internal or external stimuli. This process, termed *hypnotic induction*, allows the patient to experience greater control over sensory and physiological experiences, facilitating a greater openness and receptivity to therapeutic suggestions. Examples of such suggestions, which the therapist and patient agree on in advance, are "Your pain after the operation will be only two out of 10 or less," or "When you wake up you will feel comfortable enough to walk to the bathroom." Using the trance state to facilitate beneficial suggestions is termed *utilization of the trance state*, and it constitutes the second aspect of the process of hypnosis.

Hypnosis helps people to obtain deeper levels of relaxation, which often leads to more peaceful sleep, increased energy, and diminished pain. The patient remains in control of the process throughout the session, which reduces the risk for adverse reactions.

People vary widely in their ability to be hypnotized. About 20 percent cannot do this at all. Another 10 to 20 percent can go through surgery with only hypnosis for anesthesia. About 60 percent of people get significant benefit from hypnosis and are motivated to practice at home. Those who are unresponsive to hypnosis often do better with biofeedback, and vice versa.[24] There are many published controlled studies of the use of hypnosis in surgery. They show that surgical patients treated with hypnosis have significantly better outcomes than control groups in that they experience a reduced amount of pain, use fewer pain medications, and recover more quickly.[25] A recent review of 18 studies, designed to answer the question "How effective is hypnosis?" showed a moderate to large pain-relieving effect.[26] One study used medical hypnosis for orthopedic hand surgery, which usually results in severe postoperative pain. Compared with a "usual care" group, patients who received hypnosis had significantly less postoperative pain and anxiety. They also recovered more quickly after surgery and had fewer postoperative complications.[27]

In another study, 339 patients undergoing neck surgery for thyroid and parathyroid disorders received two types of anesthesia. One group had hypnosis along with intravenous sedation that kept them conscious; the other group had traditional general anesthesia. The hypnosis group had significantly less postoperative pain and used fewer pain medications. They also had a shorter hospital stay after surgery. The authors concluded that hypnosis is an effective technique for providing relief of pain both during and after endocrine neck surgery.[28] Of 241 patients who underwent invasive medical procedures, those who received advance instruction in self-hypnotic relaxation had less pain and anxiety than those who did not receive the hypnosis instruction.[29]

Hypnosis is also effective in children. In one study, 52 children facing surgery were randomly divided into two groups, one of which was taught guided imagery and received hypnotic suggestions for a favorable postoperative course.[30] The group who had hypnosis had a significantly reduced amount of pain after surgery and shorter hospital stays.

In 2000, a review of the field of published articles in the field of hypnosis concluded that "the clinical research to date generally substantiates the claim that hypnotic procedures can ameliorate some psychological and medical conditions."[31]

It's clear that the mind can have a tremendous influence on what the body feels. Hypnosis can demonstrate this effect very dramatically. Hypnosis and other cognitive or behavioral interventions can actually affect the body's production of endogenous opioids. A neuroimaging study of brain function, for example, yielded direct evidence that hypnosis modulates the way pain is processed in the brain.[32] While having their brain activity recorded by a PET scanner, volunteers immersed a hand in hot water. The stimuli and the scanning were repeated after the volunteers were hypnotized and told that the hot water would be less painful. In their hypnotized state, the subjects had significantly less pain–related activation in their ACC, a part of the brain that participates in the emotional experience of pain and can also influence the inhibition of pain. On the other hand, there was no decrease in activity in the primary somatosensory cortex, the region that processes the sensation of pain.

Just believing that some intervention will help can produce pain relief. This, of course, is the placebo effect, which can indeed be effective. Another PET scan study showed that pain response in specific brain regions can be modified by placebos.[33] Compared with subjects who experienced heat pain but no medication, those who received either a placebo or a potent fast–acting opioid had greater activation of both the ACC and the brain stem. This study shows that placebos can in fact cause neurochemical changes in the brain, which relieve pain.

If you are considering hypnosis for a medical problem, look for a professional who is certified by the American Society of Clinical Hypnosis, the only professional association that certifies the hypnosis training and supervision of physicians, psychologists, nurses, social workers, and dentists. On their Web site (www.asch.net) you can find a list of certified professionals as well as other useful information.

To learn more about how the mind interacts with the perception of pain, emotions, beliefs, and muscle tension, you might also look at John Sarno's book *Healing Back Pain: Using the Mind-Body Connection*.

### Eye Movement Desensitization and Reprocessing

*Maryanne, a 30-year-old woman with a kidney transplant, developed painful shingles, probably as a result of the immunosuppressant medications she took to keep her kidney from being rejected. Although she said her dose of opioid pain medication was effective, she kept running out of the drug early. Her doctor initiated a lengthy discussion about why this kept happening. Maryanne admitted that she had a morbid fear of finding herself in pain with no options, so that whenever she felt any pain coming on, she reached for another pill. She began crying as she described how following her kidney transplant she had complications that landed her in the intensive care unit (ICU) for several days. She felt helpless, in pain, unsure if she would even survive. Even now, years later, whenever her shingles pain worsened, she'd suddenly experience all those feelings she'd had in the ICU, and she felt she had to escape from that intolerable situation.*

*Maryanne's physician concluded that Maryanne was unable to tolerate an increase in her pain because it triggered symptoms of a posttraumatic stress disorder (PTSD) resulting from her traumatic experience after her kidney transplant. She referred Maryanne to a therapist specializing in eye movement desensitization and reprocessing (EMDR), a brief treatment for PTSD. Following three sessions with the therapist, Maryanne experienced relief from her symptoms, which allowed her to recognize that a transient exacerbation of her shingles pain was not a catastrophe. She was then able to manage her own pain medication more reliably and to take her pills as directed.*

Sometimes treatments whose mechanism of action isn't clearly understood can nonetheless be very useful. Acupuncture could be considered one of these. Another is EMDR. Originated by Francine Shapiro in 1989,[34] the treatment helps survivors of trauma reprocess and get relief from strong negative feelings associated with traumatic events. EMDR's unique feature is the use of eye movements done in association with suggestions made by the therapist based on prior discussions with the patient about the traumatic event. While the patient thinks about the disturbing issue or event, and ponders the thoughts and beliefs he currently has about the event, his eyes move back and forth. Sets of eye movements are continued until the memory becomes less disturbing and is associated with positive thoughts and beliefs about oneself—for example, "I did the best I could." During the session, the patient may experience intense emotions, but by the end of the session, most people report a significant reduction in the level of disturbance. Most people need three to 10 EMDR sessions to resolve their trauma.

EMDR is a powerful way of getting the brain to learn much more quickly than usual, which makes possible both rapid realization of essential truths about a situation or event and rapid recovery from the effects of acute psychological trauma, and slower but thorough recovery from the effects of chronic psychological trauma. When psychological difficulties coping with chronic pain are related to preceding trauma, EMDR can be helpful in facilitating more effective beliefs, feelings, and actions regarding the pain.

## Strategies for Improving Sleep

Many chronic pain patients have difficulty sleeping. The first strategy is often to ask the doctor for sleeping pills (see chapter 4 for a description of such medications). This may be a temporary solution to insomnia, but for a more lasting improvement, the following behavioral strategies can be effective.

- Associate your bed only with sleep or sex, not with watching TV or with worrying or planning your next day's activities. Read in bed only if it makes you sleepy.
- Maintain a regular sleep schedule: Go to bed and get up at the same time each day, 7 days a week.
- Limit daytime napping 30-60 minutes (set an alarm clock).
- Eat a light bedtime snack; don't go to bed hungry. Foods

containing tryptophan, such as milk and turkey, promote sleep. Avoid caffeine and alcohol in the late evening.

- Physical exercise is good for your body, but not at bedtime; do it at least 6 hours earlier.
- If you have to get up at night to use the bathroom, don't turn on a bright light (it's a wake-up call to the brain).
- If you can't fall asleep after 15 minutes or so, don't just lie in bed watching the clock. Get up and stay up for between 30 and 60 minutes. When you return to bed, you will likely fall asleep.

## Education

The best management for any chronic disorder requires collaboration between doctor and patient. For people with chronic pain, part of the collaboration is being an informed consumer. You obviously recognize this; after all, you are reading this book.

When someone is first injured or develops some painful condition, they often have expectations that eventually become unrealistic. One of them is that if their pain could be correctly diagnosed, then it could be cured. Unfortunately, as you have already read, one of the common features of chronic pain syndromes is that the experience of pain becomes dissociated from the cause. Even if the cause was originally clear (for example, a fractured leg, Herpes zoster infection, osteoarthritic changes in the back), with time it becomes less and less possible to truly understand why the pain persists. After all the lab and imaging tests have been done, there comes a point when the goal ceases to be diagnosis, and when you must make peace with the reality that the pain itself is a primary problem. The focus can no longer be on the diagnosis, but rather on relieving pain and improving function.

You can better help yourself by:

- developing realistic expectations of what your treatment can accomplish (for example, returning to acceptable function rather than being pain-free).
- recognizing the difference between acute and chronic pain.
- noticing that when you are involved in other activities, you are less aware of your pain; distraction is the first line of defense against pain.

- accepting that pain levels fluctuate, sometimes for no particular reason.
- learning about your medications and their risks.
- understanding that your pain perception is greatly influenced by your mood, your expectations, and your relationships with your family and friends.
- talking with others who have experienced chronic pain and learning what they have found helpful.
- learning techniques of "self-management"—that is, how you can help yourself feel better.

Finally, an important aspect of managing your chronic pain is learning more about yourself. Your temperament and your style of approaching the world strongly influence your way of coping with adverse events in your life. In the next chapter we will learn about different personality types and how each deals with life's problems.

# PART III

# THE ENNEAGRAM
# AND
# CHRONIC PAIN

# 12

## THE ENNEAGRAM PERSONALITY TYPES

### *What Type Am I?*

CHAPTER 11 DESCRIBED HOW THE MIND AND body are interconnected, how your mood and your thinking can influence your perception of pain, and how various psychotherapies can help you improve the way you deal with chronic pain. There is another area, however, that greatly impacts your reaction to stress and pain in your life, and that is your temperament or personality. It makes sense that if two people have to quit their job because of severe back pain, the one whose life revolves around his work and whose self-esteem depends on being successful might find it harder to cope than a person who is easygoing and has many other interests. The premise of this chapter is that if you have a better understanding of your personality, you will have a greater awareness of the strengths and challenges that will affect your coping ability, and greater ability to focus on the areas that need to change in order to enhance your ability to live productively with chronic pain. Reading this chapter will also help you make more sense of chapter 13.

There are many systems for identifying different personality types. You may have heard of one or another of them, such as the Myers-Briggs Type Inventory, which classifies people on the basis of several characteristics such as whether they are introverts or extroverts and whether they react to their surroundings primarily with their feelings or their thoughts. Another system, "True Colors," is roughly based on Myers-Briggs. It divides people into four colors, based on a brief questionnaire. "Gold" people put a priority on belonging; "blue" people on authenticity; "orange" people on freedom to act; and "green" people on competence in themselves and others.

Many employers offer seminars to their employees on a particular personality system, with the goal of improving their work performance and their ability to get along with their peers. All of these can be useful, because all can make you more aware of how you respond to people and situations, and whether your reactions are helping you or making it more difficult for you to deal with your health problems. You can think of your personality type as a pair of eyeglasses through which you see the world. These glasses bring some aspects of your environment into sharp focus while casting others into deep shadow. The particular personality system that you use isn't critical; what matters is that it can give you greater insight into how to help yourself.

In 2003, I decided to make a formal study of how personality influences living with chronic pain. I did this by interviewing at length more than 65 chronic pain patients, using one particular system of personality types, and then asking the patients how the strengths and challenges of their type have affected the way they deal with their chronic pain. This chapter describe the types, while chapter 13 relates how each of these types affected people's coping ability. Even if you have no particular interest in personality typing, you might still recognize yourself among the descriptions and glean some hints that can improve your own situation.

The system I used is termed the *enneagram* (pronounced ANY-uh-gram), a word with Greek roots that mean "nine types." The increasing popularity of this system has led to the availability of many books on it. Some that I particularly recommend are by Helen Palmer,[1,2] Renee Barron and Elizabeth Wagelie,[3] Michael Goldberg,[4] and Don Riso and Russ Hudson.[5] In each book you will find not only a description of the types, but suggestions for becoming emotionally healthier and overcoming the challenges of each type. The nine types have various connections, and the system is actually quite complex, but this discussion will simply describe the main features of each type. What is particularly attractive about the enneagram is that it doesn't just put people into boxes—it delves into their underlying motivations, fears, and the things to which each type pays particular attention. Of course, everyone is unique, but people of the same type have the same basic motivations and view the world in very similar ways. Each type has certain strengths and talents, but also certain difficulties. No one type is "better" than any other. In fact, people of each type may vary from very unhealthy psychologically to very healthy. At their worst, each type is manifested as a particular psychological disorder, which can be seen as carrying the core problematic issue (called "passion" or "one of the seven deadly sins plus two") by enneagram enthusiasts.

Nonetheless, after you become familiar with this way of understanding people, you will see the fundamental similarities among different people of the same type. You might also be able to identify your own type.

In the sections below you will be introduced briefly to nine different types of people. At first you may not clearly identify your own type. That's because everyone has some attributes of several types, although they are predominantly one of the nine personalities. In fact, people of each type tend to also have some features of one of the two adjacent numbers. For example, Type Ones generally exhibit some characteristics of Type Nine or Two, while Type Four will act in some ways like Type Three or Five.

The best way to gain clarity about each type is to observe and listen to others whose type you know. This is why each description below includes names of well-known people on whose personality styles enneagram experts agree. For an excellent description of enneagram types, lists of public figures and actors for each type, and summaries of films whose characters clearly demonstrate particular types, consult Tom Condon's book, *The Enneagram Movie & Video Guide*.[6]

## *Type One: The Perfectionist*

*Chief motivation:* To do things the "right" way, improve yourself and others. "I need to make myself and the world perfect."

*Chief fear or avoidance:* To be imperfect.

*Strongest positive traits:* Ethical, responsible, fair, conscientious, principled, self-disciplined, organized.

*Strongest negative traits:* Judgmental, righteous, rigid, critical of others, overly serious, controlling, anxious.

*Core issue ("passion" or "sin"):* Anger.

Perfectionists—Ones—are disciplined, conscientious, and principled. They strive to live up to their high ideals—and they want others to do the same. Perfectionists have a strong inner sense of right or wrong. They constantly compare reality to an internal set of standards. Fairness and honesty are very important to them. They notice the errors and imperfections of the world and try their hardest to correct them. They are detail-oriented, goal-oriented people, but just as important as completing the task is to do it right. Their vocabulary is peppered with "should," "must," "ought," and "it's the right thing to do." A strong inner critic is forever judging them, telling them they could do a better job. Ones are drawn to "causes," and they tend to displace their anger into righteous indignation over injustices. Another name for this type is the "Reformer" because of their attraction to solving social problems.

Ones are not wishy-washy people. They are used to having a strong sense of what's the right thing to do in a situation, and they are more comfortable when the task is clear. They generally prefer black and white to shades of gray when it comes to making decisions. Uncertainty is uncomfortable.

Perfectionists like to avoid losing self-control or violating social norms. Rather than shouting when angry, they're more likely to feel irritated or resentful. They may be perceived as inflexible, overly serious, and critical of others. It is hard for Perfectionists to have fun. Perfectionists are generally not touchy-feely people, and they are sometimes perceived as being cold. Their challenge is to lighten up, have more fun, and be easier on themselves and others.

The core issue of the Perfectionist, also called the "passion" or "sin" of the type, is Anger. Many Type Ones are not even aware of their anger. Perfectionists see direct anger as not nice, or inappropriate, so they tend to repress or stuff their anger, which then leaks out as resentment or may suddenly explode as "righteous indignation" over some misjustice.

According to Tom Condon,[6] well-known people who are Type Ones are: U.S. President Harry S. Truman; U.S. Senators Hillary Clinton, John Kerry, and Barry Goldwater; General Colin Powell; Kenneth Starr; crusader Ralph Nader; Dr. Jack Kevorkian; playwright Arthur Miller; manners mavens "Miss Manners" and Emily Post; Sir Thomas More; Martin Luther; actors Gregory Peck, Harrison Ford, Charlton Heston, Jodie Foster, and Meryl Streep.

## Type Two: The Giver

*Chief motivation:* To be loved and appreciated. "The way to get love is to give love."
*Chief fear or avoidance:* To be seen as needy.
*Strongest positive traits:* Warm, nurturing, sensitive to others' needs, loving, generous, enthusiastic, positive.
*Strongest negative traits:* Possessive, prideful, hostile, martyr-like, manipulative, hysterical.
*Core issue ("passion" or "sin"):* Pride (in being needed by others while having no needs yourself).

Givers—Twos—are warm, nurturing, and sensitive to other people's needs. They are generous, enthusiastic, and caring. They are motivated by the need to give in order to receive love; they define themselves through service to others. It is easy for Twos to give, but hard to receive; they pride themselves on having no needs, yet they crave appreciation. Twos avoid being dependent on others, and they fear disappointing others or feeling rejected or not needed. Relationships are more important to them than anything else. Givers are detail-oriented people who thrive on being "the power behind the throne" rather than the leader. When Twos get angry, it's usually in sudden emotional outbursts, accusations, and often crying.

The core issue of Twos is called Pride, a characteristic they are usually unaware of. They are out of touch with their own needs, focusing instead on making themselves indispensable to others. After they are entrenched in such a position, another aspect of their pride is the feeling that they are privileged people, entitled to the best available. Twos' challenge is to become aware of their own needs and begin to get their needs met directly rather than by manipulating others.

Well-known Type Twos include: Princess Diana; television personality Mr. Rogers; Bishop Desmond Tutu; Monica Lewinsky; Florence Nightingale; Eva Peron; Mother Teresa; actors Jerry Lewis, John Travolta, Mia Farrow, Bill Cosby, and Faye Dunaway.

## Type Three: The Achiever

*Chief motivation:* To achieve, succeed. "The way to get love is to be successful."
*Chief fear or avoidance:* Failure.
*Strongest positive traits:* Energetic, goal-oriented, self-assured, optimistic, efficient, practical.
*Strongest negative traits:* Competitive, conniving, superficial, narcissistic, deceptive, pretentious.
*Core issue ("passion" or "sin"):* Deceit (they'll turn themselves into whatever projects the image of success).

Achievers—Threes—are motivated by the need to be productive, achieve success, and avoid failure. They measure themselves by external achievements. They want to look good and project the image of someone who can handle any situation successfully. Threes are results-oriented people who are often described as workaholics. Even on vacations they are likely to bring work with them, and even illness won't keep them from doing their best to get the job done. Achievers would rather talk about their work than their feelings. Their self-worth is dependent on their accomplishments, and they believe that others judge them the same way.

The core issue of the Three is called Deceit. Achievers fool themselves at least as much as others. In order to be successful, they keep changing themselves into whatever they perceive the group wants them to be. In the course of being a chameleon, they lose track of who they really are and what they are feeling. They are much more comfortable with doing than with feeling. For Achievers, what counts is the image rather than the reality. Because of their fear of failure, they tend to put a positive spin (to themselves and others) on anything negative that happens to them. The challenge for Achievers is to slow down, recognize that they are worthwhile people even if they don't constantly accomplish things, and to get in touch with their feelings.

Famous Threes, according to Condon, include: Reverend Jesse Jackson; Henry Kissinger; Colonel Oliver North; Governor Arnold Schwartzenegger; O. J. Simpson; Oprah Winfrey; Tiger Woods; Michael Jordan; Bryant Gumbel; Diane Sawyer; Elvis Presley; actors Tom Cruise, Sylvester Stallone, Demi Moore, and Sharon Stone.

## ' *Type Four: The Romantic*

*Chief motivation:* To be understood, to be seen as special and unique.
*Chief fear or avoidance:* To be ordinary.
*Strongest positive traits:* Warm, perceptive, artistic, inspiring, compassionate, intuitive, introspective.
*Strongest negative traits:* Moody, withdrawn, guilt-ridden, stubborn, self-absorbed, self-conscious.
*Core issue ("passion" or "sin"):* Envy (others have what I want and can't get).

Romantics—Fours—are motivated by the need to experience their feelings, to be understood, to search for the meaning of life, and to avoid being ordinary. They like to be perceived as unique, and take special care to make their appearance and their surroundings special. They believe they feel more deeply than others, and what they feel often is melancholy and loss. Romantics seek peak experiences, but often feel sad or depressed. They see themselves as being very sensitive and often very creative. They tend to express themselves through music, art, theater, writing, and other creative endeavors. Fours are compassionate, warm, intuitive, introspective people who, however, can be depressed, withdrawn, and moody. Some flirt with death and may even commit suicide.

The core issue of the Romantics is Envy. They tend to notice what others have that they don't, and they envy others for having what they perceive is missing in their own lives. In relationships, they long for the unavailable person, but when they actually have a partner, they tend to push him or her away.

Among famous Fours are: Prince Charles; poet Sylvia Plath; Vincent van Gogh; Michael Jackson; Kurt Cobain; Billie Holliday; Bob Dylan; Jack Kerouac; Virginia Woolf; actors Johnny Depp, James Dean, Judy Garland, Nick Nolte, Laurence Olivier, Marlon Brando, John Malkovich, Marcello Mastroianni, and Liam Neeson.

## *Type Five: The Observer*

*Chief motivation:* To gather knowledge, to be self-sufficient. "The world is unsafe; the more information I have, the safer I'll be."

*Chief fear or avoidance:* Looking foolish, stupid.
*Strongest positive traits:* Knowledgeable, insightful, analytical, curious, sensitive, objective, persevering.
*Strongest negative traits:* Stingy, stubborn, critical of others, intellectually arrogant, negative.
*Core issue ("passion" or "sin"):* Avarice.

Observers—Fives—are motivated by the need to know and understand everything, and to be self-sufficient. They are analytical, perceptive, objective people, but they can also be intellectually arrogant, critical of others, and unassertive. They perceive the world as invasive, and they need privacy to think and to refuel their energies. Observers believe that if they only can gather enough information, they can feel safe in the world. They tend to avoid strong feelings or demanding people; they tend to experience their feelings more deeply when they are alone. Other people may see them as detached. It is more comfortable for Fives to observe than to participate. They may also be uncomfortable in social situations.

The core issue of the Five is Avarice (greed). Observers tend to be minimalists, attempting to get by with as little as possible. Observers believe that the resources of the world are limited, so that they need to hold on to those resources they have. This doesn't necessarily refer to money, as many Fives are very generous. It is more often played out in the arenas of time and emotions. Observers jealously guard their alone time and their privacy. They feel easily invaded by others, and when they find themselves among a group of people, they may need some alone time to recover afterward. They value their own space, whether that's their home, a room, or a desk, and don't want others touching those areas. Spouses of Fives often complain that Observers just don't give enough of themselves, like to spend too much time alone, don't want to talk about their feelings, and prefer to withdraw whenever any emotional problems come up. The challenge for Observers is to become more connected, to empower themselves to take action, and allow others into their emotional space.

Some well-known Fives are: Jacqueline Kennedy Onassis; Albert Einstein; Amelia Earhart; Dr. Jane Goodall; Joe DiMaggio; Bobby Fisher; Howard Hughes; Dr. Oliver Sacks; Jean-Paul Sartre; Michael Crichton; actors Richard

Chamberlain, Montgomery Clift, Daniel Day-Lewis, Ralph Fiennes, Anthony Hopkins, Jeremy Irons, Sam Neill, and Al Pacino.

## Type Six: The Detective

*Chief motivation:* Safety, security. "The world is an unsafe place. If I make every effort to notice the dangers around me, I might be able to avoid harm" (Phobic Six). "The world is an unsafe place and I have to make every effort to detect danger. If I then face the danger head on, I might be able to avoid harm" (Counterphobic Six).

*Chief fear or avoidance:* Danger.

*Strongest positive traits:* Loyal, trustworthy, warm, practical, responsible, caring.

*Strongest negative traits):* Defensive, mistrustful, second-guesses oneself, hypervigilant, testy, self-defeating, looks for potential bad outcomes of situations.

*Core issue ("passion" or "sin"):* Fear, doubt.

Sixes are called Detectives because their attention goes to potential difficulties and dangers in their environment and in other people. Their core belief is that the world is a dangerous place, and that they need to be vigilant in order to feel safe. Fear and anxiety are their frequent companions. They have two strategies to feel secure. So-called Phobic Sixes are outwardly fearful and seek approval, searching for reliable and trustworthy authority figures. They tend to seek protectors whom they can trust, who can defend them, back them up, and help them feel safe. In contrast, Counterphobic Sixes (those who move against their fears) challenge the source of their fear directly, question authority, and may deliberately participate in potentially dangerous activities in order to have a clear idea of what the risks really are. They unconsciously recognize that what is in their imagination is often more frightening than reality, so surviving dangerous situations can be reassuring. Consciously, however, they may not consider themselves fearful people, whereas Phobic Sixes are very much in touch with their fears and their need for security. Most Detectives have some combination of Phobic and Counterphobic behaviors, but are predominantly one or the other.

Sixes are extremely loyal (they are also called Loyalists), devoted to their families and friends. They can be warm, witty, practical, helpful, and responsible, but they may also be defensive, hypervigilant, suspicious, sarcastic, and skeptical of others' motives. Sixes' attention is usually focused on the possible negative outcomes of every situation, and they need to be reassured that these possibilities have been addressed before they're ready to take action. They spend a lot of time preparing for possible disasters. They may report that they can never have enough knowledge or equipment to be adequately prepared. The result may be that they seem to be procrastinators. Even after they take action, many Detectives tend to go over their decision and wonder if it was the right one. Because of this, Sixes are sometimes said to have a "doubting mind."

Some famous Phobic Sixes are: President George W. Bush; President Richard Nixon; Ellen DeGeneres; actors Woody Allen, Alan Arkin, Warren Beatty, Candice Bergen, Sally Field, Ed Harris, Jack Lemmon, Marilyn Monroe, Mary Tyler Moore, and Anthony Perkins.

Counterphobic Sixes include: Adolf Hitler; J. Edgar Hoover; Janet Reno; David Letterman; Gordon Liddy; Ted Turner; Elton John; Wynonna Judd; Spike Lee; actors Judy Davis, Carrie Fisher, Mel Gibson, Gene Hackman, Dustin Hoffman, Tommy Lee Jones, Paul Newman, Robert Redford, Julia Roberts, Susan Sarandon, and Steven Seagal.

### Type Seven: The Adventurer

*Chief motivation:* To have fun, to experience novelty and adventure.
*Chief fear or avoidance:* Suffering and pain, being hemmed in.
*Strongest positive traits:* Optimistic, energetic, lively, fun to be with, spontaneous, imaginative, charming, enthusiastic, productive.
*Strongest negative traits:* Poor follow-through, impulsive, narcissistic, undisciplined, restless, manic.
*Core issue ("passion" or "sin"):* Gluttony.

Adventurers—Sevens—are motivated by the need to be happy and plan enjoyable activities. They perceive the world as being full of opportunities and options. Sevens are positive people who look forward to future possibilities, and who assiduously avoid pain and suffering. They fill their lives with many activities, and chafe at limitations, constraints, and rules. They prefer the start-up phase of hobbies or careers rather than the follow-through, and crave variety. Sitting still or quieting their minds is hard for them, and they tend not to be introspective. They are often described as charming, spontaneous, quick-witted, with a great sense of humor. But they can also be impulsive, undisciplined, restless, rebellious, and unwilling to commit. Many gravitate to careers as comedians and other show business careers, and even if they don't do this professionally, their friends see them as funny and entertaining.

The core issue of the Adventurer is Gluttony—an endless desire for novelty and enjoyable experiences. They are always ready for new adventures, moving quickly from one to another. Along the way, Sevens may leave many unfinished projects if they are no longer interesting. They tend to have a superficial knowledge of many areas, which makes them interesting conversationalists, but what they have in variety they may lack in depth of experience. They tend to be creative, imaginative people who leave the details and the grunt work to others. The life of many Adventurers includes multiple jobs, relationships, residences—a life full of changes.

Famous Sevens include: President John F. Kennedy; Sarah Ferguson; the Duke of Windsor; Magic Johnson; Ram Dass; Steve Allen; Jack Benny; Victor Borge; Allan King; Francis Ford Coppola; Federico Fellini; Steven Spielberg; Franco Zeffirelli; Larry King; Regis Philbin; Sonny Bono; Dizzy Gillespie; Loretta Lynn; Linda Ronstadt; actors Kenneth Branagh, Michael Caine, Michael J. Fox, Tom Hanks, Goldie Hawn, Michael Keaton, Dudley Moore, Jack Nicholson, Brad Pitt, Dennis Quaid, Martin Short, Barbra Streisand, Lily Tomlin, Robin Williams.

## Type Eight: The Leader; the Boss

*Chief motivation:* To be strong, powerful, self-reliant. "The world is a dangerous place, and I have to get them before they get me."

*Chief fear or avoidance:* To show weakness.

*Strongest positive traits:* Self-confident, energetic, self-reliant, protective, direct, authoritative.

*Strongest negative traits:* Controlling, domineering, self-centered, aggressive, rebellious, insensitive, explosively angry.

*Core issue:* Lust.

Leaders (also called Bosses or Asserters)—Eights—are motivated by the need to be self-reliant and strong and to make an impact on the world. They are very protective of themselves, family, and friends, and do so in an aggressive, often combative way. Leaders are comfortable with overt anger. They welcome confrontation—they like to get things out in the open. They are take-charge people who love to be in control; feeling weak or dependent is anathema to them. They are loyal, direct, energetic, blunt, self-confident people. Eights are often gregarious, and love to swap stories with others. They can also be insensitive, domineering, and controlling. They tend to overindulge in food, sex, or drugs, living by the principle that "If some is good, more is better." Leaders hate to depend on other people. In showing that they care for others, they are much better at doing things for them than in sitting with them and listening to their feelings. Eights prefer action to introspection.

Leaders are often more in touch with their anger than any other emotion. If they are afraid or sad, it will emerge as anger. They perceive other emotions as signs of weakness. Whereas several other types (especially Perfectionists and Mediators) are uncomfortable around anger, Leaders welcome confrontation, believing that this is the way to truly get the measure of another person. They are easy to anger, but easily return to their positive, outgoing behavior. Having just blasted someone else with their over-the-top anger, they may not understand why an hour later that person is still upset with them.

Eights are sometimes initially confused with Counterphobic Sixes. However, whereas Detectives are driven by fear, repeatedly run tapes in their minds about the potential negative consequences of any action, and endlessly analyze decisions before making them, Leaders tend to charge ahead, take control, and rarely second-guess their actions.

The core issue of the Eight is Lust, which manifests itself as lust for life. They truly believe that when some is good, more is better. Unlike Adventurers, who want more variety and novelty, Leaders want more quantity—more food, more sex, more money, more power.

Tom Condon lists the following famous Eights: Napoleon Bonaparte; Fidel Castro; John Gotti; Saddam Hussein; Mao Tse-tung; Golda Meir; Donald Trump; John McEnroe; F. Lee Bailey; Alan Dershowitz; Norman Mailer; Evil Knievel; Frank Sinatra; Barbara Walters; Mike Wallace; actors Humphrey Bogart, Charles Bronson, Sean Connery, Russell Crowe, Matt

Damon, Brian Dennehy, Danny DeVito, Michael Douglas, Sean Penn, Julianne Phillips, Queen Latifah, Charlize Theron, Denzel Washington, John Wayne, and Debra Winger.

## Type Nine: The Mediator

*Chief motivation:* To keep the peace, to obtain consensus.
*Chief fear or avoidance:* Conflict.
*Strongest positive traits:* Good-natured, supportive of others, generous, empathic, patient, open-minded, diplomatic.
*Strongest negative traits:* Unassertive, stubborn, forgetful, procrastinating, easily distracted, passive-aggressive.
*Core issue:* Sloth.

Mediators—Nines—are motivated by the need to keep the peace, to avoid conflict, and to go along with others. Also called Peacemakers, they can easily see all points of view, which makes them skilled at helping others resolve conflicts. Mediators' friends generally see them as easygoing, peaceful, nonjudgmental, and agreeable. In a group, they'll go along with whatever the other people want to do. They tend to be very well-liked by their many friends. They are generous, giving people who (unlike Twos [Givers]) are not looking to get something out of it. Nines are very uncomfortable with anger. When they are upset, they are likely to keep quiet or react in some indirect way.

The ability to see all sides of every issue sometimes makes it difficult for Nines to make decisions or to take action. They are very easily distracted from the task at hand, and sometimes have difficulty setting priorities. It's hard for them to say no, so they may find themselves with more commitments than they can fulfill. When faced with a problem, Nines tend to ignore it or put it off, hoping that somehow the problem will go away or solve itself.

Mediators tend to defer action until the last minute. They are so used to focusing on others that sometimes it's hard for them to know what they really want; it's easier for them to know what they *don't* want. Uncomfortable with overt anger, Mediators are more likely to be stubborn or passive-aggressive when they are unhappy with a situation. Mediators are afraid of being invisible, but they somehow seem to "forget" themselves, and their friendly, unassuming, undemanding demeanor may make it easy for others to assume that they'll agree to anything.

The core issue of the Nine is Sloth, which consists of being easily distracted from the important things they have decided to do for themselves. They feel overwhelmed by life's details and distractions to the point that it's almost impossible for them to work on themselves, or even know what they want. It's easier for them to continue doing whatever they're doing rather than getting to the important things.

Some well-known Nines are: President Bill Clinton; President Abraham Lincoln; President Ronald Reagan; Queen Elizabeth II; King Hussein of Jordan; Tony Bennett; Nancy Kerrigan; Connie Chung; actors Jennifer Aniston, Antonio Banderas, Annette Bening, Tom Berenger, Matthew Broderick, Sandra Bullock, Kevin Costner, Clint Eastwood, Peter Falk, John Goodman, Anjelica Huston, Lisa Kudrow, Jennifer Jason Leigh, Jerry Seinfeld, Garry Shandling, Martin Sheen, Mary Steenburgen, and Billy Bob Thornton.

Now that you've been introduced to the nine types of the enneagram, you're ready to see how these types play out, in the words of individuals of each group. In the next chapter, you will learn the specific challenges people of your personality type face when they develop chronic pain, and how they use their strengths to live constructively with their pain.

# 13

# How
# Personality Types
# Cope with Pain

## *Advice and Challenges*

HAVING READ CHAPTER 12, YOU PROBABLY HAVE a sense of where you might fit among the nine enneagram types. Many people are still unsure at this point, because just reading about these types doesn't bring them to life. The best way to learn what your type is to have a "typing interview" with someone knowledgeable in the enneagram, or to listen to people of known types talking about their goals, fears, and what they pay attention to. Another method, of course, is to read some of the books I recommended in chapter 12. Even without reading those books, you might be more certain of your type when you finish this chapter.

Whereas the prior chapter was a theoretical introduction to the types, chapter 13 shows how they play out in the life of chronic pain patients.

### *Type One: The Perfectionist*
MY STORY. As a One myself, I experienced ongoing pain when I sustained a severe fracture of the middle of my femur (thigh bone),

which required two operations over a year before it healed. In addition to the pain, what was very upsetting to me was the upheaval to my orderly life. It was very frustrating, because for a while I couldn't go to work, and at first I was so depressed I couldn't concentrate on anything for long—not even reading or watching TV. I was so used to being efficient, and for weeks I wasn't doing anything productive. I like things to be organized, but my house was a mess.

Also, it was hard for me to accept help. I was used to being very independent, self-sufficient, and competent, and at that time I needed help to cook meals, to make the bed, to get items from upstairs (I was living downstairs because I couldn't climb upstairs to my bedroom), and to get food from the grocery store. I felt guilty asking my friends to do things for me. I didn't want to impose on them, and I thought they'd eventually become resentful.

My commitment to doing the right thing helped me in my treatment. I never missed a physical therapy session, I used the prescribed exercise machine at home 6 hours a day exactly as I was instructed, and I did the home exercises. I wanted to do whatever I could to get myself better. But when my fracture didn't heal after many months, I felt very agitated about what to do next. I didn't know what the right course of action was, and this was particularly difficult for me as a physician; I'm much more comfortable when there's a clear direction to go. I spoke with a dozen bone specialists to get their expert advice and I got two different opinions about the type of operation to have next, which only made me more uncertain and upset. I dislike uncertainty.

Some positive things did come out of my experience: In the end, I had to let go of my need to have all the answers in advance. I finally decided to go with the recommendation of my local specialist, and to have the simpler procedure. I came to an inner peace about the reality that if this operation didn't make the bone heal, I'd still have to have the other operation, the more complicated one. I learned to take this fracture one day at a time and to live with uncertainty without constantly trying to get all the answers or control the future. Another thing I learned was that it's okay to accept help. I saw that my friends felt good about helping me, and now it's easier for me to ask.

My advice to a younger Perfectionist is: There are a lot of gray areas when your body isn't working perfectly. If you focus on having the exact diagnosis, or predicting and controlling the outcome, you'll only destroy your inner peace. Take it one day at a time and have realistic expectations of yourself, meaning accept that you can't do everything you're used to doing, that you need more help, and that you may need to cut corners to get done what has to get done. Ask for help—it gets easier to ask the more you do it!

If you are a Perfectionist, you might be able to relate to the following Type One patients' stories.

## HOW THE PERFECTIONISTS' STRENGTHS HELPED THEM COPE

**SAMANTHA,** 51, executive secretary to several lawyers:

*Three years ago, I developed debilitating back pain. The most difficult part for me was getting to accept that it won't go away. The first couple of years I was very angry and frustrated. I kept looking for an explanation of why this happened to me. I'm still looking for an explanation, although my expectations of finding it have changed.*

*The pain affects my ability to function; I can't do normal things. I'm very moody when in pain, impatient and snappish. I'm like Dr. Jekyll and Mr. Hyde. I've had to let go of being neat. I'm less hard on myself. Otherwise I'd make myself crazy. I don't pick on myself as much as I used to, and I don't complain as much. In some ways I enjoy life more now. I'm more appreciative of the things I can do, of the things I used to take for granted. I have increased gratitude.*

*I'm more tolerant of other people, of things I used to roll my eyes at. I'm much more empathetic with people and their problems. I didn't understand before, and I thought they were probably pretending or milking it for sympathy. I knew a woman who had migraine headaches and missed a lot of work. At the time I thought she was faking it, but now my perception has changed. People can't see my pain either, so now the shoe is on the other foot.*

*I'm a much more grateful person now. My advice to another Perfectionist with pain would be to let go of the anger, work on it. Accept the situation. Find out as many answers as you can, but work on the acceptance. Get help through physical therapy, stress management, depression treatment. Ask for what you feel you need.*

Like Samantha and myself, Perfectionists desire to do things right, to control the outcomes, to be independent. With time comes an acceptance of reality and a letting go of the need to have everything "just so."

GLORIA, a 50-year-old former teacher, has ongoing pain in her temporomandibular joints (TMJ) related to a car accident; severe asthma has also restricted her activities:

> *The worst trait I have has helped me the most—I'm very stubborn. I refuse to give in to this. It's not going to control my life; I'm going to control my life. Also, I now allow myself to give myself a little more care, to say to myself, okay, I need some pampering today. I've never told another person I need to be pampered, not even my husband.*

FIONA, a 59-year-old businesswoman:

> *I'm a detail person with good follow-through and perseverance. I have a strong sense of the right way to do things. My strengths have helped me to research my disease [interstitial cystitis] and to know how to cope with it. I started a support group—I wanted to do it right. No one should have to deal with this alone. My perseverance has helped me to be tough, not letting the disease win.*

SANDRA, an introverted 62-year-old retired pediatrician, has had pain in her neck, shoulders, and jaws for many years:

> *My personality kept me looking for solutions for my pain. I explored different ways—acupuncture, physical therapy. I've been open to alternative treatments. My strength helped me tolerate the pain. I persist, I don't give up easily. So instead of being hysterical about having pain, I'm able to put up with a lot.*

The strengths that help Perfectionists deal with their pain are their persistence, desire not to give in, good follow-through, willingness to follow instructions and try recommended treatments, and their detail orientation, which pushes them to pursue multiple solutions to their medical problems.

## CHALLENGES FOR THE PERFECTIONISTS
GLORIA:

> *It's hard for me to ask for help. If I'm not sure how to do something, I'll ask for help in a heartbeat. But if it's something you should know how to do, or I was capable of doing before but can't do now, it's very hard to ask for help. Because I have such high standards for myself, it makes it hard for me to cope when I can't meet them. It gets very frustrating.*

FIONA:

> It bothers me that I can't do things right and I can't do what I should. I can't keep my house as clean as it should be. I don't have the energy to deal with it. It makes me less content, because I still have those "shoulds" in my head. I'm more irritable than I would be otherwise, which hurts my relationships.
>
> I'm not as sure of myself as I used to be, more depressed. I've had to decrease my expectations of myself big-time. If I focus on what I could have done, then I feel down, but if I focus on what I've learned, then it's okay.
>
> It's hard for me to ask for help, and I don't do it much. It's such a hard thing for me to do. If I'm asking, I must be defective in some way. I don't want to admit I'm not perfect.

BETH, 48, a former emergency room physician:

> Not being in control of my body is intolerable. I do everything right, and my body still fails me. I'm so self-critical that I can't live up to my own standards. I was very judgmental: When people broke the rules I'd get angry and resentful—it's unfair. They did this and they don't have to answer for it.
>
> I'm angry much of the time. I'm angry at myself, and the pain has made me irritable. I'm angry at my inability to do the things I want to do. I can't even play the piano. I want to get past the anger and into acceptance.

The biggest challenge for Perfectionists with chronic pain is the discrepancy between their high internal standards and the reality of their current lives. This leads to frequent self-criticism over their inability to live up to their standards. They have difficulty asking for help because their internal critic keeps telling them they should be able to do better, they shouldn't have to impose on others, and they just should try harder. Another frequent theme is feeling anger, often described as "irritability" or "frustration," at their limitations. Anger about their pain problem occurs in people of all personality types, but since many Ones don't perceive themselves as getting angry and don't think they *should* get angry (unless it's for a righteous cause), this is another source of self-criticism and disappointment in oneself.

## LESSONS PERFECTIONISTS LEARNED
### GLORIA:

*It's made me accept that I can't always have the perfection that I demand from myself. Because of that I've learned to accept flaws or mistakes a little more graciously than I used to.*

### SANDRA:

*For the longest time I wanted to be rid of the pain, so I fought it very hard. What's helped me is acceptance, surrendering to it, learning to live with it. I've come to accept the pain, and also my recurrent depression. It's taught me an acceptance of life, a realization that there are a lot of things I can't control. I've let go of the tight control I used to need to have. With the acceptance came less pain.*

*The pain pushed me into dealing with the emotional stuff that's behind it. It gave me a lot of compassion for other people in pain. It made very clear to me the association between mind and body. I meditate frequently now, and it helps.*

In the stories of how these Perfectionists have learned to deal with their chronic pain, the concept of acceptance comes up again and again. Ones speak of surrendering the struggle to be in control, to have all the answers, to do it perfectly. Ones, in particular, also need to learn compassion—both with themselves and with others. Coming initially from a position of "If you'd done it right, you wouldn't be in this situation," eventually they come to realize that getting things done isn't all about will. Bad things do happen, even if you follow the rules and do everything right.

## HOW OTHERS CAN HELP PERFECTIONISTS

Perfectionists care a lot about what others think of them. When they can no longer do the job (whatever the job is, from homemaker to CEO), they worry that others will see them as flakes and will no longer respect them. Perfectionists are very responsible, good people. What they basically want from others, as described by the Ones quoted above, is validation and respect. They want others to mirror for them that they *are* being responsible and good, and are trying their best. It is important for Perfectionists that others acknowledge that Ones are not shirking their responsibilities, that they are not flakes.

Perfectionists have spent years demonstrating to friends and coworkers that they are rational, competent, and independent. Not surprisingly, friends and family may underestimate the emotional support Perfectionists need in dealing with their chronic pain. Others can help Perfectionists by recognizing that they are experiencing strong emotions about their situation, by initiating contact to offer empathy and by talking with them about feelings rather than focusing on plans.

### Ones' Advice to Other Perfectionists

DORIS, 54, who's had long-standing back pain, advises:

*Stop blaming yourself and realize it wasn't your fault.*

FRANCINE, 63, developed chronic back pain following an accident. She recalled:

*I used to get very angry at myself. I'd be thinking, "If I hadn't done this or that, it wouldn't have happened." What I'd like to say to another Perfectionist is: First, keep a journal. I used my journal as a sounding board. It was a way of handling my anger. Next, try to hang on to the friendships you have, because it's hard to make new friends under these circumstances. Your friends know the kind of person you used to be before the accident.*

NORA, 52, a former teacher, has fibromyalgia exacerbated by chronic hepatitis C. She told me:

*I didn't do anger; I usually went right into sad. My advice is to stay focused on the positives. Focus on gratitude and stay away from depression; it's worse than the pain.*

TRESSA, a petite introvert with chronic back pain, advises:

*First look inside yourself and look at your limitations and give in. Pick your battles. The mental pain is sometimes worse than the physical.*

This was echoed by KELLY, 62, who has chronic back pain:

*Try to give yourself a break. Don't try to be so perfect. It's not possible, and it's not good for you.*

The main messages here are: Don't blame yourself for your problem, let go of the need to be perfect, pick your battles, and stay connected to your friends.

## *Type Two: The Giver*

### HOW THE GIVERS' STRENGTHS HELPED THEM COPE

Givers are positive, action-oriented people who feel good when helping others. Although caring for oneself is important in dealing with chronic pain, the other-focus can be harnessed toward the same goal.

WILL is a 56-year-old former military officer, the older of two sons, an extrovert. He describes himself as formerly happy, loving, giving, active in his church, and always concerned about family and community:

> *Eleven years ago, the cable snapped on an elevator I was in, and I broke multiple vertebrae in the fall. I've had ongoing back pain ever since. I ended up losing my wife and couldn't do my job well. The only piece of my identity that was left was my work, and I could no longer please my supervisor. I survived hell. I was all alone with a body that was going crazy. My outside looked unchanged, but nothing was working right.*
>
> *What helped was my belief in God, and some friends. God is some-one to talk to 24/7. My friends and doctors kept me from "going postal" because I didn't want to disappoint them. I tell myself that I must be going through this because someday I'm going to meet someone who'll need to talk to someone who's been through the war like I have.*

CHRIS, a 52-year-old Giver, has chronic knee pain stemming from a wound sustained in Vietnam. Recently the knee became increasingly painful. Given his usual pattern of ignoring his own needs and staying very busy helping others, he delayed seeking medical help. Chris finally consulted an orthopedic surgeon, but never got around to making the physical therapy appointments the surgeon advised. Eventually, Chris convinced himself to begin taking care of his body:

> *It's hard for me to treat myself as my own best friend, but when the chips are down, I can do it, I can look to get the best care. That's what happened with my knee. I told myself, "I have to be in good shape to help others. I have to take care of myself so I can be there for others. I need to get it taken care of so I can get back to my life. Once I've experienced this, I can connect with others in a more empathic way and help others." Turning it around in that way, I finally motivated myself to take the time to help my knee.*

LETICIA, a 48-year-old, has ongoing knee and back pain from a car accident:

> *Except for times when I can't, I mostly go on even if it's hurting. I see other people who are in more pain and I think, "I really hurt, but I imagine they're hurting even more."*

The strength of Givers is their interest and ability to help others. Being able to reframe their own experience and needs in a context of helping others motivated several Givers to get help and survive their misery. Chris, whose knee injury limited his locomotion, told himself that taking care of the injury would let him move freely again and help others more effectively. Will told himself that God was putting him through his ordeal in order to better prepare him to help another person in dealing with a similar experience. More than one Giver reported that his or her own experience made him or her more empathetic of others in pain. Focusing on others' needs allowed several Givers to divert their attention from their own pain. If they couldn't get around, they used the phone or e-mail. Givers are very relationship-oriented people, and some of them reported that strengthening their relationship with God was a big help to them.

## CHALLENGES FOR THE GIVERS

Twos pride themselves on giving to others, while projecting the image of not needing help themselves. Consequently, asking for help (or even accepting it) is one of their biggest challenges.

WILL, 56, who injured his back in an elevator fall, recalled:

> *What's hard for someone like me is when you have a can-do attitude in life and suddenly everything changes. I was so used to saying, "I can do that, everything's okay, that I was my own worst enemy. People asked, "How are you doing today?" and I'd say, "Fine." I didn't know how to communicate. If the doctor says, "How are you doing?" and the patient answers, "Fine," the doctor has to realize that the patient was responding socially, not medically. Also, if I recognized that the doctor wasn't having a good day, I'd find myself trying to cheer her up instead of thinking about myself.*

**DENISE:**

> *Because I'm very strong, it's very hard for me to be unable to do what I used to. I get very angry, not at myself, but just anger and frustration that I can't do what I want to. I was always the one who helped everyone. Everyone was used to seeing me able to help. I shouldn't have to depend on anyone. I wouldn't want people to think I'm a failure or can't handle it myself. It's hard for me to receive help. I don't deserve it.*

Givers' biggest challenge is asking for or even accepting help. Their identity is based on giving and they—consciously or unconsciously—feel pride at having no needs while being essential to others. Deep down, however, Givers believe that the way to get love is to give, so even though they don't want to ask for help, they would like others to somehow know that they need assistance. They may think, "Why aren't people helping me? After all I've done for others, people *should* be helping me." On the other hand, if they are unable to help other people, they may feel they don't deserve other people's assistance. Many Givers, in fact, don't even recognize their own feelings and their own needs. And if they do, their pride keeps them from asking for help. Health care providers and friends of Givers need to be aware of Givers' tendency to turn attention to the other person, and they need to bring the focus back to the needs of the Giver.

### LESSONS GIVERS LEARNED

**LEILA,** 33 years old, who has chronic pelvic pain:

> *When I was younger, I always felt I wanted to be accepted, to be needed. I tend to be a doormat for people. They can always rely on me to help them, but when I need something, sometimes they're not there for me. It can hurt. I don't feel comfortable asking for help. I don't want to bother people; I'd rather do it myself than bother someone else. I keep my feelings to myself. I used to keep a journal. Now I let my feelings out with my husband and close friend. I need to talk about things. I'm more emotional.*

A lesson Givers need to learn in better handling their chronic pain is to be more open with others about their feelings and their needs. Givers search for love through giving. When chronic pain puts their own needs on the front burner, Givers face their primary paradox: They are focused on giving, but are very uncomfortable receiving help, and as a result they deprive others of the same opportunities [to give] that they constantly seek themselves. Several Givers reported having learned that other people were very willing to help, and that they felt supported when others helped them.

## How Others Can Help the Giver

HANNAH had a brain tumor and still has chronic pain in her head:

*When I agree to babysit my grandson, it would help if my family could bring him to my house instead of me driving over there. It would help if they'd have me take him for fewer hours at a time, because I get exhausted. But of course, I haven't asked them to do this. . . .*

Based on Givers' past behavior, others may come to expect them to have no needs and to be able to handle everything by themselves. That's why Twos want others to understand that they really do have pain and need help. What makes it hard for others to understand that the Giver's ability to give is limited, is that Twos are reluctant to state their needs. They want others to understand without being told. An important lesson they need to learn is to spell it out.

TULA, a 47-year-old woman with long-term abdominal pain related to Crohn's disease, describes herself as someone who wants to make people happy and likes to care for others. "Relationships are the most important thing in my life," she asserts. At the same time, she admits that others tell her she doesn't take care of herself as she should. Her advice to other Givers is:

*Seek help, especially for the emotional effects of being ill. Don't try to do it yourself. At times I tried to do it alone, and you can't; you need strong support from your family or someone else.*

LEILA, who has chronic pelvic pain:

*Share your problem with people. I tried to hide it for a long time, because I thought it was a weakness to be sick, that people would think less of me. I still feel somewhat that way. I'd shut people out. I recommend that you let them help you and become part of the solution.*

Givers may need assistance recognizing that it's okay for them to ask for help, and that others, just like themselves, can feel good by giving. Some patients were able to ask for help by reframing it as a way to ultimately help others. Eventually, however, they need to learn to focus on themselves *for* themselves instead of just in order to be able ultimately to better help others. A good strategy for a counselor or other person working with a Two is to suggest that you "Treat yourself as your own best friend." A good question to the Giver is "If your best friend were in this situation, what would you encourage your friend to do?"

Givers can get very prideful in resisting asking for help. Counselors need to respect their position and pride. Twos need encouragement not to distract themselves by helping others, and reassurance that they themselves deserve to get their own needs met.

Givers who wallow in resentment and who blame others for not helping them need encouragement to take responsibility for helping themselves, including asking others to help them. The best way for Twos to "get back" at a particularly unhelpful person whom they resent is to move on with their lives.

## Type Three: The Achiever
### HOW THE ACHIEVERS' STRENGTHS HAVE HELPED THEM COPE
ERIC, a 56-year-old retired high-level military officer:

> I was the oldest child in my family, and I was a "third parent" to my younger sister. Performance got me approval in childhood. I was always independent. I participated in many sports—track, wrestling—and I was a National Merit Scholarship finalist. In college I had part-time jobs, and then I joined the military. Work was the most important thing in my life. I liked active vacations, like skiing. I relaxed by working on my finances— I invested for fun. I read only nonfiction books. It was hard for me to express my feelings.

In the midst of a successful career, Eric developed abdominal pain, but he waited until it was excruciating to see a doctor, because he feared the impact on his career—he couldn't be a leader of people if he was disabled. By the time he sought medical help, he required major surgery, developed chronic pain, fatigue, and weakness, and eventually was forced to retire. Although his wife is very supportive, Eric still finds it difficult to tell her—or anyone—that he's in pain. But over several years, he came to terms with his limitations:

*At first I was severely depressed, because I couldn't do anything except deal with my medical issues. . . . I've had to change my expectations for myself: I can't go back to skiing or skydiving or running.*

*Now I spend a lot of time evaluating portfolios for my friends and family. These days I'm doing more around the house because my wife is ill. I don't feel as good about myself as I used to, but I'm thinking about a new hobby—woodworking. It feels very good that I can do things for my wife; she did a lot for me for so long.*

Eric's case demonstrates how much it takes to get Achievers to their knees. Their initial response is often to ignore the problem, to try to continue their previous activities despite the pain. When they are finally forced to stop, their self-esteem is likely to suffer because they are no longer able to earn love through professional accomplishments. Eric has been able to find self-esteem in more sedentary activities that are valued by his friends and family and by keeping himself busy with productive pursuits. Initially depressed, he became more accepting of his limitations by changing his expectations.

DEBORAH, a 57-year-old school administrator who is still working full-time despite years of progressive back pain:

*I do yoga, take warm baths, sometimes use ice, drink herbal tea, and I take walks to get past it. I use everything I can get my hands on to learn how to deal with it. I've learned more about myself, that I have a strong and positive character. My work is with children. I can turn my problem into compassion for people who suffer, and also to let them know that you can do something about it.*

The strengths Achievers bring to their recovery from their medical problems include their tenacity and goal-orientation, their problem-solving skills, and their positive attitude. They described being active participants in their rehabilitation and in searching for solutions.

## The Challenges for Achievers

The biggest challenge for Achievers is the adverse effect of their chronic pain on their ability to be successful.

**Valerie,** a 51-year-old former TV producer, now disabled with fibromyalgia:

> *When I quit my job, I lost my identity. I fulfilled my needs through my work, because people loved my work. My work brought me love and gratification. I only took vacations that were related to my work—I barely could get my mind off work. The fibromyalgia interrupted my work. I had to skip work. I was always afraid to lose my job. I used up all my vacation and sick time and struggled to go to work. When I had to quit work, I felt worthless.*

**Hillary,** 60, works full-time despite leg pain:

> *Some days I'd be better off lying down and getting relief, but I don't because I don't want to give up control. I never tell people—I rarely complain . . . I think that if I do less, they'll admire me less.*

It's important for Achievers to maintain an image of success, and sometimes doing so exacts a high price from them. They are likely to keep going, covering up their pain, until they absolutely cannot continue. As long as they're able to do this, they may find themselves unsympathetic to the physical complaints of others. They don't ask for help, because admitting they need it will destroy the image that is so important to them.

## Lessons Achievers Have Learned

**Helen,** a retired physician with chronic headaches:

> *A lot of my self-esteem came from my work. Now it's from my friends. I still have all the friends I had before. None of my friends cared as much about my accomplishments as about the person I am. Even my ex-husband wrote me a nice letter outlining all my positive characteristics, and he said I still have all those except for my job. Also I have two very good friends who are also disabled. They were also successful women. We help each other.*

TERESA, an outgoing Achiever whose focus was always her home and family:

*I'd have 20 or 30 friends over, and I'd do all the cooking. I sewed almost all my clothes—I'd start in the morning and have it done by afternoon. My friends thought of me as someone who was always going. My house was immaculate. I was also self-employed—my husband had a business, and I scheduled calls and did book work. I separated my personal life from my business. I felt if I let my emotions take over, I couldn't get my work done. I've always been in control of my emotions.*

*One of the most difficult things [after the back pain started] for me was to learn my limitations. I had to set up my priorities. I can deal with it now, but the first 3 to 4 years I was very angry. I used to be a stickler for a shiny kitchen floor. Now I have to be content with just a light mopping. I've had to learn the Serenity Prayer.*

Teresa still gets her self-esteem from doing the best job she can for her family, but she's been able to come to terms with her disability by changing her definition of success.

VALERIE, the former TV producer, joined a 12-step group (a self-help program based on Alcoholics Anonymous) for her eating disorder and experienced a "spiritual awakening":

*I've gotten a closer relationship with God. It came as a real blessing to me as I realized I'm not going to get better. For the first 2 years that I was on disability I was very depressed, but now I feel more like a normal person. I have more time to learn to be who I am, to talk with God, to talk with people about what's happened to me. I have more time to get in touch with my inner self. I don't think I knew my feelings before. I didn't think about feelings. Now it's second nature. I don't feel like "poor me" so much. Workaholic that I am, I believe I'll do something one day to help people—maybe write something.*

*I have a wonderful boyfriend who's really caring, and I have my dog. I have the relationship I've always wanted, and I don't even work. God took away what I thought was my most important relationship—with my work—and I found what I really wanted.*

The chief lesson that Achievers with chronic pain need to learn is to let go of their image of success, to become more authentic and to recognize their limitations. They also need to find other ways to meet their self-esteem needs.

## HOW OTHERS CAN HELP THE ACHIEVER

Each personality type sets up expectations about their behavior in relationship to other people, but is then distressed when others continue to have these same expectations of them. For Achievers, their friends and family have seen them as active go-getters, and sometimes find it hard to realize that the Three can no longer accomplish as much. Threes want understanding and compassion from others.

### VALERIE:

*The best thing they can do is ask me every once in a while, "How are you feeling?" I want them just to acknowledge I have this problem. When I'm not functioning well, when I'm tired, instead of saying something derogatory, they should say, "You've been running and running. You need to take care of yourself. Get some rest." Some of my friends don't understand if we're on vacation together that I can't join them in all-day activities. The hardest thing about this disease is that people don't understand.*

### HILLARY:

*My friends could help by not expecting as much from me. Christmas was really hard. I've been trying for 2 years to say, "I can't do all this baking— I can't stand so long." I don't just lie around, so maybe they don't realize I need to do less. This year my husband said I should do less, but I still ended up doing everything. Then I get angry and I need more pain medicine. I think that if I do less, they'll admire me less.*

Part of the reason that friends and fellow workers continue to have unrealistic expectations of disabled Achievers is that Threes want to look good and look successful, so they find it hard to accept and admit their limitations. Achievers need to first recognize and accept that they can no longer do everything they did before, and then admit and explain their limitations to their friends and family. This, of course, is not easy for them.

## ACHIEVERS' ADVICE TO OTHER ACHIEVERS

VALERIE, 51, the former TV producer, said:

*Your life has changed. You may not be able to do your work, but it's not the end of the world; you can still have a life. Talk to people who've gone through it. You can be happy. If in the past you got your self-worth from your work, you can now get plenty of self-worth from realizing what you go through with your disease, and getting through it.*

**HELEN,** the physician who had to retire because of migraine headaches, said:
*I would suggest to them to start thinking about broadening their interests, activities, and hobbies. If sports and other physical activities were very important to them, they need to develop less physically demanding hobbies—sewing, knitting, reading, and other constructive activities. They need to develop their friendships.*

**HILLARY,** whose chronic leg pain following an injury hasn't stopped her from working, advised:
*You can have pain, but it doesn't have to have you. Don't give in to it to the point that you can't enjoy life. Even if you're somewhat limited, it doesn't mean you can't be happy and productive. Read about the problem. Do whatever you need to do medically to improve your condition. But fighting it every day is not the answer; at some point you need to accept it, recognize that it's part of your life, not expect it to go away. I was so busy trying to find what it was and getting rid of it that it became an obsession, and I didn't pay attention to anything else.*

The biggest challenge for Threes whose lives are limited by chronic pain is how to maintain their self-esteem when they can no longer win love through their professional accomplishments. Early on, Achievers report feeling a loss of self-esteem, accompanied by anger and/or depression. Achievers who were able to overcome these feelings did so by:
- Ramping down their definition of success in light of their limitations. This can include working part-time, getting a more sedentary job, or developing projects at home that keep them busy and accomplishing things.
- Redefining their priorities. One example is developing their relationship with their family, an area that is often neglected by Achievers. Another is beginning to pay attention to their own needs and to work on personal growth.

Other helpful strategies for Achievers included:
- Harnessing the strengths of their type—positive outlook, goal-orientation, and energy—toward active participation in their diagnosis, treatment, and physical exercise.
- Forming a support system that includes others who have had similar experiences, and talking with these other people about their feelings.
- Willingness to explain their limitations to friends and colleagues, and to ask for help when needed.
- Developing a spiritual life. This means that instead of relying only on their own abilities to achieve their goals, they are helped by developing a connection with other people and with a higher power and allow themselves to be helped by such resources outside of themselves.

Seeing a psychologist or counselor can be very helpful to an Achiever if he or she is willing to look inward, recognize and focus on feelings, and stay with the process. Threes in therapy often come "to get their tires rotated and drive away"—in other words, they seek the quick solution that will give them a course of action to take. Seeing a psychologist or counselor can be very helpful to an Achiever if she is willing to look inward, recognize and focus on her feelings, and stay with the process.

## Type Four: The Romantic

BRENDA, an introverted 40-year-old with a 20-year history of fibromyalgia and chronic fatigue:

*I was a very sensitive child who absorbed the negative or positive energy that was around me. Sadness has played a large role in my life. I'd have times of depression and hopelessness. I was labeled the creative one. I went to Europe dancing in a ballet company. When I came home at age 20, I developed severe neck and back pain. Eventually, I could hardly get out of bed.*

*When I help friends, I can help them feel better, but I can take on their emotions and feel worse. When I watch the news, I can put myself in the people's situation and feel what they feel.*

*Beauty and art are very important to me. I need beautiful surroundings. I love paintings.*

*I'm a very private person. When I'm out, I can be perky, but it takes a lot of energy and I prefer being alone. To feel better, I need lots of quiet time alone. I need to be alone to be creative. I write, draw.*

*What has helped me is that I can still go on and have my dreams. As a child living through all the fighting in my family, I was very emotional, but I persevered. I still have a positive attitude. Children and animals love me; they've helped me not complain. I don't complain to people about how I feel.*

## HOW THE STRENGTHS OF ROMANTICS HELPED THEM COPE

KATHARINE, an active 47-year-old Romantic with a history of child abuse, depression, and years of abdominal pain and problems related to inflammatory bowel disease; she has worked hard all her life, and currently works in a group home while caring for a disabled son:

*I enjoy working with the people I'm working with now. It makes me feel good inside because these people enjoy seeing me. One homeless man kept waving at me. People just want to be acknowledged. I saw the recognition in him and I waved back. Before, the busier I kept, the less I thought about things and the more I thought I was avoiding the pain. I was nearly killing myself by working so hard to make money. Now I've been doing more thinking and dealing with my issues.*

Romantics can be very strong, very persevering people, who can apply their perseverance to dealing with their chronic pain. For some of them, their familiarity with suffering makes them better able to cope with pain. Relationships—having understanding people in their lives—can also help them heal. As Katharine said, the greatest desire of Romantics is to be truly "seen," to be understood. I recently asked a healthy Romantic what strengths she thought might help her cope if she developed chronic pain. Her reply: "I think I might cope better than other people, because I know how to do pain—I've done it for much of my life."

## THE CHALLENGES FOR ROMANTICS

WINONA, a 59-year-old introverted retired social worker, loves to write poetry and has struggled for years with chronic muscle and joint pain:

*I have a very low tolerance for pain—sensitive people probably do. We feel things so strongly. I need quite a bit of time alone, but not as much as I now have. The worst part of my situation is the social isolation. I don't have the energy to go out. I haven't been on a date in 2 years. I can't concentrate on writing poetry. I don't go out and ask for the support and love I need. I feel very alone. I'm not getting what I need emotionally. I feel a bitterness and anger I've never had before.*

LINDSAY, a 36-year-old woman, has undergone multiple surgical procedures during years of endometriosis-related pelvic pain:

*Because I'm very sensitive and emotional, I get my feelings hurt. Many people don't know what to say, and they say things that hurt: "Oh, you look good, so you must be feeling better." They have no idea how bad I'm feeling. Or they say, "Take this herb." They're offering medical advice, but they don't know. They don't see me struggling, they don't know the real me.*

*My husband, my mother, and my best friend are the only ones I let see me when I'm down and out .... I used to think people would think less of me if I were sick, that it's a defect. I still feel that way somewhat.*

KATHARINE:

*When I get really stressed out, I close in on myself. I don't call people back, I don't go out. No one has listened to me anyway. No one really wants to hear your problems. I'm a great listener to other people's problems. Sometimes all I need is to be able to vent, but if people keep telling you to shut up, how can you vent?*

Unfulfilled dreams, depression, and difficulty asking for what they need are the major challenges for Romantics. Abandonment is another huge issue. For some, like Winona, the social abandonment her illness has created is undoubtedly stirring up previous feelings of abandonment.

Romantics are caught in a difficult double bind. As another Romantic told me, "Fours are very concerned with identity, and having your identity be a sick person rather than an artist is potentially devastating." Lindsay, above, expressed her concern that others would see her illness as a "defect." As a result, Romantics are motivated to hide their illness from all but close friends. Many lead a double life: In public, they continue to be as active and achieving as they can manage, while in private life the loss and sadness crashes in on them.

The dilemma for the Romantic is that on the one hand, they want to maintain their artist image in public, which keeps them from admitting their limitations; on the other hand, they seek to be really known and understood. When Lindsay's effort to project a healthy image was successful and she was told, "You look good so you must be feeling better," she didn't feel understood; she felt demeaned and perceived as ordinary, as though her friend were saying, "Cheer up, you'll get over it." Romantics don't want to be cheered up; they want to be seen where they're really at.

Another challenge for Romantics is their perfectionism. They tend to be as critical of themselves as are Ones (Perfectionists). It is difficult for them when their pain prevents them from living up to their own expectations.

Finally, Fours have an intimate understanding of sadness and depression. It is easy for them to fall into a black hole of hopelessness.

## LESSONS ROMANTICS HAVE LEARNED
### WINONA:

*I've become much better at requesting help than I ever was before. I can be sensitive and compassionate to myself. I used to push myself and then get sick; now I've learned to treat myself the way that, as a social worker, I used to tell people to treat others.*

Romantics have a tendency to be self-absorbed. Being helpful to others, both people and animals, helps them to get out of their own dark hole. Empathizing with others, listening to them, and doing things for them, can help Romantics feel better.

This was echoed by **LINDSAY,** who related:

*I probably wouldn't be as feeling for people as I am now. I'm a lot more empathetic to others. I can relate better. I'm a better listener, a more caring person.*

## HOW OTHERS CAN HELP ROMANTICS
**SERENA,** a psychotherapist and a Romantic, has been through major illnesses in her own life:

*What Romantics need more than anything else is to be showered with understanding and empathy. That is so important, feeling understood! No one can solve our problems, but if the people trying were aware that they could certainly help alleviate pain with good listening skills, it would simplify their lives, too. A sick person can be a real pain to live with. But the*

*depression, the manipulative gloom, can be lifted amazingly easily if the
friend or spouse makes the decision to sit down and listen. Reflective
listening, mirroring, really listening, and letting the sick person know
you're understanding, is invaluable. A few times a day would be wonderful if it's someone you live with. End with "How can I help?"*

*Understanding and genuine compliments can work miracles. I'd say,
"I'm impressed with how well you're handling this problem. A lot of people would be totally defeated and depressed. While I know you do feel
both of those from time to time, you're still plugging away, trying to get
better. Emotionally you must feel like you've been run over by a fire
engine, and you're in intensive care with every bone in your body crushed.
No wonder you're hurting! Anyone would be. At least pat yourself on the
back at how strong you are in your desire to feel good again. You know
you're doing the very best you can, and with that kind of determination,
you're sure to see improvement. I know it's discouraging that it doesn't
happen as quickly as you want it to. I wish I could give you a magic pill
that would make that happen." A Romantic hearing that kind of understanding and encouragement would feel an appreciable rise in self-esteem
and a proportionate lessening of fatigue and pain.*

Romantics appreciate a positive, optimistic attitude, as long as it's not
patronizing, preachy, or insistent on particular solutions. Adventurers
(Type Seven) have it just right: They can stand shoulder to shoulder with
the Romantic, empathizing and encouraging, without blaming the
Romantic for their sadness, never advising them to get over it and put
on a happy face, and don't insist on optimism and solutions.

## ROMANTICS' ADVICE TO OTHER ROMANTICS
A 30-YEAR-OLD WOMAN, interviewed a year before her death from colon
cancer, advised other Romantics on how to handle the simultaneous need
to project a good public image while obtaining needed support:

*Go easy on yourself. You don't need to tell the whole world about your pain,
but have a small group of confidants whom you can tell, who will just listen
without trying to make you seek additional, possibly unnecessary medical care
because they can't handle knowing you are in pain. If your pain waxes and
wanes, and if you feel hopeless when it gets worse, keep reminding yourself
that it has gotten better before and it will get better again.*

WINONA:

> *Don't allow your illness to totally define your personality. Don't keep reminders: I keep my pillbox out of sight. Don't make your home look like a hospital room.*

One of the challenges for Romantics is to maintain their connections despite their pain and limited lifestyle. They feel their losses deeply, want to be really understood and comforted, but have difficulty letting others in because of their desire to project a unique and attractive public image. Romantics' advice to other Fours on dealing with their ongoing pain focused more on having empathetic friends, and less on taking action. A listening ear and permission to vent are indeed crucial to them. But so is involvement in the real world—helping others and taking action for themselves.

Fours' trap is to fall into isolation and self-absorption. They need to avoid developing a sense of specialness through having their illness. They can get caught in endless research designed to uncover a unique or special cure for their disorder. They need to look for ordinary, practical solutions. They need to create structure for themselves—a plan, a regimen of exercise, physical activity, meetings with friends, and follow-through in a disciplined way. Structure *is* ordinary, but it will help.

## *Type Five: The Observer*

WALTER (see beginning of chapter 5), a 32-year-old former computer programmer now on disability because of chronic pain that began as repetitive stress injury to his hands:

> *As a child, I was a loner. I spent a lot of time in my room on the computer or reading science fiction or doing math puzzles. I liked playing the piano and playing chess on the computer. I had a hard time in college, because I was socially clueless.*
>
> *Privacy is very important to me. Being alone is easier than being with people, although it makes me lonely. Interacting with people is stressful; being alone is not. The thinking side of me questions and doubts, because I have a lot of fears. I don't like conflict, and prefer to walk away from it. It takes a lot for me to get angry, but when I do, I do it very strongly.*

*Before finding a doctor who was willing to provide enough pain medication for me, I had several very difficult years. Now that I have a life again, I am feeling much more optimistic. Recently, I applied to graduate school and have begun playing the piano again.*

*What helped me cope the most was my intensity, by which I mean an inner strength in adversity. I'm naturally a problem-solver, and I have an unwillingness to give up.*

Like Walter, other Observers tend to isolate but have a hunger to connect with others. They are natural problem-solvers and are very determined. They tend to get sidetracked with minutiae, but when they get on track, they are very effective. Other typical characteristics of Observers are their impatience with incompetence, and their ability to block out pain through mental processes (mind over matter).

## How Observers' Strengths Helped Them Cope

BETTY, 48, gave up her job after developing a painful bladder disorder, interstitial cystitis:

*Once I've made up my mind about something, I follow through. For example, one day three years ago I said, "This is my last cigarette," and I never smoked again. Also, my imagination, my mind, has helped. I imagine that good things are possible, that one day this problem won't be here and I will be able to do things.*

GEORGE, 55, describes himself as shy and reclusive most of the time, but in fact he has a thriving practice as a psychologist and has used hypnosis to help many people who have chronic pain. Following a car accident 4 years ago, he developed severe neck pain and headaches, which still have a significant impact on his life. An Observer, he uses thinking to cope with exacerbations of his pain:

*Instead of reacting emotionally, I talk to myself. I say, let it go, it's only temporary, it will pass.*

The strengths that help Observers cope include determination, stoicism, problem-solving skills, and the ability to distract themselves mentally.

## THE CHALLENGES OF THE OBSERVER TYPE
### WALTER:

*It's hard for me to ask for help, because of my fear. It's the same fear I have when talking to people. I'm afraid of their judgment, of them thinking negatively of me, that they'll think I'm too demanding.*

### BETTY:

*It's hard for me to trust people. My social anxiety keeps me at home, and makes me more aware of my pain problem.*

Although Observers tend to behave as though they are out of touch with their feelings, they are actually very sensitive people who are easily overwhelmed. They are sensitive to criticism. They have very permeable boundaries, meaning that they experience the world as invasive; their only defense is to retreat. Self-sufficiency is a very strong characteristic of Observers, which makes it difficult for them to ask for help.

## LESSONS OBSERVERS HAVE LEARNED
### WALTER:

*One of the positive outcomes of my chronic pain situation has been an increased confidence in my ability to handle change. In the past, I tended to get stuck by obstacles and run away from them. But being in a situation like my pain, where I couldn't do that, allowed me to find the strength to overcome them. For example, in the past I was very afraid to travel because there were so many unknowns. I was afraid that something terrible would happen, and I'd freak out and couldn't deal with it. But having gone through the experience of being constantly in situations and being overwhelmed, I learned what my basic needs were and how to meet them, and that gave me the confidence to travel.*

### PENNY, a former teacher:

*I can now understand other people's pain better. I'm stronger in dealing with it. Once I take my medication, I get very involved in things and when my mind is busy, then I don't think about the pain.*

Observers, who tend to be isolated people, report increased compassion for and empathy with other people. They also gained experience in coping with difficult situations.

## How Others Can Help the Observer
WALTER:

*I want them to be present with me, to not let me suffer alone. I often feel that people don't give me enough emotional support. If I'm doing well they want to hang out with me, but if I'm not, they don't want to have to deal with the problem.*

PENNY:

*Just being there—letting me vent when I need to. Offering to help me physically, since I don't like to ask for help.*

Like other personality types, Observers want to be understood, listened to, and believed. People assume that Observers don't really need anyone or don't need emotional support because they are generally so self-sufficient and in their heads. When Observers are suffering, however, they may welcome people being nearby to give them emotional support.

## Observer's Advice to Other Observers
NANCY:

*Ask for help sooner. Don't just grit your teeth. Also, it helps to use other techniques. If the pain increases, do self-calming to deal with the panic that comes with pain. Having a pet, having someone else to take care of, helps. I like to be alone, but not totally alone. A dog gives you unconditional love.*

Getting out of oneself and caring for another person—or an animal—is an excellent strategy for Observers. A pet can alleviate loneliness while making few demands. As for "other techniques," meditation and other self-calming techniques can quiet the Observer's active mind, fear, and tendency to intellectualize everything. A sense of humor, supportive friends, and awareness of the good things in one's life are all highly recommended by Observers. For those who find it hard to socialize, joining a support group on the Internet is an excellent way of overcoming isolation and finding support.

As for knowing about one's illness, some knowledge is definitely good, but it's easy for the Observer to turn the research into an endless project, an intellectual exercise. Some fall into the trap of becoming hypochondriacal—they may look up everything about their disorder on the Internet and then take on all those symptoms.

Distraction is a good coping mechanism for everyone, but can be particularly effective for Observers, who enjoy being involved in intellectual pursuits. This is a natural approach for them, but the trap is that it can lead them down the wrong path—away from their body and their feelings.

Equally useful is for Observers to get out of their heads. One way is meditation, which teaches them to get away from constant thoughts. Another way is to get into their bodies. Physical activity—walking, massage, stretching exercises, or whatever their pain allows them to do—will help them feel better both physically and emotionally.

Because their perceived world is one of scarcity, Observers find it hard to indulge themselves. Watching movies, taking hot baths, participating in nonproductive enjoyable activities—all these will help them feel better.

Their overarching emphasis on self-sufficiency makes it hard for Observers to ask for help. Even harder is to share their feelings with others. Learning to do so will help them feel supported.

The need to be in control is another huge obstacle for Observers. When they get angry, it is often about feeling out of control. Spiritual growth for the Observer includes letting go of control and giving it into the hands of a higher power.

Finally, it is helpful to Observers to get out of themselves by learning to be generous of spirit. Give to others—help a neighbor, do volunteer work.

## Type Six: The Detective

In chapter 12, you learned that understanding the Detective can be a little harder than other types because Sixes have two very different ways of dealing with their fear. The assertive, at times aggressive, way that Counterphobic Sixes handle their core belief that the world is a very fearful place, makes them seem very different from Phobic Sixes. The latter tend to placate others and seek a protector to keep them safe. To give you a flavor of the two approaches—and their underlying similarities—here are descriptions of two patients.

MICHAEL, 63, a retired Army officer who has chronic neck and shoulder pain:
*As a young man I was constantly angry; my wife has helped me to control my temper, but I still get upset at other drivers. My family—my wife,*

*six children, and many grandchildren—are the focal point of my life. I have a strong belief in God and Christ. All my life I've strived for financial security.*

*I'm a stay-at-home person, an introvert, uncomfortable in large groups. My wife says I'm a very negative person. I often sit around worrying about things, such as what if something would happen to the kids. It's hard for me to trust others. Someone has to prove themselves beyond a doubt for me to trust. If you expect the worst of people, you'll never be disappointed.*

*I have a hard time making decisions. I look at all the alternatives, and it takes me forever to decide. Yes, this was a handicap in the Army. So was my problem with authority figures. I resented being told what to do. I just didn't have any respect for authority. I expressed my opinion, and I always questioned. This got me in trouble a few times. I always sympathized with the underdog—I felt I was one of them.*

GRACE, a divorced 58-year-old woman, works as a house cleaner:

*I have extreme fear that can go into terror. A lot of time I fear I'm in a war zone and I have to be hypervigilant. I'm always checking people for cues, to know what they're about. Authority figures can be terrifying to me. At times, I've gotten into their face, but mostly I want to blend in and not make any waves. I'm loyal to a fault—in relationships and at work. Sometimes I let people walk over me. If I feel betrayed—for example if someone was dishonest with me—I feel crushed. It's very easy for me to think of worst-case scenarios; I think they're really going to happen.*

*I have an over-the-top need for safety and security. I like to have structure. I like to know where I'm going and with whom. I scan the environment for danger and I scan people's faces. Am I safe physically and emotionally?*

*For the past 15 years, I've had intermittent severe pain in my joints and muscles. If I catch a cold or get a sinus infection, I develop excruciating pain in my jaws and eyes. This happens to me several times a year, unpredictably. My doctor can fit in only two patients per day on an urgent basis. So I worry, "Am I going to be able to get in to see the doctor if I get this pain?"*

*What makes it hard for me to cope is that I go right to the worst-case scenario. How will I survive? How will I pay the bills?*

Michael and Grace are very different, but both are very loyal, find it hard to trust people, have difficulty with authority figures, and are worriers who tend to see the glass half empty rather than half full and to expect the worst. Both are hard workers. Counterphobic Michael, however, has difficulty controlling his anger, tends to get into people's faces with his views, is fiercely independent, and in his youth was a risk taker. Phobic Grace is much more compliant, less likely to confront others, and seems to have fewer strategies for managing her fears, which are constantly in the forefront of her thinking.

## HOW THE DETECTIVES' STRENGTHS HELPED THEM COPE

MICHAEL, the retired Army officer:

*I can still help other people. When a friend needed help moving, I didn't think about the pain while helping him. When I do what I enjoy, I have less pain.*

JENNIFER, a married 34-year-old who developed fibromyalgia 2 years ago:

*I'm persistent. That helped me find the treatment and help that I needed when I wasn't getting it from my regular doctor. Since I'm loyal, I still think she's an excellent doctor, but I kept searching.*

Detectives' persistence makes them persevere in finding solutions. Their dutifulness helps them follow through with the treatment plans, and their questioning nature means that if something doesn't make sense to them, or isn't helping, they will let the doctor know and seek a different path.

## THE CHALLENGES FOR THE DETECTIVES

NELSON, 26, an outgoing, personable, and very polite young man, is married and the father of three children. The veteran of multiple injuries and multiple surgeries related to past high-risk activities such as rodeo bull-riding, he already has osteoarthritis in his neck and back, and chronic back pain:

*I'm still working on being able to ask outsiders for help. I'm better in asking my family—my wife and my kids. I was conditioned not to let on about my weaknesses; when you're a cowboy, you don't expose your weaknesses. Now I live a different lifestyle, and I don't need to have that mentality. But I still don't trust people and I'll never expose myself to danger and risks.*

URI, 49, was a stubborn and headstrong rebellious risk-taker in his youth. He raced motorcycles, played football in high school, and drove his cars fast. After suffering for the past 5 years with peripheral neuropathic pain secondary to diabetes, his life is very different:

*It's hard for me to talk to doctors. I say, "Everything's fine," when it isn't. In my own mind I was invincible, and I didn't want to tell anyone I wasn't. Now I'm trying to be more open. If you don't tell the doctors, they can't help you.*

Counterphobic Detectives are extremely reluctant to ask for help. This is based partly on their unwillingness to impose on others, but also because of their fierce independence as well as their distrust of others' intentions. They may find it hard to state their concerns even to a physician or nurse because they don't want to appear weak. Phobic Sixes, in contrast, have less difficulty asking help of those they trust. In fact, they are one of the very few enneagram types for whom asking for help is easy. However, they may fear questioning authority even when it's appropriate, so they have difficulty advocating for themselves.

## LESSONS DETECTIVES HAVE LEARNED
NELSON:

*I've learned a lot about myself physically. I've become stronger mentally. I was raised with "If you have pain, you stick it out." But with this pain, you can't. I ended up in the hospital by ignoring it. So I've learned you have to ask for help. I've learned not to be so hardheaded and independent.*

JENNIFER:

*I'm more tolerant of people and less demanding of people in terms of my expectations of them. I'm less judgmental of others. I'm also less fearful of people and less afraid of conflict. Taking Paxil [paroxetine, an SSRI antidepressant that is also effective against anxiety] has really helped, especially in social situations. I'm not as sensitive to everything going on around me. It's easier to relax and feel that people are just people. Before, I was constantly worried about what they were thinking of me or that they were judging me negatively.*

> *I joined a support group in my church for people with chronic illness.
> I write in my journal, and I talk with my husband a lot about feelings.*

Jennifer's fears about being judged by others, her anxiety in social situations, and her constant worries about what others are thinking are very typical of Phobic Sixes. The adverse effect of this keeps Detectives isolated. The use of Paxil, and some positive self-talk, allowed Jennifer to benefit from a support group.

## HOW OTHERS CAN HELP DETECTIVES
MICHAEL:

> *I think my kids believe I'm using my pain as a crutch, to avoid doing home projects. It would help if they understood that I'm not using this as an excuse. I was always a good provider. I'm really ashamed that I've given in to this.*

Detectives have a tendency to question other people's motives. Understandably, they project this quality onto others, and assume that others will doubt the reality of their disease. Others can help Detectives by reassuring them that they are believed.

The big issue for Detectives who struggle with chronic pain is trust. Their fear of others' underlying motivations and the desire to find safety and security can cause them to isolate at the very time that they most need to include other people in their lives and to ask for their help. Counterphobic Sixes believe there is safety in their own strength, so they are reluctant to admit their vulnerability. At the same time that they are reluctant to admit their limitations, the most common type of support that Sixes want from their family and friends is the understanding that they really cannot do the things they used to be able to do and would like to be able to do. Detectives who spoke about the lessons they'd learned emphasized asking for help, talking about their problems with others, and avoiding isolation. Phobic Sixes, on the other hand, are very willing to ask for help from those they trust. In a way, they see themselves as small children who need a protector. After they find him or her, they are comfortable making their needs known.

Detectives commonly become isolated and depressed when they are not well. The goal for Sixes is to overcome their distrust and develop courage—which, in the case of Counterphobic Sixes living with chronic pain, is the courage to turn to others. This is the best way for them to get both physical and emotional relief.

### DETECTIVES' ADVICE TO OTHER DETECTIVES
Sixes' main difficulty is trust. Not surprisingly, then, their advice to other Sixes focused on overcoming fear and learning to trust.

GRIFFIN, a 49-year-old Counterphobic Six with chronic neck pain, suggested:

> *Try to stand up straight and make yourself do things, and not just give up. Trust the doctors and work with them. Accept that there are some limitations to what you can do, but don't stop trying.*

## Type Seven: The Adventurer

TAMARA is a bubbly, outgoing 58-year-old who lives with chronic back and shoulder pain. She is very active in the Alcoholics Anonymous community. Tamara recalls:

> *Drugs and alcohol have always been a part of my life. My mother was an alcoholic. In my twenties, I was a hippie in California, taking acid and turning tricks to make money. I moved a lot. I was open to different lifestyles. I loved adventure. I had lots of life experience. I was outgoing, and I could make people laugh. Rules? I didn't pay attention to them! Later, I spent several years at Synanon [an addiction treatment facility] getting clean and sober, and ended up being their best fund-raiser. I worked as a drug and alcohol counselor for many years. I was well respected. I enjoyed working with people. I'd make them laugh. I'm still the eternal optimist—I always think things will be better.*
>
> *Ten years ago, I developed back and shoulder pain, which still severely limit my activities. When my friends are going somewhere late at night, I'm too tired and in pain. What's helped me cope with it is that I make jokes about it. Other people can identify with me.*

### HOW ADVENTURERS' STRENGTHS HELPED THEM COPE
STEVE, 50 and on Social Security Disability for chronic abdominal pain, can no longer be as active as in his youth:

*Having fun is very important to me. If I couldn't have fun, it wouldn't be worth being around. I used to do a lot of traveling. I used to be the city golf champion. Now I play golf with my father on a regular basis, I play guitar, and I follow the stock market and the world news. A lot of it now is at home. I also take care of my animals—a 2-foot-long lizard, four birds, and an old cat. I don't waste a lot of time getting frustrated—that would just be negative. I'd rather be positive.*

BURT, a 64-year-old retired car dealer, has been slowed down by peripheral neuropathic pain in his legs:

*I've always been a high-energy person. There wasn't time enough to do everything in life I wanted to do. I always had to have a challenge; I did lots of different things. I was a real optimist. I still am. When I catch myself in a negative thought, I take a deep breath and go outside and get fresh air and think positive. I still have a lot of new ideas. I'm about to venture into a whole new project working with my son to renovate old homes.*

Adventurers want to enjoy a busy, fun-filled existence. Their strengths are their optimism and positive attitude, their future-orientation, their determination to have fun, and their creativity in problem-solving and in bringing about their goals. Even when slowed down by chronic pain, they can creatively find fun activities and maintain their optimism.

### CHALLENGES FOR THE ADVENTURER

TROY is an extroverted 50-year-old man who used to be an "excitement junkie." He traveled extensively in his youth, held a series of jobs, and is now retired. He's had many years of abdominal pain related to chronic pancreatitis:

*The worst thing is it's hard to plan things because I don't know how I'm going to feel. I might be having a good time, but then I feel crummy.*

TAMARA:

*I hate the limitations. I have trouble working on my yard. Sometimes I push myself to get something done right away when I should have waited until someone came over to help. It's hard for me to ask for help.*

By nature, Adventurers do their best to avoid pain, whether physical or emotional. They have been called the "monkey mind" because of their tendency to escape into fantasy, mental gymnastics, and endless planning. Adventurers do not like introspection—they prefer planning and action. Their biggest challenge is that when an injury or illness puts a stop to their activities, they are forced to face reality, confront their feelings, and find it harder to enjoy themselves. Sometimes they become very depressed until they can throw themselves into something new that can replace the adventures they can no longer have.

The usual role of Adventurers among their family and friends is to be upbeat and entertaining. They are reluctant to ask for help, because they don't want to seem like wet blankets.

### LESSONS ADVENTURERS HAVE LEARNED
Adventurers tend to be impulsive, to focus more on having a good time and less on other people's needs. Being slowed down by chronic pain can actually make some positive changes in these areas.

### STEVE:
*It's made me more compassionate. It's made me think a little more about pain and about people who have pain, about other people. It's slowed me down and made me think about consequences, about things I wouldn't have thought about before.*

JULIAN, 54, whose severe back pain keeps him horizontal much of the time:
*I used to be very impatient; my lesson in life has been patience. I do yoga, which helps me relax and focus. I get my needs for novelty met by writing music; I'm going to send a package to Eric Clapton. On the Internet, the world is at my fingertips. I get on it about twice a week.*

The biggest lessons that chronic pain taught the Sevens are to be more compassionate toward others (many Adventurers are rather narcissistic), to slow down and become more introspective (to quiet their "monkey mind"), and to find novelty and enjoyment among the activities they are still able to do.

## How Others Can Help the Adventurer

Adventurers don't want to dwell on the negative. Most of them don't want to dissect their feelings; what they *want* from others is action; what some of them *don't want* is any attention brought to their pain. For example, Burt reported, "My family can help me by not ever asking me about my painful feet or how it feels. I don't want to drag them down." Adventurers like their family and friends to do concrete tasks for them rather than inquire about their pain.

As is true for other personality types, Sevens bring about expectations from their friends and family. For Adventurers, it's that they will always be ready for action. One of the ways others can help Adventurers is recognizing that they have changed.

PATTY, whose fibromyalgia limits her activities:
> In the beginning my family encouraged me to take it easier than I did, but some of my friends didn't understand why I didn't want to go out Friday or Saturday night. They used to say, "Come on, once we get there you'll feel better. " I think they've learned over the years to take advantage of the good days, and if I say I don't want to go out, they understand.

TROY:
> Don't be too hard on yourself. Try to keep a sense of humor. Cultivate your family and relationships—they're very important. Have a "never say die" attitude.

MELISSA, a tiny 56-year-old woman who's had multiple operations because of rheumatoid arthritis:
> I'd tell them not to feel sorry for themselves, to learn that they have limitations but can still do some things. Get together with friends. Get a doctor that believes them and believes in them.

JULIAN, a tall 56-year-old man whose hunched-over posture attests to his chronic back pain of 15 years stemming from a car accident:
> Be patient. My lesson in life has been patience. I used to be very impatient. You'll have setbacks and you'll never be the same, but you can get better.

Adventurers are optimistic, enjoy laughter and fun, have a penchant for trying new things, don't like to take no for an answer, and can persevere in searching for solutions. These positive traits can be of great service in enabling them to cope with chronic pain. Adventurers are fun to be around. In relation to others, their script is to entertain and pump up their friends. When they can no longer do so, their friends are understandably disappointed. Adventurers need to let go of the expectation that their job is to uplift their friends—and others need to recognize this, too.

Pain and deprivation are a huge challenge for this group. Limitation is hard for them. Similar to the Achiever (Type Three), Adventurers need to accept their physical limitations and to find other ways to fulfill their need for action. Surfing the Internet, reading, and finding sedentary hobbies may provide enough variety for them to be able to enjoy life.

Adventurers tend to lack follow-through. They need to discipline themselves to do what is recommended and to stick to their treatment, even if it's routine. They also need to get more in touch with their feelings, to become more introspective and let themselves grieve their loss. They need to gain acceptance that they cannot live their previous life and find ways to enjoy their current stage of life.

## Type Eight: The Leader

DAVID, 64 years old, did heavy physical work all his life, until an accident changed everything. He relates:

*When I was young, I was very athletic. I went hunting and fishing, played softball and baseball, and coached Little League. I was definitely a leader—I don't like to follow anybody. I had a quick temper—I'd yell and curse, and then later I'd be sorry. I headed straight for conflict. I was a positive person. I've been married for 42 years—I raised a family with 2 kids, and I never worried much about the future. Working and feeding my family was the most important thing to me. I was a truck driver for a while, then I worked as a smelter for over 40 years. I always used tools and lifted heavy things.*

*That was until I had an accident 4 years ago. I fell off a ladder hitting my back and neck. I've had pain ever since. I can no longer hike or enjoy the country. Even walking hurts. Some days I'm in so much pain that I just sit in a chair and watch TV. I try to blank it out of my mind as much as possible. I think about things I'm going to do—cut the grass, go to the city. I try to keep my mind busy. I never used to worry about health, but I've had so many operations that I worry about my future.*

*I've always done everything for myself. It's very hard for me to ask for help. I only ask my sons. They do everything for me—they take me to the doctor, they bring me home from the hospital. They're very supportive of me.*

*I would tell other people who have chronic pain to stay as busy as possible. Don't dwell on the pain or it'll just get worse.*

David's story demonstrates the strong denial of the Leader. They tend to block out feelings, deny the illness, and exhaust themselves. Leaders prefer to keep moving, to keep busy, to problem solve with action.

### How the Strengths of the Leader Helped Them Cope

KAYLA, 43 years old, has had disabling pain in her left foot for 6 years:
*My strength helped me from giving in to the pain and saying I can't do it anymore. I thought a lot about ending my life, but I thought it was weak and selfish to do so.*

RHONDA, 49, used to be an independent, take-charge person who held a responsible administrative job. Following a medical procedure called an angiogram, she developed reflex sympathetic dystrophy (RSD) in one arm and had to leave her job:
*I come from an alcoholic family. Fifteen years ago I was headed for alcoholism myself and began attending 12-step meetings. I'm glad I was in recovery before this started. Because of my strengths I'm not suicidal and I have confidence that something will work for the pain. I'm still looking ahead and seeing myself getting better. Before the angiogram, I was the independent one, helping others. It's still hard to acknowledge at times that I can't do it alone. But I believe that God doesn't give you more than you can handle, so He must have a lot of confidence in me.*

Note how Rhonda reframes her medical problems: God had confidence in her that she can still be strong and in charge. The strengths of the Eights—their positive outlook, action-orientation, and confidence in their ability to conquer adversity—helps them cope.

## CHALLENGES FOR THE LEADER
### KAYLA:

> *I was very reactive. I got angry a lot when I was really feeling sadness and pain. I was tired all the time, but the pain kept me from sleeping. I felt like a burden a lot. It was hard to ask for help—I wanted to do anything I could for others, but I didn't want help. I considered it weak to ask for help; I wanted to think I didn't need it.*

TOM, 55, was a truck driver until 3 years ago when he injured his foot and underwent several operations and is now on disability. He can hardly wait to get off of his opioid medications so that he can get back to his truck, but pain prevents him from doing so:

> *I've been hurt a lot through the years. I've read* The Power of Positive Thinking *and that helped a lot. In the past, I was able not to take pain pills except for a short time after each injury. It really bothers me now that I can't get off them. It means I'm not strong enough to get through it myself—I've tried to be Mr. Macho all my life. I've had to accept that I have to take the medication [opioids]. I could take more and be more comfortable, but I don't want to.*
>
> *I don't like asking for help; I've never wanted to. I'd rather do it myself. I don't like to admit I'm fallible or weak. It seems weak to have to take pain meds to get around. Sometimes I have to ask my wife to help me get dressed. Knowing that she loves me and won't tell anyone, I do ask her to help me get up or take a shower. But in public I don't want to show my weakness. I'm embarrassed in public because I walk funny. I don't want to have to explain to anyone. I feel like I'm sitting on a foot stool on a big stage and everyone's watching me.*
>
> *My friends don't criticize me, but I feel they think I'm weak. I imagine them thinking, "Why don't you just get up and go to work?"*

Tom's reluctance to take pills emanates from his reluctance to be dominated by anyone or anything—and that includes pain and medications. It's difficult for him to admit his weakness or vulnerability.

The biggest challenge for Leaders, who are used to running the show as well as their bodies, is the loss of control they experience with their chronic pain. They dread appearing weak, yet their need for help shows that they indeed are vulnerable. They can no longer enjoy the abundance of the good things in life, and often they can't even do the simple things they enjoyed such as take long walks or participate in sports. Their self-image undergoes a drastic readjustment for the worse. They are generally impatient and not introspective, and the emotion they are most comfortable with is anger, so early on they may feel lost in understanding how to deal with the new reality of their life.

## LESSONS LEADERS HAVE LEARNED

**WANDA,** who had polio in early childhood and now has progressive post-polio syndrome:

> *What has helped me is a great faith in the Lord. And an excellent relationship with my husband, because we've both chosen to work on it. I've somehow become more patient. I've learned to appreciate the important things, the relationships with people rather than what I can accomplish. I've learned the value of a quality of life. I can continue to have a good life, with satisfaction and contentment, even if I get worse.*
>
> *I've also learned that grieving is real—you have to grieve the losses and then get up and go. What has helped is allowing myself to just be who I am. If all I can do is stay in bed and watch soap operas that day, so be it! I'm accepting myself more. A therapist helped me.*
>
> *Early on, I carried a lot of anger that I didn't realize. Dealing with the anger and facing the issues, I've become more relaxed and accepting of life and people.*

In this account, Wanda demonstrates how Eights can soften in therapy. This is hard work for them, but they can learn to overcome their denial and become more introspective.

## KAYLA:

> *The worst part was that I lost so much of myself. My creative, loving, joyous parts went away. I was almost numb. My relationship with my husband and children suffered. I felt very isolated. When I wasn't in pain, I was worried about being in pain. I felt guilty.*
>
> *Pain management changed it. Now that I'm on the other side of it, I can say I'm more aware of my good qualities. I'm a lot less reactive and judgmental than I used to be. The sharp edges of my personality have really smoothed out.*

RHONDA:

> *I'm more accepting of people's help than I was before the pain problem. I let them in more. Because so many people have been praying for me, I'm much more grateful, and I see much more of the graciousness and grace of people than I saw before.*

TOM:

> *I suppose it's made me a stronger person. At least I have three people who love me—my wife and kids. My wife is solidly beside me, and I realize she really loves me. I feel very fortunate.*

Tom's comment is typical of Eights, who want to know where people stand in relation to them. They are more comfortable when someone else's loyalty is clear.

## HOW OTHERS CAN HELP THE LEADER

WANDA:

> *When my polio-affected muscles got weaker, they thought I was just lazy. It helps me if people validate my reality, the reality of my limitations. They can also help me physically by doing what they can for me.*

RHONDA:

> *By being there for me when I call them and want to cry or talk. They send me money unasked.*

OLIVER:

> *Just understand that I have this pain problem and it gets to me after a while. Be patient.*

Because of their denial, Leaders are often not good advocates for themselves. (They share this with Twos.) Eights need others to give them a reality check, to validate that they in fact have needs. If others don't do this, it feeds into the Eights' denial and makes it more difficult for them to ask for help.

## LEADERS' ADVICE TO OTHER LEADERS

WANDA:

> *First, to accept that wherever they are, that's okay. If they're very angry,*

*that's where they're at. Get others to validate your feelings—the more val-*
*idated, the less you have to fight the reality if you can't get out of bed. Five*
*years ago I'd have suggested finding a hobby and read, but now I think*
*that's just busy work. The most important thing is to accept yourself.*

Like other personality types, Leaders bring about expectations from others, and then have difficulty when they can't fulfill those expectations. For Eights, the expectation is that of strength and of being able to manage everything. As Wanda said, validation from others that you do have needs helps Leaders accept themselves as they are.

RHONDA:

*Let people in. Feel the feelings. Have a strong support network, and—this*
*is really important—you are your own doctor; you are responsible for get-*
*ting better. You need to constantly make sure that what your doctors are*
*doing for you is in your best interest. Don't hesitate to question them.*

Eights' underlying motivation is to control and be strong. They want to dominate, although their perception rather is that they do not want to *be* dominated. In their relationship with chronic pain or illness, their position is not to give in, not to let it control and dominate their lives. Even if they are handicapped, they want still to be in charge. But Eights' dilemma is that they can't just be their own doctor—they must also be willing to surrender at some point and go with the doctor's recommended treatment.

Leaders' difficulty in asking for help comes from their fear of appearing weak and vulnerable. Loyal, supportive family and friends can be a great help. The Eight who is willing to work with a counselor can learn to soften, to get through the denial, and to access feelings. The Eight needs to reframe strength as the ability to get through the challenges of life rather than to control and overpower others.

## *Type Nine: The Mediator*

WARREN, a 32-year-old muscular, healthy young man walks with a slight limp because he has a leg prosthesis:

*When I was growing up I was the quiet type; I didn't draw any attention to myself. If there was any trouble, I'd walk away. I always hated arguing and fighting. Even today, I'd rather leave than fight. I'm still pretty quiet with people I don't know. It takes a lot to get me mad, but when I do, I explode. I yell, I stomp around, but it's not often. I'm a good listener, and I bend over backwards to help a friend.*

*Procrastination is a big problem for me. If there's something I need to get done, I'll do everything and anything else instead. I'll get busy with other things. Sometimes it's hard for me if there's more than one thing going on around me. I tend to start something, and then I won't finish it because I get distracted. Sometimes it's hard for me to make up my mind. If there's something I want and there are several choices, I might decide and then change my mind two or three times, thinking that maybe something else would be better.*

*I don't like having stress in my life. Comfort is very important to me. Other people take problems more seriously than I do. To me, it's no big deal—it'll just work out. I really like nature. I like the quiet. When I was a kid, we used to go trout fishing. I loved it. You could smell the pine trees, it was quiet. You could hear the river running.*

*When I was 19, a car hit me head-on while I was riding my motorcycle. I lost my leg and had a nerve injury to my arm, so I can no longer lift it. After the crash, I was depressed for a while, but then I started doing things and moving on. Now I ride my horse, and help my father with his work. I'm physically active. The worst part of my life is being in pain all the time—I have phantom limb pain in my leg. When it hurts, I go crazy. I still get down sometimes. What helps is to start thinking of something else, and then I go on. I do a lot of thinking inside me. I've learned that, yes, this happened and I can't change it, so I have to keep going on.*

Warren's story illustrates his search for consensus and comfort, difficulty with getting things done, and his problem-solving strategy by distracting himself.

## How the Strengths of the Mediator Type Helped Them Cope

ROBERTA, a 54-year-old schoolteacher, has had increasing hip and knee pain in the past few years because of osteoarthritis:

*The worst thing is that it's hampered my teaching, my driving. I can no longer dance or hike. In the classroom, I have to sit most of the time. What's helped is that I'm a very patient person, and I've been patient with the pain and I've made peace with it. I never complain.*

STACY, a shy, slender, petite 47-year-old divorced woman, has been living with both fibromyalgia-related pain and schizophrenia, which was diagnosed in her twenties:

*People often tell me I seem so calm and easygoing, but everything inside me seems to be going at hyperspeed. Sometimes I may seem calm on the outside, but inside I'm trying to figure out what to do. I procrastinate a lot about doing things, which is a real problem because there are so many papers I need to organize. Making a decision is hard because once I decide, I might find out something that might make me feel different about it.*

*What's helped me cope with my fibromyalgia pain is my patience. If I'm having a really bad night, rather than just dreading it or thinking how horrible it is, I'll try to talk to myself in a positive way—that I've had bad flare-ups before and they went away, that if I'm having a bad time, that will change.*

Mediators seem to have an enormous capacity for putting up with pain and disability. Their ability to be patient and accepting of whatever befalls them can be a real strength. They do this by recognizing that others are worse off, by minimizing the situation, by telling themselves that somehow things will be better, and by tuning out with self-soothing activities. Unfortunately, these characteristics can also create their biggest challenges.

## CHALLENGES FOR THE MEDIATOR
ROBERTA:

*My patience kept me in pain for a long time without doing anything about it. A side of me cried because I knew there was help and yet I didn't do anything. I beat myself up about it, but I still didn't do anything. I hate to admit I'm such a sloth. My shyness was another problem. I have some irrational fears of calling for appointments. I don't make decisions when I should. My mom took me by the hand and helped me get a divorce. My sister had to grab my hand and take me to the doctor. I just lived with it, and I'm so sorry now!*

DONALD, who lives with severe back pain and migraine headaches:
*When I could no longer work, I got depressed. But when I'd see a doctor, I'd have a smile on my face and not show my depression. At times, I did more damage to myself by acting happy. Of course, sometimes when I'm going to see a doctor I feel better because I think I'm going to get help.*

Mediators have very little experience in making their own needs known; it may be hard for them to even recognize what they need. The same qualities that give them patience with the pain also prevent them from getting needed assistance. It's easier for the Mediator to tune out with an attitude that he or she is helpless to make any changes, than to take action, even if the action is beneficial. In the service of maintaining a constant emotional and physical status quo, with no ups and downs, Mediators will understate their symptoms when asked by their physician, turn down friends' efforts to help, and thereby miss opportunities for improvement.

BENITA, the Leader wife of a Mediator man who's had bone cancer for several years, gives a different perspective on the challenges of being a Nine with chronic pain and illness:
*Bryce was unwell for quite a while—he was tired, his body swelled—but he didn't seem aware of it, he was so out of touch with himself. By the time he got diagnosed with bone cancer he was very ill. Nines have a fear of being overlooked. When Bryce was healthy and felt I was ignoring him, he'd withdraw, turn on the TV, and tune out. But now, when he has serious reason to get attention from nurses in the hospital or from me at home, if he's ignored he gets irritable, impatient, and angry. But most of the time he's been a wonderful patient—he doesn't chafe at his inactivity. He's comfortable with a sluggish routine. He's very agreeable. The primary avoidance of the Nine is conflict—you don't have to rise to meet other people's needs, just adjust to your situation.*

*When I don't interfere, my husband tends to vegetate. He likes to be in a comfortable twilight zone, not challenging anything. In his cancer support group, he's been the least physically active person there. For a while, all he did was sleep, eat, and play bridge. I finally had enough! I was feeling like I was tending a rock garden, there was no relationship, he wasn't doing anything for himself, he just wanted to be taken care of. So one day when he didn't get up until 2 P.M., I said to him, "This isn't good for you, and it isn't working for me. It's important for you to exercise and keep your bones strong. These are choices you're making, like not to get up." It had never occurred to him that his disease was stressful to me. The next day, after he had time to assimilate what I'd said, he had a 180-degree turn. Ever since then he's been setting his alarm and getting up at a reasonable time. He said, "It just never occurred to me I had choices." Until then, he just thought of himself as a victim. He's thanked me dozens of times for that conversation.*

Benita's description illustrates two of the major challenges of the Mediator. One is the dilemma of sloth versus illness. For Bryce, the fatigue of his illness provided an excuse for falling into the sloth of the Nine, whereas what was required for his health was regular activity. It may be difficult for Mediators themselves to sort out the reason for their reluctance to take action; stimulation and encouragement by a spouse or friend can be very helpful. So can being reminded that doing nothing is a definite choice, and that there are better choices.

The second challenge is the self-negation of the Nine. They tell themselves, "Nothing bothers me," "Nothing makes me uncomfortable," including situations in which it would be in their self-interest to present a more reality-connected account of their pain or illness. This makes it difficult for Mediators to advocate for themselves in terms of their health care.

## LESSONS MEDIATORS HAVE LEARNED
Several Mediators described being better able to understand others and to empathize with them (qualities they already have in spades). Others reported, "I've tried to see my inability to work in a positive light," and "I've learned about hanging in there, to be gracious and kind even if I'm in a lot of pain."

STACY, who has fibromyalgia and schizophrenia, was the only one who talked of positive action:

*I definitely know there's no more fooling around with my health. I know that I have to treat my body well or I'll suffer for it. I no longer take chances—like staying out too late. It's still hard for me to ask for help, but now I do it.*

Mediators tend to accept their lot rather than be proactive. Clearly, they need others to advocate for them, stimulate them, and energize them into action.

## HOW OTHERS CAN HELP THE MEDIATOR

Family and friends of Mediators need to be aware of Nines' difficulty in bringing attention to themselves and their needs.

DONALD, a single father who's disabled because of his back:

> *I couldn't have gotten through this without my family and friends. They are very concerned about me, because I've withdrawn a lot from the pain and depression. They call to check on me if they haven't heard from me. They are loving.*

Nines have a fear of being invisible; it helps them if others who offer help follow through. According to Barbara, "It's hard for me to ask for help. If people offer to do things and then don't, I get mad." This was exactly what Benita, the wife of an ill Mediator, reported above.

At the same time, it's hard for Nines to admit when they *don't* want advice or help. Others need to be proactive in asking the Mediator what they want or don't want.

ROBERTA:

> *My sister yells at me for not making appointments. She says, "You're not taking care of yourself! Use your cane! You're doing too much!" Right now, I wish my family would back off. But I wouldn't tell them, or they'd be hurt. Before, I wanted their help. I appreciated it. It helped me to move, to do something about my pain. They initiated my getting help.*

## MEDIATORS' ADVICE TO OTHER MEDIATORS

WARREN:

> *I'd tell him, "No matter what, don't give up. It will get better. It's not the end of the world. You will get back to life." I'd tell him, "I'm active, I do as much as I can, you have to adapt to things."*

ROBERTA:

> *I'd say get help. I know people at school who have pain. I befriend them,*

*I give them your card, I encourage them, but I don't push them, or they'd probably hide! I'm there for them—I'm empathetic and compassionate.*

STACY:

*A really important thing I'd tell her is to make it her job to take care of her health. Don't do anything that's bad for your health. Avoid people who are bad for your health—someone who's pessimistic, cynical, or mean. Keep looking for answers, keep reading. Keep your hope alive.*

It's interesting that so many people in this survey were able to advise others of the same enneagram type to do exactly the things that were most difficult for them. In the case of Mediators, the good advice included to be physically active, to encourage Nines—without pushing them—to get the help they need, and to pay attention to their emotional and physical health needs.

## How Personality Type Affects Chronic Pain

Regardless of a person's personality type, chronic pain causes some predictable challenges; the person must learn to live with the pain itself, as well as the limitations in activities and the resultant life changes. Almost everyone I interviewed had difficulty asking for help, regardless of type. But each type presents its own specific challenges, as I found out in the interviews. Counselors and family members who work or live with a chronic pain sufferer can learn from this study how to be more effective in helping the patient cope with their often unremitting pain problem.

The different types, however, faced specific challenges in adjusting to their new physical state and its effects on their job and relationships. For Ones, the challenge is to become less self-critical about their inability to do a perfect job and more accepting of the unfairness and imperfections of the world. Twos have to figure out how to feel loved when they can no longer spend all their time giving. Threes have to find meaning in their life without their high-powered jobs. Fours, faced with physical problems that could be depressing to anyone, have to find some positive focus in their life that can help them feel better emotionally. Fives need to let others help them without feeling invaded. Sixes, having received confirmation that the world is a dangerous place, have to learn to trust others to help them. Sevens need to let go of many of their fun activities, and craft new ways of meeting their needs for novelty and variety. A challenge for both Sevens and Eights is to face their losses directly and develop the ability to be more introspective. Eights with debilitating chronic pain have to make peace with their loss of power and control and redefine the meaning of strength in their life. Nines' challenge is to empower themselves in their own healing and overcome their tendency to be passively accepting and self-forgetting.

# PART IV

## COPING
## WITH
## CHRONIC PAIN

# 14

# THE COSTS
# OF CHRONIC PAIN

## *Treatment and Insurance*

W E LIVE IN A CHANGED MEDICAL ENVIRO-nment—in the United States, cost issues intrude into every aspect of medical care. How the costs are paid changed drastically in the twentieth century compared with earlier times. Before, the financial relationship between doctor and patient was like that of any other provider of services: The consumer (the patient) was free to choose a physician—or a plumber, or a piano teacher. Physicians set their own fees, which the patients paid directly to them. No third party was involved. Today, technological advances, rising malpractice costs, and other factors have made health care so costly that it is no longer practical for most people to pay the full cost of their medical care out-of-pocket. Most people have health insurance, provided by insurance companies that, depending on the type of health plan you have, may have a large voice in determining which physicians and other health care providers you can use, which hospitals you can go to, and which medications you can take. Getting insurance company approval for services and medications outside their lists may be possible, but it involves extra time and paperwork for the physician's office, and can add hours to her weekly workload.

Even your choice of insurance companies is often limited. Most health insurance today is provided as part of an employer's benefit package. People who work for small companies that do not provide health insurance benefits, or who are self-employed, often buy health insurance through their business or professional associations. Employers and associations strike deals with insurance companies in order to obtain group rates that are more favorable than what individuals have to pay on their own. They then offer their employees or members one or a few insurance options.

## Types of Health Insurance

PRIVATE HEALTH INSURANCE. There are two types of private health insurance—fee-for-service and managed care. Fee-for-service policies let you choose your own physician and pay most (usually 80 percent) of the bill. They also pay some percentage—or all—of your medication costs. This is the most expensive type of health insurance. Managed care policies don't cost as much, but limit your choice of physicians, hospitals, and medications. Managed care providers fall into two categories—health maintenance organizations (HMOs) and preferred provider organizations (PPOs).

> **HMOs**, the least expensive type of health insurance, work through a "gatekeeper" system. You choose your physician, now called a "primary care provider," from a limited list. This internist or family practitioner coordinates your care and decides if you should be referred to a specialist or have a particular test. Many services, such as imaging studies or physical therapy, require prior authorization from the HMO.

> **PPOs** are groups of physicians (and/or hospitals) who arrange with employers to provide medical services at a discount if the employer agrees to offer only those services to their employees. Employees then pay a small co-pay or a relatively small percentage of the costs, perhaps 10 to 20 percent. The employee may use a physician (or hospital) outside the network, but in that case the patient pays a greater percentage of the costs, perhaps 30 percent.

Insurance plans, whether fee-for-service or managed care, limit to a greater or lesser extent the services they cover. For example, alternative treatments such as hypnosis, acupuncture, and massage therapy are usually not covered. Some insurance plans pay for chiropractic care, but others don't. Managed care plans are usually more restrictive than fee-for-service. Read your own insurance information to learn what services are covered by your plan.

## Government Insurance and Prescription Costs

Some people who are not employed may be eligible for government health insurance (Medicare). This includes most people older than 65, who can apply for Medicare. Medicare has two parts: inpatient hospital insurance (Part A), which is paid during the working years as part of Social Security taxes; and outpatient doctors' services (Part B), which costs extra but is inexpensive. The big deficiency in Medicare is prescription costs, which currently are borne by the patient. In 2003, a new law added some prescription benefits to Medicare, but this will not take effect until 2006. To ease the burden until then, Medicare recently began contracting with private companies to offer Medicare-approved drug discount cards, which entitle the bearers to pharmacy discounts on medications. Supposedly, the cards will produce discounts of 15 to 25 percent on medications. The cards cost no more than $30 per year. In addition, Medicare-eligible people whose annual income in 2004 is no more than $12,569 for a single person, or $16,862 for a married couple, may qualify for a $600 credit on the Medicare-approved drug discount card they choose. Obtaining the cards was initially confusing, but in April 2004 Medicare announced it will provide a standard application form to simplify the process.

Also in April 2004, Medicare began publishing detailed information comparing the prices of most prescription drugs. This information, available on the Medicare Web site, www.medicare.gov, is intended to help Medicare beneficiaries, but is also immensely useful to other consumers. The site lists the prices charged for various dosages of specific drugs at retail pharmacies in or near a given ZIP code, as well as online pharmacies, mail-order pharmacies, and Canadian drugstores. If a brand-name drug has generic equivalents, their prices are displayed as well. The Web site also shows prices for competing brand-name drugs used to treat the same condition. The Web site listings are updated weekly. This listing makes it much simpler for consumers, especially those who have to pay out-of-pocket for their drugs, to find the lowest prices. If, like many older people, you are not comfortable using the Internet, you can call a toll-free number, 1–800–MEDICARE, to obtain the prices.

Unfortunately, as of May 2004, what the Web site showed was problems with the discount cards. One finding was significant disparities in the cost of the same drug at the same pharmacy depending on the particular discount card. It was also evident that the discount cards give fewer benefits than touted; sometimes they do not give any savings at all in comparison to online pharmacies. For example, the table below shows the prices on May 2, 2004, for a 1-month (60 tablets) supply of four drugs commonly prescribed twice a day for chronic pain. The table shows first the retail price that day at Walgreens, a large drugstore chain, then the price with three discount cards as listed on www.medicare.com, and finally the price shown on the Web site of a popular online pharmacy, Drugstore.com:

### DRUG PRICES ON MAY 2, 2004

| PHARMACY NAME | CELEBREX 100 MG | MS ER 30 MG | NEURONTIN 600 MG | OXYCONTIN 10 MG |
|---|---|---|---|---|
| Walgreens retail price | $118.00 | $92.19 | $163.79 | $105.19 |
| Walgreens Discount card | $101.61 | $70.46 | $189.66 | $82.81 |
| AARP Discount card | $165.21 | $81.87 | $190.67 | $83.81 |
| Rx Savings Discount card | $172.04 | $92.28 | $222.11 | $79.12 |
| Drugstore.com | $91.99 | UNAVAIL | $207.99 | UNAVAIL |

You will notice several interesting things about this table. For Celebrex, the three discount cards had significant differences in their price. In fact, the retail price at Walgreens was significantly less than that of two of the discount cards. Moreover, the online pharmacy price without any card was less than that of any of the cards. For Neurontin, on the other hand, the online pharmacy charged more than two of the three discount cards. Amazingly, the Walgreens retail price was the least of all of them, and $25 less than the Walgreens discount card listed on the Medicare Web site. This seemed so improbable that I asked the pharmacist at Walgreens what his computer said is the Walgreens discount card price. He told me it was $145.41, which is $44 less than the price listed for the Walgreens discount card on the Medicare Web site. Finally, you cannot purchase any controlled drugs (such as opioids) on www.drugstore.com.

What are the lessons to be learned from this experiment? The most important one is that if you want to get the best price for your medications, you need to do your own research. Check the prices on the Medicare Web site, which is easy to navigate, and check the prices of at least one online pharmacy. If you have a Medicare discount card, don't assume that the prices listed on www.medicare.com are correct; ask your pharmacist what she is actually going to charge you.

Senior citizens are not the only people eligible for government insurance. Disabled persons of any age can apply for Social Security Disability Insurance (SSDI). If you are applying for SSDI or any other type of disability payments, you will need your doctor to fill out supporting documents. Most patients simply leave the papers at the doctor's office, hoping the physician will eventually have the time to fill them out. This is not the way to get the most effective evaluation. The forms ask for information about your specific limitations that may not be readily available in your medical chart, such as how many minutes or hours you can sit at a desk, how many minutes you can walk, how many pounds you can lift, or how many minutes or hours you can stand. The physician may make educated guesses or leave items blank. I recommend that you make an appointment with your physician specifically to fill out your forms.

Social Security typically denies a patient's initial application. Don't be discouraged if this happens. The next step for many people is to consult an attorney who specializes in disability. If your physician has a number of disabled patients, she is likely to know which reputable lawyers in the community handle such cases.

Another government insurance is Medicaid, a federal-state health program for people with very low income and assets. This program is called by different names in some states.

## Medication Woes

Both HMOs and PPOs limit their medication costs by creating a formulary, which is a list of drugs they will pay for. Some plans will not pay for brand-name drugs, that is, a drug whose patent has not yet expired and that is therefore manufactured by only one company. After the drug's patent expires, other pharmaceutical companies are free to make cheaper versions of the drug, which are usually less expensive and equally effective. For formulary drugs, patients pay a relatively small co-pay per prescription, and the insurance company will pay the rest. Prescription quantities are limited to a 30-day supply.

If several similar drugs exist in the same drug class, another cost-saving strategy for the insurance company is to work out a discount with the manufacturer of one of those drugs and permit you to purchase only that drug. Additionally, they often divide the drugs in their formulary into categories, and each category requires you to pay a different co-pay. For example, the formulary may designate its generic drugs as "first-tier," for which you pay a $10 co-pay; a preferred branded drug as "second-tier," a $25 co-pay; and the remaining medications as "third-tier," a $45 co-pay. Yet another wrinkle, as I found out when I tried to fill a prescription for 30 Ambien (zolpidem, a sleeping pill), is to permit only a smaller quantity—despite the prescription for 30 tablets, I was given only 15 tablets for my $45 co-pay. (I chose instead to pay $75 cash at a local discount pharmacy for the 30 tablets, a $15 savings.)

Operating within a formulary system can create several problems for both the patient and physician. First, the physician is limited in which drugs he can prescribe. This can be a real problem for patients with chronic pain. Some insurance plans permit drugs to be prescribed only for indications that have been approved by the FDA, even if the drug is widely used for other indications. The drug gabapentin (Neurontin, see chapter 4) is a good example. This drug was originally FDA-approved for treating seizure disorders, and more recently it was approved for treatment of post-herpetic neuralgia (shingles). However, it is now considered a first-line treatment for various types of chronic neuropathic pain (see chapter 4). But because it's not specifically approved for these other pain disorders, some insurance plans won't pay for prescriptions written for nondiabetic neuropathic pain. The doses of Neurontin needed to give relief for neuropathic pain are quite high, and so is the cost of these high doses. Unless you have unlimited financial resources, it may be a stretch to pay out-of-pocket for this drug.

The same problem has been encountered with modafinil (Provigil), a new non-amphetamine medication that fights drowsiness and is useful for patients who have residual sleepiness from opioids. Because it is FDA-approved primarily for narcolepsy, an uncommon sleep disorder that causes daytime drowsiness, the insurance company may decline to pay for it for a chronic pain patient.

If the insurance company will pay only for generic drugs, a physician who wants to prescribe a long-acting opioid for a chronic pain patient will be restricted to methadone and sustained-release morphine. These are excellent drugs, but morphine has a greater probability of causing itching than do synthetic opioids such as oxycodone and fentanyl, and methadone has some characteristics that make it tricky to use (see chapter 5). The branded long-acting opioids OxyContin (oxycodone), Duragesic (fentanyl), and Avinza (a once-a-day morphine), as well as the breakthrough pain lozenge Actiq (fentanyl), will be unavailable to that patient. The 80-mg dose of sustained-release oxycodone recently became available as a less expensive generic, but many patients are complaining of decreased efficacy and duration of action, suggesting possible problems with this particular formulation.

Another problem for physicians treating chronic pain patients is that some pain medications have been touted by their manufacturers as providing pain relief for a longer period of time than they actually do for some patients. Because the Duragesic patch lasts 72 hours for most patients and OxyContin 12 hours, the insurance company may authorize only 10 Duragesic patches or 60 OxyContin per month. But the reality is that about 25 percent of patients require a new Duragesic patch after only 2 days or an additional dose of OxyContin after 8 hours. If you bring a prescription for 15 Duragesic patches or 90 OxyContin tablets to your pharmacist, you may learn that the drugstore can give you only part of your prescription. In this situation, the physician can sometimes get an override by submitting a written request to the insurance company.

## The Law and Increased Number of Co-pays

Most insurance plans require the patient to pay a co-pay for every prescription, no matter for how many days it covers. For example, if you cut your hand while cooking and need stitches, the emergency room doctor may give you a prescription for a few pain pills for the short time that you are expected to have pain. For that prescription you will have to pay the same co-pay as for a 30-day supply of the same drug.

The DEA, which controls the prescribing of medications it considers liable to be abused (these are called "scheduled drugs"), has created regulations for the filling of prescriptions for these drugs. Legal drugs that the DEA believes have the highest potential for abuse—Schedule II drugs—have the most stringent regulations. Such medications, which include morphine, methadone, oxycodone, fentanyl, and methylphenidate (Ritalin), can't be phoned in; they must be written. Prescriptions for Schedule II drugs cannot have refills. And if the pharmacist does not have the total number of pills the doctor prescribed, a new prescription must be presented by the patient later for the balance of the pills. Depending on your insurance plan, you may have to pay a second co-pay to get the rest of your pills. This situation will also cost your doctor money, as well: The office will need to take your phone call or the pharmacy's asking for a new prescription, the staff will need to pull your chart for the physician, and the doctor will need to take time to write the additional prescription and to document the reason for it.

## What if You Have No Medication Coverage?

Chronic pain patients are often on a cocktail of pain medications, which can include an anti-inflammatory (NSAID), opioid, muscle relaxant, sleeping pill, and anticonvulsant. The total cost can easily run to hundreds of dollars a month. If your financial resources are inadequate to support extensive prescription drug payments, there are a couple of ways you can work around this. One is to talk with your physician about substituting a less costly medication in the same drug class as you are already taking. Unfortunately, this is often not possible. However, if you are on an opioid that costs several dollars a pill, your physician might switch you to methadone, which costs only pennies per tablet.

Another possibility is to apply to the maker of your drug for help. You may not realize that most large pharmaceutical companies have patient-assistance programs, which provide free medications to patients whose income and assets are below a certain level. Your doctor or pharmacist can give you the name of the drug's manufacturer so that you can contact the company, and your doctor may be able to obtain an application form for you. The application has a section for your doctor to enter your medical and prescription information, and for you to delineate your financial resources.

# 1 5

# TO THE FAMILY
# AND FRIENDS

## *How to Help*

*Ever since Paul's accident 5 years ago, he doesn't drive, so I've been taking
him to doctors' appointments. I'm always there in the examining room with
him. When the doctor asks me a question, it's always about how Paul is
doing. My life, too, was changed drastically by the accident. At home it's prac-
tically a full-time job taking care of him. In the doctor's office, I feel like I'm
invisible as a person. No one asks me how I'm coping, or what my life is like!
Counseling would really have helped us, but no doctor ever suggested it to us.*
—PATTY, 50 YEARS OLD

WHEN A PERSON DEVELOPS A CHRONIC PAIN PROBLEM,
her life may change significantly. What is often forgotten
is that the life of the spouse and family also changes, as do
friendships. The patients in a pain specialist's practice are often
accompanied by a spouse, partner, or close friend. In many cases, this
person is the most significant member of the patient's treatment team,
sometimes the only reason the disabled person is able to lead a mean-
ingful life at home. A supportive partner can make a huge difference in
someone's ability to cope with chronic pain; an unsupportive spouse can
make it that much harder. This chapter, based on interviews with
involved spouses, describes their reactions, their challenges, and what

they are doing to obtain the support and nurturance that they need for themselves. If you are a spouse, partner, or friend, you may identify with some of the feelings expressed in this chapter.

## Arnold's Story

ARNOLD, 67, has been married for 20 years. He raised his children alone after his first wife left, so he has experience being a caregiver. His wife has had severe fibromyalgia pain for 4 years:

*We used to have a motor home, but we got rid of it because it hurt her too much to sleep in it. We used to walk on the beach, but she can't walk long distances. We no longer take bicycle rides. We spend a lot of time in the backyard. She used to grow vegetables, but her hands hurt too much to do any potting. At times, she gets irritable. She tries to do things, lift a pot, and I know it's gonna be a problem later. She was always an active person, and now she can't. I understand her frustrations. She can't even play with the grandchildren. I do all the shopping, the housecleaning, everything she used to help with. I try not to show her when I'm frustrated. I just walk away or change the subject. Once I go outside for a bit, it's okay. I don't want to argue with her.*

*It gets frustrating for me. But I've learned to be a little more patient. I used to try to do too much for her. Now I try to let her do more, so she gets more movement. I've learned to adjust to it. It doesn't depress me. It makes me feel bad because I can't do anything. Sometimes I try to be overly helpful.*

*Since she got sick, seems like our friends have disappeared. Part of it, I'm sure, is that we can't plan anything. For example, I was going to fly with my wife to California for a surprise birthday party for my son. She had a plane ticket and reservations at a motel. The day before her flight she hurt so bad, she couldn't do it.*

*I don't really have any men friends, and don't go out with the guys. Before she was sick we spent a lot of time together, so I didn't go out without her. Now she'll have some coffee and cereal and go back to bed, and I won't see her for most of the day. We're in the same house, and I still feel the closeness, and I understand what she's going through, so I just live with it. When she has a good day and does what she likes to do, it brings me up, too.*

*Sometimes during the day, I'm gone for a couple of hours. I go to the bank or shopping for food. I've always been a pretty easygoing guy. I'm happy at home. Spending time with her means more to me than going out with the guys. I don't go to movies alone, because I don't want to be away too long. I worry about her passing out. She's sometimes unsteady on her feet. We watch movies on TV. Sex is few and far between, but we've always been very affectionate. Whenever we go to a store we hold hands. Half the time we know what the other person is thinking. We get a lot of enjoyment out of each other.*

*Recently, we went shopping for clothes. It's hard for her to go to the dressing room and change, so I went in to help her. Then a voice on the loudspeaker announced, "There's a man in the women's dressing room." They wouldn't let me help her. We ended up taking the clothes home to try on, and then bring them back if she doesn't want them.*

*As for the future, I foresee it getting worse, in terms of what she can do. But we try to take it day by day. We tell each other there are a lot of people who are worse off. We feel lucky that we can do what we can do. We hope things will get better. We try to think positive.*

*I'd do anything for her, even if I had to change her diaper. I keep putting myself in her place. I feel she would do the same for me.*

Arnold is an extremely supportive and loving husband. He's old enough to be comfortably retired, and his easygoing personality helps him accept his situation. His story brings up several themes that recur throughout the experiences of other caregivers. As a spouse or partner, you may have grappled with these issues yourself. These include:
- the effect on your life—including friendships.
- the effect on the relationship—including sex and affection.
- how much of your feelings to share with your spouse.
- when to take charge and when to back off.
- how to get support and nurturing for yourself.

Each of these aspects is discussed in the following sections.

## The Effect on Your Life

When your partner develops a chronic pain problem, your life can change dramatically as well (see box on p. 294). You may have to take over the housekeeping, run errands, do all the driving, and perhaps even give up your job. You may have to decrease or give up enjoyable activities with your spouse—traveling, hiking, playing tennis, even going to a movie or restaurant. Your partner may become increasingly irritable and unsociable. And you may find yourself with an unanticipated career change.

CHRISTINE, now 40, whose husband developed debilitating back pain that was unrelieved by several operations:

> *Ever since I was a little girl I dreamed of getting married, having children, and being a housewife. I didn't go to college. I planned on staying home and raising kids. I married this gorgeous guy who had a good career. But after Cal's second operation, which was shortly after my second child was born, it became clear that I needed to get a job. It was overwhelming for me to take care of the two babies and him, and to work, too. I was very depressed for a long time. I'd cry and cry when I was alone, so the kids and Cal wouldn't see it. He was very depressed, too, about losing his life. He was in so much more pain after the surgery. He lost his mobility, his function was minimal. He couldn't be the dad he wanted to be.*

## When Your Own Health Isn't Great

BILLIE, 66, describes how her life changed after her husband hurt his back 5 years ago:

> *I've had a lot of operations, too. I wait on him more than I used to. Bob doesn't expect it, but that's how I am. I think it's a woman's place to help a man. We used to eat at the table, but now he likes to eat in a chair, and I serve him. When we're going on a trip to visit the kids, I'm the one who packs everything and loads up the car. Sometimes my bones hurt, I get tired, and I can't do things, so I just let it go.*

## Helplessness

Watching your partner experience pain and suffering can be very difficult. Just as patients so often decry their helplessness and their need to ask others for assistance, so one of the most common feelings in spouses is also helplessness at their inability to solve the problem.

DUSTIN, a construction supervisor, describes what happened 5 years ago, when his wife injured her leg and ended up with painful RSD (reflex sympathetic dystrophy):

> *Deslie injured her leg and was almost bed-bound for 2 years, with several operations and infections. Before that she'd been always so active and full of life. Afterward she couldn't do much for herself. She was so weak and didn't feel well. I hated to see the change in her. It was hard for her, and hard for me to see. I felt very helpless when she'd have another setback, another infection, another operation.*
>
> *My escape was my work. The closest to home I work is 100 miles. I enjoy what I do, but while I was gone I'd worry. One day I was at work when I got a call from a friend that Deslie had to go to the emergency room. I felt so helpless! I was 3 hours away. By the time I got there she was in the midst of emergency surgery.*

## Anger and Resentment

HAROLD LEAR was a urologist who was stricken by a massive heart attack in 1974, when medical and surgical options were less advanced than now. His wife, Martha, watched him struggle for 4 years as he became weaker and weaker. Although he did not have chronic pain, Lear experienced similar losses of his career, ability to function, ability to travel, even to walk. In her book *Heartsounds*, Martha Lear describes her feelings as she became more and more a caregiver for her husband:

> *I used to resent only strange men walking briskly in the street. Now I feel the old resentment swelling and extending to all healthy men, healthy friends, healthy husbands of friends. I find myself hating muscles, displays of strength. And listening now to Alex [a friend who had successful heart surgery] speaking of health—of how great he is feeling and how well he is working and how long he jogged last week—I start to cry. Suddenly, bitterly.*
>
> *I despise this pettiness in myself. Sometimes I have confessed it, abashedly, to Hal [Harold], ". . .and I get this feeling—Why you? Why not Alex, or Lewis, or David or Bob—why you?" And he chastised me: "Oh, come on. That's awful. That's mean-spirited."*
>
> *Is this genuine? Does no faint vapor of resentment seep out of his own bones?*
>
> *It has comforted me to learn that my feelings are shared. Normal, I am told. Normal, they keep assuring me: It's okay to feel what you feel because that is what you feel, so it's okay.*[1]

When your partner has a chronic pain problem, it's hard to watch him or her suffer. It's hard to sit by as he or she tries to deal with the many losses. You may find yourself feeling angry at healthy people who don't have such problems. You are also likely to feel some anger at your spouse for the losses *you* have experienced as a result of the chronic pain problem. And if part of your spouse's way of coping is to be short-tempered and irritable with you, it makes it all the harder for you. That's why it's so important to have a support system of your own.

## Invisible Symptoms

If your spouse has a disability that is evident—such as a leg deformity resulting from an injury—it's not hard to remember their pain problem. But what about the person with an invisible disorder such as fibromyalgia? Your spouse may look perfectly healthy, so it's easy to forget that some simple jobs, like reaching into the dryer to take out clothes, may be very painful. You may find yourself feeling resentful (and then feeling guilty for those feelings!) when she keeps asking you to help in ordinary tasks. On the other hand, she may feel guilty constantly asking you for help and instead do too much, with the result that the pain level may rise.

## Friendships

It's easy for friends to empathize with someone who has an acute pain problem, but hearing about chronic pain quickly gets old. When conversation with friends repeatedly turns to one's chronic pain problem, friends tend to fall away. This problem is made worse if your partner's pain and fatigue are unpredictable. You are likely to find yourself making excuses to friends at times when the spouse in pain does not want company at home or doesn't feel up to travel. You may find yourself becoming isolated. It's important for you to maintain connections with at least some friends and relatives.

## The Effect on the Relationship

Chronic pain often has a major impact on a couple's relationship. Both may experience significant losses. They can no longer share many of the enjoyable things they had shared in the past. Their conversation may be focused on medical problems, doctors' appointments, and financial concerns. For the pain patient, sex may be very uncomfortable physically, or depression or medications may decrease the libido. Many men believe that if you can't have intercourse, your sex life is over. Sometimes they cease all forms of affection. The spouse may feel unfulfilled sexually or even rejected.

Emily's husband, ERNEST, developed back pain that the couple was told would be a lifelong problem. Emily went into a prolonged depression, one that improved only after extensive counseling:

> *My depression was about grieving for what we lost. I still love him with all my heart, but we haven't had sex for 3 years [she begins to cry]. We were very sexually active, and the change is hard to live with. He thinks if you can't have intercourse, you don't even kiss. I've tried talking with him, but he doesn't seem to understand. I've been thinking maybe if we could go to the counselor together, but it's difficult to talk about sex with someone else. This loss isn't something that you just get over. I thought I was okay, but it's obvious to me now that I still have strong feelings about these things and need to go back to the counselor.*

If a couple is willing to see a counselor, they can learn that sexual gratification is possible even without intercourse. Even if no form of sexual activity is feasible, people still crave physical affection. Hugging, kissing, touching, all transmit the message, "I care."

## Parent-child Interactions

Another potential problem for couples is that some gradually transition from an adult-adult to a parent-child relationship, a transformation that makes for a difficult marriage situation. This is especially likely if affection is minimal, and their interactions are primarily ones of giving and receiving care. Ernest's mobility became very limited so that Emily had to help him in many ways:

> *When someone becomes dependent on you, you tend to start treating him like a child. You have to be careful to remember that even though he's dependent on you, he's still an adult. I get impatient with him. I want him to be like he used to be, but he's not.*

The parent-child dynamic is particularly a problem when the chronic pain patient experienced a head injury that affects his or her judgment.

HAYLEY, 40, whose husband, Hal, has a head injury:
> *I feel frustrated, I feel angry, and then I feel guilty. Hal looks so normal, but then he forgets what he just said. Last week we were out and he got lost, and these other people just laughed at him, and I got so angry! His forgetfulness has gradually gotten worse. He has an emotionally child-like quality. I'm a professional, and I try to educate Hal, but it's hard for him to learn. I work the night shift, and I try to be around when he's awake. I never go out without him. I spoke with another woman whose husband had a head injury, and it was very helpful. She'd say, "Yes, my husband's the same way; it's the head injury."*

JESSICA, 45, has similar feelings:
> *Since his head injury, it's like dealing with a child. We went to the store, and he started opening packages. I told him he shouldn't, and he got upset with me. We both got angry with each other. Also, he feels angry with me because I'm no longer interested in sex. We need counseling for this. We have to come to terms with it. But we've been too busy up to now.*

Going to a counselor and/or a support group would be very helpful, but the challenge for caregivers is that the more attention the chronic pain patient needs, and the more the family is now financially dependent on the healthy spouse's career, the less time she has for the counselor or support group.

When the relationship changes from adult-adult to caregiver-patient, the partnership that is the essence of a marriage tends to disintegrate. Sometimes a spouse may make choices that are later regretted.

MARIA, whose husband had a progressive painful neuromuscular disease and eventually died:
> *Matt was very weak. I knew he had little energy for daily life. Since I didn't want to interfere with his energy, I stopped sharing any of my feelings with him. I did not share any of my personal, physical, or household needs with him. In doing so, I cut him out of my life. I no longer felt like we were living*

*as husband and wife. I was there as his caregiver. I could have been a hired person. Now, as I look back, I can see how that separated us on an emotional level. Our relationship didn't feel close. It felt like we were just existing. After his death, I grieved the last months that we lost.*

Balancing the patient's needs, your own needs, and the needs of an intimate relationship is a huge challenge for caregivers.

## When to Take Charge and When to Step Back

When a person is living with chronic pain, the spouse wants to help. It feels good to be helpful and makes you feel you have some control over the difficult situation the patient is in. To feel helpless to remedy the situation is very uncomfortable. A big problem for spouses is knowing when to intervene, and when to allow the patient to make his own decisions and deal with the consequences. Typical scenarios are when you (the loving partner) see the patient being too active, not doing enough, or not being compliant with medications.

EMILY:

*The most frustrating thing for me was Ernest still trying to do more than he was capable of. When that happened, then all of us had to pay the price. Like climbing ladders, knowing it was going to aggravate his back. He's better now, so he can do more, and this is less of a problem.*

Emily's dilemma was figuring out when to step in and ask Ernest to do less, and when to keep silent when she felt he was overdoing it.

A similar experience was reported by PATTY, who had been married for 30 years when her husband Paul developed severe back pain that persisted after surgery and largely disabled him:

*It was very frustrating for me to see Paul try to do physical things that were dangerous for him, like climbing ladders. That's exactly what he tried to do when a friend came over to fix our cooler. We had to physically pull him off the ladder. He couldn't stand the thought that he was not in shape to get up on the roof. He was really in denial about his condition.*

Just as common is the opposite situation—when, as a caregiver, you are tempted to do too much, especially when you know activity is painful for your spouse.

MARIA:

> *Even getting dressed was painful for Matt. He couldn't reach his feet, so I helped him with his trousers. But he was able to get his shirt on, although it hurt. I couldn't stay in the room when he was getting dressed. If I watched, it was extremely difficult not to help him. Yet, I knew, the squirming to get the shirt over his head was good exercise for him, and it was important for him to feel some independence.*

KAREN, a 60-year-old psychotherapist, is married to an older man who was very independent all his life. He now has multiple medical problems, but still doesn't like to take advice. Her challenge, too, was knowing when to step in and when to back off:

> *The best advice I can give others in my situation is to stay out of the mix unless invited. I tend to be a "doer," rolling up my sleeves and solving problems. In this case, it's his problem. I have found over time that unless he is in an emergency situation or asks for my help, it is best that I keep my help to myself. However, I have also taken the position with him that I find it difficult to hear his continual, repetitive complaints unless we are going to engage together in problem-solving. I have encouraged him to complain/vent to a therapist or someone else who does not live in our household. These changes on my part make for a more harmonious marriage.*

Finding a balance between intervening and stepping back is difficult. You may find yourself wondering if your spouse is really doing as much as possible to take more control in alleviating the pain. At times, encouragement from you may be just what is needed to get your loved one out of a default mode of helplessness and giving in to the disease. Helping him to feel hope about the future may empower your spouse to take more responsibility for healing.

## The Relationship Can Improve

Couples may develop greater emotional intimacy, greater appreciation for what they do have.

CHRISTINE:

*You lose some things, you gain others. Cal is my friend. We may not be able to have sex or go fishing, but Cal is extremely supportive, he's always been there for me, he holds me when I'm feeling down. We talk sometimes for hours. I share intimate thoughts and feelings with him like you would a girlfriend. We have a very good relationship despite his disability. Plus, I always try to learn something good out of something bad, and change the situation to our benefit. One of the benefits we really see of Cal's being disabled is that he's there all the time for the children. Most kids never see their dad 'cause they're working. My children have a wonderful relationship with their father.*

*In the beginning, I dwelt on the bad. Then two things happened that gave me a different perspective. One was when I had palpitations, blacked out, and was briefly hospitalized. That's when I realized how good I had it. I began to maintain a positive attitude. I look for what is good. I'm grateful for the things we have, and I don't wish for what's unrealistic. I'm grateful I have a house, just little things. When Cal almost died in an operation, I started reading spiritual books, found more inner strength, and found a new outlook on life. Every day is a special day. Life is so short and so precious. We don't know when we're going to lose each other.*

When couples don't communicate, the relationship can also suffer.

DUSTIN:

*When Deslie was going through her ordeal, I didn't tell anyone how I felt. I think it was a defense—I was so worried about losing her that I put a wall up, so it wouldn't be so bad if I lost her. I didn't want her to know how upsetting it was and how worried I was. The man is supposed to be strong, but if you're that way too much it can backfire. She started getting the feeling I didn't care.*

*One night we were watching a movie in which the man's wife dies. As I watched I lost it, crying. I remember that movie so well, how upsetting it was. That's when we both realized that I'd put a wall up out of fear, and trying to be so strong and not show weakness or worry or sadness, it looked like not caring. That really turned things around for me, and for her, too. She realized I did care, and that I'd overcompensated.*

*My advice? You've got to be honest with your spouse about your feelings. If you're worried, you have to let her know! Otherwise, she can end up thinking you don't care.*

## Your Feelings

When your partner develops chronic pain, disability, or illness, you are affected as well. You are likely to develop strong feelings about your situation—sadness, resentment, anger—and then develop guilt about having these feelings! After all, it's not your spouse's fault that he or she was injured! Your feelings are legitimate, but what do you do with them?

BILLIE:

*When Bob gets frustrated, I get a little tense, but I try not to say anything. He can't help it. I talk with my daughter—it helps get it off my mind.*

IRA, whose wife has chronic back pain:

*My wife can't go places with me anymore, or do things with me. I almost lead a single life. I go camping with my friend, go to a movie with my daughter. When I feel frustration or resentment, I just bury those feelings. I don't resent Ilene—it wasn't her fault! I have frustrations, but I married her for better or worse. It isn't how I thought my life would be, but I just deal with it. How? I just suck it up. I don't bitch with my friends about it. I guess I'm used to it by now. I don't think about it on a daily basis.*

Women often have friends or family they can unload on, but many men tend to hold those feelings in and remain isolated.

DUSTIN:

*I never talked to anyone. Most people would say, "That's too bad—I saw a really good football game yesterday." They'd change the subject. I don't think anyone really understands unless they've been through it. Now I'd tell someone else in the same boat to find someone to talk to—it would really help. Let them know how you're feeling.*

GERALD, 65 years old, has been married for 36 years to a woman who had chronic back pain. Recently she developed an additional progressive back disorder. He relates:

*I've been a giver all my life. I have a big willingness to give to others. If I feel myself getting angry I usually just back off and find something else to do. Yes, the feeling does come back, and what I then do is the same—I just put it inside my head. I hold it in. I try not to jump on her for her problems. I hold the resentments to myself. I resent not her but the situation. No, I don't have any outlet for my feelings, not really. I use reason—I can't do anything, so why make it worse by complaining about it? It's not going to help anything.*

*I'm a man of my word. I said, "I'll stick with you," and I do. There are many ups and downs. A doctor suggested I hook up with a counselor, and I'd have had no problem with it, but I had no time, I had to make money.*

One man was fortunate in being surrounded by others in the same boat. This was FRANK, whose wife developed severe painful osteoarthritis of the neck and could no longer drive:

*At first, when she became quite dependent on me, it bothered me. I didn't tell her, because she was having her own battles with pain, so I just kind of sucked it up and went my way. We live in a senior citizens' park, and most of our acquaintances also have medical problems. We talk and, over time, you learn to put aside your own things and concentrate on the disabled person. I've learned to do that—I don't mind.*

Frank's decision to say nothing to his wife about his feelings illustrates the dilemma faced by many spouses of ill or disabled persons. This is discussed in the next section.

The sidebar on page 294 summarizes the lifestyle and emotional consequences of chronic pain for the spouse. I want to emphasize that the emotions listed negative under—grief, anger, resentment, guilt—are normal and expected. But one must develop coping strategies to deal with them. The next section addresses some of these.

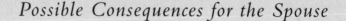

## Possible Consequences for the Spouse

NEGATIVE
- Grief over the loss of your previous life
- Feelings of anger, resentment, and guilt
- Additional responsibilities at home
- Unanticipated change in career—give it up, or go to work
- Decreased social life and recreational activities
- Friendships fade away/increased isolation
- Decreased sex life
- Relationships can change from peer–peer to parent–child

POSITIVE
- Increased closeness with spouse
- Disabled person has more time at home, with family
- Increased appreciation for what's really important

## Nurturing Yourself and Getting Support

Families of chronic pain patients have a real dilemma: They may feel frustration, anger, and grief because of the patient's illness or disability, but the patient is often not the best person with whom to vent. On the one hand, it's not healthy to constantly pretend that everything is fine while in fact you are experiencing strong emotions about your situation. But on the other hand, you know it's not your spouse's fault, that she would prefer to be healthy rather than in pain, and that if you frequently complain about your own resultant burden, you will not be helping your spouse or the relationship.

The solution is to seek a balance. It's good to have open discussions with your spouse about your fears and about your efforts to work through your losses, but venting your feelings about the situation frequently to her is not so good. Yet you need to let your feelings out, to work through them. The question is where to find an appropriate forum. This is often not easy to find. Several spouses reported that the time commitment involved in caring for the patient and the difficulty making plans to see friends resulted in a falling away of friends, with resulting isolation. Others found communication with family difficult. A woman whose husband was already disabled when she married him related about this very problem.

*I'm afraid to go to his family. I think they know I'm frustrated and unhappy right now, but if I said anything to them directly, they'd accuse me of being disloyal. I've tried talking with my mother, but she says, "I told you so, but you married him anyway."*

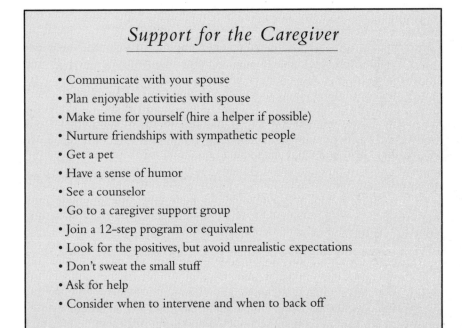

## Support for the Caregiver

- Communicate with your spouse
- Plan enjoyable activities with spouse
- Make time for yourself (hire a helper if possible)
- Nurture friendships with sympathetic people
- Get a pet
- Have a sense of humor
- See a counselor
- Go to a caregiver support group
- Join a 12-step program or equivalent
- Look for the positives, but avoid unrealistic expectations
- Don't sweat the small stuff
- Ask for help
- Consider when to intervene and when to back off

One of the most moving situations a physician witnesses is the many times that people support and assist their spouses who have a chronic illness, injury, or disability. It's as though over the years, each member of the couple has built up a positive bank account full of shared experiences, loving gestures, and positive feelings about their life together. The well partner draws on that account to give to the other who is in need. But if the account is not replenished, the well partner risks "caregiver burnout," a feeling of discouragement, anger, and depletion. It's important for the caregivers to nurture themselves so that the account doesn't dry up. How can this be done?

The box above lists some strategies to avoid this all-too-common problem. Several of these have already been mentioned in this chapter. One is the recognition that you can't be an effective caregiver 24/7. You need to take some time out for yourself. Go to a movie, have a meal with a friend, take a short trip. Plan to do this on a regular basis. Do this even if it means asking for help if you feel uncomfortable leaving your spouse alone. You may need to ask a friend or relative to stay with your spouse, or you may even need to hire someone.

Talking with others who are going through a similar experience to yours can also be extremely beneficial. Hearing from others that they have the same feelings as you—including the negative ones—can alleviate your guilt and normalize your experience. That is, it will help you realize that what you are feeling in your situation is normal and expected. Learning what has helped another person might result in solutions you never even considered.

In my city, a caregiver support group has been going strong for many years. Led by a professional, the group provides a safe place to vent and an audience who really understands and can give helpful feedback. Members can learn what has helped others to cope with their situation, and they can see that others—who may appear to have it worse—have found ways to focus on the positives in their situation.

A WOMAN whose husband died of pancreatic cancer after months of pain:

> I think getting therapy is critical for the caregiver. Watching your loved one suffer (as you know) is almost unbearable. Those pictures are burned into your brain, and you feel the need to speak about it. Sometimes I would yell at the top of my voice in the car or wherever I felt safe in doing so. Counseling helped because I could repeat my complaints at the unfairness of it all, but I didn't get counseling until Bob was gone.

Some people who were already attending self-help groups such as Al-Anon, for family and friends of alcoholics, found help in those groups for living with someone who is ill or has chronic pain. Al-Anon, which is an offshoot of Alcoholics Anonymous (AA), uses the same 12-step program as in AA, and teaches family members to focus on their own needs, feelings, and actions rather than on those of the addict. In Al-

Anon, people learn that they cannot control another person, and they learn to discern when they can actually change something and when they need to let go. This is encapsulated in the Serenity Prayer of AA, which can be very useful for spouses of people with chronic pain:

God grant me the serenity to accept the things I cannot change,
The courage to change the things I can,
And the wisdom to know the difference.

Offshoots of AA are now available for many other addictions, including gambling, compulsive overeating, and compulsive sexual behaviors—and each of these has a related program for family members.

When considering joining a support group, be sure that the focus of the group is on the members of the group rather than the needs of the patient.

MARIA:

*I first went to a group for family members of people with my husband's disease. But the trouble was, the people who came were only able to focus on the ill person. They did not understand the need to take care of their own needs. They acted like I was selfish when I talked about my feelings. Where I really got help was my 12-step support group for my family addiction. There, I was able to talk about all my losses, my loneliness about my decision to not share my burdens with him, my anger about my losses, my anger about my relentless, unending duties to him. I am sure I would not have survived otherwise. I certainly couldn't have taken care of him at home. The right support group can make all the difference in the world.*

## A Final Word to Friends

Good friends can make a huge difference in the ability of a chronic pain patient to cope with pain and limitations. This is especially true for people living alone. A back injury, worsening arthritis of the knee, or a car accident can turn a previously very independent person into someone who now has new physical and emotional needs. When my broken leg gave me ongoing pain and made me unable to drive for months, friends transported me to appointments, went shopping for food, brought meals over, and lent a listening ear when I felt depressed and in need of empa-thy. Looking back, I don't think I could have gotten through that period without my friends.

Unfortunately, many friends tend to disengage when a chronic pain problem or illness goes on and on. If your friendship was based on shared sports activities, traveling, or going to the theater, you may feel you no longer have anything in common with a person who now has difficulty moving around. Especially in the early months, when your friend is try-ing to adjust to what may be a significantly altered lifestyle with ongo-ing pain, limitations in activities, and perhaps inability to work, his or her conversation may be full of discouragement, complaints, and medical stories that you really don't want to know. You might feel that you no longer want to be around this negative person.

Another problem might be that it's hard for your friend to commit to an activity because there's no predicting if she will feel well enough to go when the time comes.

Your friend might also push you away. If you phone or e-mail, she might not return your message. When you finally do speak, she might not want to tell you about her health problems and might not have the energy for any social interactions. It's easy in such situations to take your friend's word for it and cease contact.

Too many people with chronic pain become isolated, in part because of their own actions and behavior. Yet they need friends more than ever, although it may be more difficult to be friends with them. If you have a friend you care about, consider what other options you have besides going your separate ways. Some suggestions are listed below:

- You may be able to find enjoyable activities to do with your friend at home to replace the ones he can't do right now. You can watch sports or movies on TV, surf the Internet, listen to music, take a home course, or sew or knit.
- If the pain or fatigue is variable so that it's hard for your friend to commit to an activity, plan to include him in something you intend to do with other people, anyway, or in an activity you'd still enjoy going to alone, such as a movie. Offer to pick your friend up if driving is a problem, and plan to phone an hour or two beforehand to confirm. If you don't count on your friend's participation, you won't be annoyed or put out if he can't

accompany you.

- Remember that people in chronic pain may look normal. Unlike the person with acute pain, your friend may not be groaning or writhing or making faces. He may be smiling and carrying on a conversation. If your friend is then not up to going somewhere with you or needs to take a nap, his normal appearance doesn't mean there's not significant pain or fatigue.

- Consider the current situation an opportunity to get to know your friend in a different way. Perhaps before, you shared more activities than conversations. You might find that your friend has had interesting experiences you hadn't heard about, or is now more willing to talk about feelings.

- If your friend doesn't return your call, or doesn't feel well enough to visit with you, don't take it personally. When people feel pain or fatigue, they might be less pleasant than you'd like. This isn't about you, it's about your friend. Remember that this is how she feels *right now*. Your phone call or company might be welcome tomorrow. Don't give up easily. Your friend will undoubtedly feel grateful for your persistence.

- Most people feel good when they help others. At the same time, most people are reluctant to ask for help. Offer to help your friend in some concrete way when you see a need—a ride, an errand, empathic listening, walking the dog. At the same time, give your friend an opportunity to be helpful to you. When she is up to it, ask for an opinion on some situation that's troubling you, or ask for assistance on some subject your friend has some knowledge about.

- You will be less likely to bow out of the friendship if you take care of yourself. If your friend tends to self-pity or endlessly talk about her aches, listen empathetically for a short while and then change the subject, get off the phone, or leave. If your friend can't reliably commit to doing things, don't make plans that depend on her company or that would be difficult to change.

- If you are exhausted and had planned to do something for your friend but just can't, explain why you can't do it right now and rest instead.

Finally, here are some simple tools for pain control that you can use with your spouse or friend if there is a flare-up of pain or trouble relax-ing or sleeping. This list was suggested by James Dillard, M.D., in his excellent book, *The Chronic Pain Solution*.[2]

- Touch: Hold the sufferer's hand, rub her back, or give her a leg massage. Ask her first what would help.
- Guided imagery: Take her mentally on a trip to some place she enjoyed visiting before, a trip you already know something about. If it's on the beach in Hawaii, talk about the smell of the ocean, the sound of the breeze blowing through the palm trees, the feel of the sand between your toes. Describe the scene in as much detail as possible, using all five senses to evoke the place once again. This is a wonderful way to diminish a person's suf-fering.
- Breathing exercises: Learn some, and do them together with her. Breathing exercises are very calming.
- Distraction: There are many ways of distracting a person's atten-tion so that it is less focused on the pain. All the techniques described above are forms of distraction. So are listening to music, hearing an interesting story or a joke, talking to a friend on the phone, watching an interesting TV program, or listening to you read the newspaper or a book aloud to her.
- A heating pad or ice pack.

# 1 6

# CURRENT RESEARCH
# AND TRENDS

## New Developments
## in Surgery, Postoperative
## Analgesia, and Opioids

PAIN HAS UNDOUBTEDLY BEEN AROUND FOR MILLIONS of years, ever since animals evolved into multicelled creatures. Man has surely experienced pain since humans first walked on this earth. Effective treatments for pain, however, are relatively new in the history of man, probably only for the past several hundred years. Morphine was first extracted from poppies only 200 years ago. Painless surgery became a reality only about 150 years ago. You may have noticed as you read this book that most of the references are rather new—much of the research in the understanding and treatment of chronic pain has been published within the last few years. It is evident that interest in chronic pain has been accelerating.

This chapter describes only a few of the new treatments that are currently under investigation in the areas of surgery and pain medications.

### Surgery

One of the trends that will surely continue is the development of increasingly less invasive ways of surgically correcting problems. Hernias are often fixed by outpatient procedures, gall bladder surgery is routinely done laparoscopically with only an overnight hospital stay and a quick recovery, and the same is true of many back operations. Even knee and hip replacements, as you read in chapter 8, are now sometimes being done by means of "mini" procedures. In the next few years, as new techniques are perfected, more surgical patients will experience a reduced amount of pain, fewer dysfunctions, and less downtime.

Another active research area concerns new materials to replace body parts. Orthopedic surgery often involves the use of pieces of bones. Traditionally these are obtained from the patient. A patient who has a back fusion using his own (termed *autologous*) bone may have more pain afterward from the area in the hip from which bone was removed than from the back, the original source of pain. The same is true when autologous bone is used in the repair of complicated fractures.

Soon, there will be less need to use the patient's bone. Cadaver bone is already being used in some cases. Various types of synthetic bone graft material are being developed and tested. In clinical trials, recently discovered natural proteins, termed *bone morphogenic proteins* (BMP), that stimulate bone growth are being tested. Once they are widely available, they will likely diminish the need for using the patient's own bone.

Other artificial parts are also being developed. Artificial disks to replace damaged intervertebral disks in the neck and back is an active area of research. Several different designs, consisting of combinations of metal, polyethylene, and polyurethane, are undergoing clinical trials. A disk made of cobalt and chrome may be available within a year or two.

## Postoperative Analgesia

As you learned in chapter 8, postoperative pain relief is receiving more and more attention. Patient-controlled analgesia (PCA) was a major improvement over the need to ring for a nurse whenever there is pain, but PCA pumps require the patient to be stuck with a needle so that the pump can be connected via tubing to the patient's vein or spinal canal. If the patient can get up, she has to drag the PCA pump around. It would be more convenient to have a transdermal pain–medication delivery system that, like a PCA pump, can be activated when it's needed, but which would also be completely self-contained.

Such a system is being tested now. It consists of a patch, about half the size of a credit card, which contains both a reservoir of fentanyl, and a combination of chemicals that produce a low-level electric current. The patch is applied to the upper arm or chest. When the patient needs more pain medication, pressing a button on the patch activates the current, which forces a measured dose of pain medication across the skin. A built-in lockout feature prevents self-administration of more pain medication than is prescribed. In a trial of more than 600 adults coming out of surgery, half were randomly assigned to intravenous morphine via a PCA pump, and half were given the patient-controlled transdermal fentanyl.[1] Unlike a conventional PCA pump, the patient can even be sent home with this transdermal PCA system. This exciting new development, however, is still investigational.

## Opioids for Chronic Pain

Another active research area is in providing new delivery systems for opioids. As was explained in chapter 5, taking a long-acting opioid for chronic pain is preferable to an immediate-release drug. This is because the long-acting preparation gives more even blood levels, resulting in better pain relief and less likelihood of mood alteration. Additionally, it provides longer relief, so you can get a good night's sleep rather than being awakened with pain in the middle of the night. The choice of long-acting and sustained-release opioids currently available is small: sustained-release morphine (generics, Oramorph, MS Contin, Kadian, Avinza); sustained-release oxycodone (OxyContin and a generic); methadone; and fentanyl transdermal patches (Duragesic).

At this time, the powerful opioid hydromorphone, five times as potent as morphine, is available only in an immediate-release tablet. However, a sustained-release is undergoing clinical trials. When this product becomes available, it will add to the short list of sustained-release opioids available. A sustained-release form of oxymorphone, another powerful opioid, is also in development.

Many health care providers are reluctant to prescribe any opioids for chronic non-cancer pain because they fear the drugs may be abused by the patient, or else diverted to drug abusers. Research is actively going on into developing a way to make opioids less abusable.

Abuse of opioids requires disrupting their delivery system. They are also frequently introduced into the body in ways other than intended. An example of such misuse would be crushing a tablet and then inhaling or injecting the contents. One way of discouraging abuse is to compound the opioid together with an antagonist that counteracts its effect. The idea, of course, is to produce a combination in which the antagonist doesn't take effect if the product is used as intended. A prototype for such a combination is already available for treatment of narcotic addicts. Called Suboxone, this product is a combination of the opioid buprenorphine and the opioid-antagonist naloxone (Narcan). Naloxone binds to the same opioid receptors as does buprenorphine and prevents the buprenorphine from having any effects. Suboxone is a sublingual preparation; when put under the tongue, only the buprenorphine is absorbed. But if it is crushed and then injected or otherwise misused, both chemicals are absorbed, and will neutralize each other. Not only that, but if the person is addicted to opioids, the naloxone, if absorbed, will cause very unpleasant withdrawal symptoms. As a result of this safety mechanism, people are unlikely to abuse Suboxone.

Pharmaceutical companies are actively researching combinations of their opioids and opioid-antagonists in order to make them less abusable. They are also working on better delivery systems for their existing drugs. The transdermal fentanyl patch (Duragesic) is a clever alternative to oral opioids. However, the patches come in only a few strengths, and the patches can't be cut if intermediate doses are needed. Physicians have long wished for additional dosage strength, especially because the lowest dose currently available, 25 mcg per hour, is still too high for many people who aren't used to taking such a powerful medication. A 12.5 mcg per hour patch will soon be available. In addition, a new type of fentanyl patch is now being developed in which the medication is embedded in tiny spheres distributed throughout the patch. Such a patch can be cut without altering its sustained-release properties, allowing for much greater flexibility in dosing.

# GLOSSARY OF TERMS

**ADDICTION:** a primary, chronic, neurobiological disease, with genetic, psychosocial, and environmental factors influencing its development and manifestations. It is characterized by behaviors that include: impaired control over drug use (compulsive use), continued use despite harm, and craving. (AAPM/APS/ASAM consensus document, 2001). According to the Diagnostic and Statistical Manual of Mental Disorders, 4th Edition, addictions are characterized by (1) loss of control, (2) continuation despite significant adverse consequences, and (3) preoccupation or obsession with obtaining and using the drug.

**AFFERENT SIGNALS:** Electrical and chemical signals that travel from peripheral nerves to the central nervous system.

**ALLODYNIA:** A sensation of pain resulting from a normally nonpainful stimulus (e.g. light touch, clothing, or air movement, or an ordinarily nonpainful warm or cold stimulus).

**ANALGESIA:** Absence of pain in response to a normally painful stimulus.

**ANALGESIC:** Pain-relieving, or a pain reliever.

**ANESTHESIA:** Total or partial loss of sensation. This may be deliberately produced—by acupuncture or an anesthetic—or an undesirable effect of disease or injury.

**ANESTHETIC:** A drug that produces loss of consciousness (general anesthetic) or loss of sensation in one part of the body (regional or local anesthetic).

**ANTINOCICEPTIVE:** A drug or procedure that blocks pain sensations or the transmission of pain signals.

**BIOFEEDBACK:** A training technique for enabling a person to voluntarily control an autonomic body function, such as breathing, brain waves, or skin temperature.

**BREAKTHROUGH PAIN:** Intermittent exacerbation of pain that can be brought on with increased activity or may occur spontaneously.

**CENTRAL NERVOUS SYSTEM:** The brain and spinal cord.

**CENTRAL PAIN:** Pain resulting from nerve injury or abnormal function of nerves in the brain and/or spinal cord.

**CENTRAL SENSITIZATION:** Changes in the central nervous system that increase its sensitivity to pain signals. A state of spinal neuron hyperexcitability caused by inflammation, aberrant neural input, or both, which is maintained by ongoing nociceptive input.

**DORSAL HORN:** The part of the spinal cord through which pain signals are processed and transmitted.

**DOUBLE-BLIND STUDY:** A study in which neither the experimenter nor the subject knows whether he or she is getting the real medication or a placebo.

**EFFERENT SIGNALS:** Electrical and chemical signals that travel from the central nervous system to peripheral nerves.

**ENDOGENOUS:** Originating within the body.

**ENDORPHINS:** A group of opioids that are synthesized in the body. They can bind to opioid receptors and can produce pain relief and euphoria.

**ENKEPHALINS:** Another group of opioids that are synthesized in the body.

**EPIDURAL:** Located in the spinal canal, outside the thick membrane that surrounds the spinal cord (the dura mater).

**EXOGENOUS:** Originating outside the body.

**GATE THEORY:** A theory proposed by Wall and Melzack that describes a functional "gate" within the spinal cord that allows or blocks pain impulses from proceeding upward to the brain.

**HYPERALGESIA:** Increased sensitivity to pain. An exaggerated painful response to a mildly noxious stimulus, either mechanical or thermal.

**HYPERSENSITIVITY:** Increased sensitivity.

**HYPNOSIS:** A state of increased focus and heightened sensitivity that can be used to reduce or eliminate pain.

**META-ANALYSIS:** Combining the results of more than one study of the same subject (such as a new drug or procedure) so as to draw more definitive conclusions.

**NERVE BLOCK:** A procedure to relieve pain in which an anesthetic is injected into or near a nerve.

**NEURON:** Nerve cell.

**MODULATION:** Affecting the intensity of pain signals.

**NEUROPATHIC PAIN:** Pain that results from malfunction of or direct injury to a nerve.

**NEUROTRANSMITTER:** A chemical that transmits information between nerve cells.

**NOCICEPTIVE:** Pain-producing.

**NOCICEPTOR:** A nerve cell that detects injury and transmits pain signals.

**NON-STEROIDAL ANTI-INFLAMMATORY DRUG (NSAID):** A drug that acts like aspirin in its ability to reduce pain and inflammation that arises from injured tissue.

**OPIATE:** A natural pain-killing drug derived from morphine.

**OPIOID:** A drug with morphine-like effects. It may be natural or synthetic.

**PAIN THRESHOLD:** The point at which a stimulus is perceived as painful.

**PERIPHERAL NERVOUS SYSTEM:** The network of nerves that includes the entire body except for the spinal cord and brain.

**PERIPHERAL NEUROPATHY:** Pain along the distribution of one or more peripheral nerves caused by nerve damage. Examples are diabetic neuropathy, carpal tunnel syndrome, and post-herpetic neuralgia.

**PHYSICAL DEPENDENCE:** A state of adaptation that is manifested by a drug class–specific withdrawal syndrome that can be produced by abrupt cessation, rapid dose reduction, decreasing blood level of the drug, and/or administration of an antagonist ((AAPM/APS/ASAM consensus document, 2001).

**PLACEBO:** A drug or treatment that contains no active ingredient.

**PLACEBO-CONTROLLED STUDY:** A study in which some patients get the active drug or treatment, the others a placebo. It's important to compare an active drug to a placebo because the placebo may have beneficial effects just because people believe they're receiving treatment.

**PROSPECTIVE STUDY:** A study in which the investigators plan in advance how to treat patients or survey them at baseline and then again later to see what happens in the meantime. This type of study is considered of higher quality than a retrospective study (see below).

**RECEPTOR:** A "lock" or site on the surface of a cell into which a chemical such as a drug or neurotransmitter fits like a key.

**REFERRED PAIN:** Pain felt at a site different from the injured or diseased body part.

**RETROSPECTIVE STUDY:** A study in which the investigators review past records or ask the participants questions about their past experiences.

**SOMATIC PAIN:** Pain involving structures in the body such as muscles, bones, tendons, and ligaments.

**SYNERGISM:** The ability of two medications to interact in a way that the total effect of the drugs is more than the sum of both.

**TOLERANCE:** A state of adaptation in which exposure to a drug induces changes that result in a decrease of one or more of the drug's effects over time (AAPM/APS/ASAM consensus document, 2001). Simply put, a given dose of the drug has less effect over time so that more is needed to get the same effect.

**TRANSDERMAL:** Through the skin. A popular way to give some drugs.

# References

## PREFACE

1. MDs struggle to treat chronic pain. *The Quality Indicator Compendium on Pain*, Nov. 2002, pp. 9-10.
2. Hill, C.S. *JAMA* 274:1881-1882, 1995.

## CHAPTER ONE

1. Merksey, H., and Bogduk, N. (Eds) *Classification of chronic pain – Descriptions of chronic pain syndromes, and definitions of pain terms*, 2nd Edition. Seattle: IASP Press, 1994. pp 40-43.
2. Fishbain, D., Cole, B., and Cutler, R. Is pain fatiguing? Abstract 620 at the 2003 meeting of the American Pain Society, March 20-23, 2003.
3. Stewart, W.F., Ricci, J.A., Chee, E., Morganstein, D., and Lipton, R. Lost productive time and cost due to common pain conditions in the U.S. workforce. *Journal of the American Medical Association* 290:2443-2454, 2003.
4. Apfelbaum, J.L., Chen, C., Mehta, S.S., and Gan, T.J. Postoperative pain experience: Results from a national survey suggest postoperative pain continues to be under-managed. *Anesthesia and Analgesia* 97:534-540, 2003.
5. Foley, K.M. "Europe against pain: Current program and new epidemiologic data." Presentation at the 6th International Conference on Pain and Chemical Dependency, New York, Feb. 5, 2004.
6. Lanes, T.C., Gauron, E.F., Spratt, K.F., et al. Long-term follow-up of patients with chronic back pain treated in a multidisciplinary rehabilitation program. *Spine* 20:801-806, 1995; Deardorff, W.W., Rubin, H.S., and Scott, D.W.. Comprehensive multidisciplinary treatment of chronic pain: a follow-up study of treated and non-treated groups. *Pain* 45:35-43, 1991.
7. Dworkin, H.R., Backonja, M., Rowbotham, M.C., Allen, R.R., Argoff, C.R., Bennett, G.J., et al. Advances in neuropathic pain: diagnosis, mechanisms, and treatment recommendations. *Archives of Neurology* 60:1524-1534, 2003.
8. Waxman, R., Tennant, A., and Helliwell, P.A. Prospective follow-up study of low back pain in the community. *Spine* 25:2085-2090, 2000.
9. Kolata, G. With costs rising, treating back pain often seems futile. *New York Times* Feb. 9, 2004, p. A1.
10. Deyo, R.A., and Weinstein, J.N. Low back pain. *New England Journal of Medicine* 344:363-370, 2001.
11. Wiesel, S.W., Tsourmas, N., Feffer, H.L., Citrin, C.M., and Patronas, N. A study of computer-assisted tomography. I. The incidence of positive CAT scans in an asymptomatic group of patients. *Spine* 9:549-551, 1984.
12. Deyo, R.A., and Tsui-Wu, Y.J. Descriptive epidemiology of low-back pain and its related medical care in the United States. *Spine* 12:264-268, 1987.
13. Biering-Sorenson, F. Physical measurements as risk factors in low back trouble over a one-year period. *Spine* 9:106, 1984.
14. Lawrence, R.C., Hochberg, M.C., Kelsey, J.L., et al. Estimates of the prevalence of selected arthritis and musculoskeletal diseases in the United States. *Journal of Rheumatology* 16:427-441, 1989.
15. Boden, S.D., Davis, D.O., Dina, T.S., Patronas, N.J., and Wiesel, S.W. Abnormal magnetic-resonance scans of the lumbar spine in asymptomatic subjects: A prospective investigation. *Journal of Bone and Joint Surgery* 72A:403-408, 1990.
16. Cook, D., Lange, G., Coccone, D., Liu, W., Steffener, J., and Natelson, B. Functioning imaging of pain in patients with primary fibromyalgia. *The Journal of Rheumatology* 31:364-378, 2004.

17. Durham, P.L. CGRP-receptor antagonists—a fresh approach to migraine therapy? *New England Journal of Medicine* 350:1073-1075, 2004.

18. Olesen, J., Diener, H-C., Husstedt, I.W., Goadsby, P.J., Hall, D., Meier, U., Pollentier, S., and Lesko, L.M. Calcitonin gene-related peptide receptor antagonist BIBN 4096 BS for the acute treatment of migraine. *New England Journal of Medicine* 350:1104-1110, 2004.

19. JCAHO. *Pain Assessment and Management: An Organizational Approach.* Oakbrook Terrace, IL: JCAHO, 2000.

CHAPTER TWO

1. Melzack, R., and Wall, P.D. Pain mechanisms: a new theory. *Science* 150:971-979, 1965.

2. Travell, J. Myofascial trigger points: clinical view. Bonica, J.J., and Albe-Fessard, D. (Eds.) *Advances in Pain Research and Therapy* 1:919-926, 1976.

3. Calderone, K.L. The influence of gender on the frequency of pain and sedative medication administered to postoperative patients. *Sex Roles* 23:713-725, 1990.

4. Fillingim, R.B. Sex, gender, and pain: women and men really are different. *Current Review of Pain* 4:24-30, 2000.

5. Fillingim, R.B., Maixner, W., Kincaid, S., and Silva, S. Sex differences in temporal summation but not sensory-discriminative processing of thermal pain. *Pain* 75:121-127, 1998.

6. Zubieta, J-K., Smith, Y.R., Bueller, J.A., Xu, Y., Kilbourn, M.R., Jewett, D.M., Meyer, C.R., Koeppe, R.A., and Stohler, C.S. Mu-opioid receptor-mediated antinociceptive responses differ in men and women. *Journal of Neurosciences* 22:5100-5107, 2002.

7. Flores, C.M., and Mogil, J.S. The pharmacogenetics of analgesia: toward a genetically-based approach to pain management *Pharmacogenomics* 2:177-194, 2001.

8. Gear, R.W., Miaskowski, C., Gordon, N.C., Paul, S.M., Heller, P.H., and Levine, J.D. Kappa-opioids produce significantly greater analgesia in women than in men. *Nature Medicine* 2:1248-1250, 1996.

9. Fillingim, R.B., and Edwards, R.R. The association of hormone replacement therapy with experimental pain responses in postmenopausal women. *Pain* 92:229-234, 2001.

10. Anderberg, U.M., Martinsdottir, I., Hallman, J., and Bakcstrom, T., et al. Symptom perception in relation to hormonal status in women with fibromyalgia. *Journal of Musculoskeletal Pain* 7:21-38, 1999.

11. Riley, J.L. III, Robinson, M.E., Wise, E.A., and Price, D.D. A meta-analytic review of pain perception across the menstrual cycle. *Pain* 81:225-235, 1999.

12. Unger, J., Cady, R.K., and Farmer-Cady, K. Migraine headaches, Part 3: Hormonal factors. *The Female Patient* 28:31-34, 2003.

13. Bergh, I., Steen, G., Waern, M., Johansson, B., Oden, A., Sjostrom, B., and Steen, B. Pain and its relation to cognitive function and depressive symptoms: a Swedish population study of 70-year-old men and women. *Journal of Pain and Symptom Management* 26:903-912, 2003.

14. Andrews, K., and Fitzgerald, M. Cutaneous flexion reflex in human neonates: a quantitative study of threshold and stimulus–response characteristics after single and repeated stimuli. *Develop Medical Child Neurology* 41:696-703, 1999.

15. Fitzgerald, M., and Beggs, S. The neurobiology of pain: developmental aspects. *Neuroscientist* 7:246-257, 2001.

16. Scholz, J., and Woolf, C.J. Can we conquer pain? *Nature Neuroscience* 5(suppl):1-62-1067, 2002. Anand, K.J. Pain, plasticity, and premature birth: a prescription for permanent suffering? *Nature Medicine* 6:971-973, 2000.

17. Simons, S.H.P., Van Kijk, M., Anand, K.S., Roofthooft, D., Van Lingen, R.A., and Tibboel, D. Do we still hurt newborn babies? A prospective study of procedural pain and analgesia in neonates. *Archives of Pediatrics and Adolescent Medicine* 157:1058-1064, 2003.

18. Taddio, A., Katz, J., Ilersich, A., and Koren, G. Effect of neonatal circumcision on pain response during subsequent routine vaccination. *Lancet* 349:599-603, 1997.

19. Weisman, S.J., Bernstein, B., and Schechter, N.L. Consequences of inadequate analgesia during

painful procedures in children. *Archives of Pediatric and Adolescent Medicine* 152:147-149, 1998.

20. Buskila, D., Neumann, L., Zmora, E., Feldman, M., Bolotin, A., and Press, J. Pain sensitivity in prematurely born adolescents. *Archives of Pediatrics and Adolescent Medicine* 117:1079-1083, 2003.

21. Howard, R.F. Current status of pain management in children. *Journal of the American Medical Association* 290:2464-1469, 2003.

22. Malleson, P.N., Connell, H., Bennett, S.M., and Eccleston, C. Chronic musculoskeletal and other idiopathic pain syndromes. *Archives of Diseases in Children* 84:189-192, 2001.

23. Ferrell, B.A. Pain evaluation and management in the nursing home. *Annals of Internal Medicine* 123:681-687, 1995.

24. Bergh, I., Steen, G., Waern, M., Johansson, B., Oden, A., Sjostrom, B., and Steen, B. Pain and its relation to cognitive function and depressive symptoms: A Swedish population study of 70-year-old men and women. *Journal of Pain and Symptom Management* 26:903-912, 2003.

25. Cleeland, C.S., Gonin, initials Hatfield, A.K., et al. Pain and its treatment in outpatients with metastatic cancer. *New England Journal of Medicine* 330:592-596, 1994.

26. The management of persistent pain in older persons. AGS Panel on Persistent Pain in Older Persons. *Journal of the American Geriatric Society* 50:S205-224, 2002

27. Wright, D., Barrow, S., Fisher, A.D., Horsley, S.D., and Jayson M.I. Influence of physical, psychological and behavioural factors on consultations for back pain. *British Journal of Rheumatology* 34:156-161, 1995.

28. Palmer, K.T., Syddall, H., Cooper, C., and Coggon, D. Smoking and musculoskeletal disorders: Findings from a British national survey, 2003.

29. Andersson, H., Ejlertsson, G., and Leden, I. Widespread musculoskeletal chronic pain associated with smoking. An epidemiological study in a general rural population. *Scandinavian Journal of Rehabilitation Medicine* 30:185-191, 1998.

30. Eriksen, W.B., Brage, S., and Bruusgaard, D. Does smoking aggravate musculoskeletal pain? *Scandinavian Journal of Rheumatology* 26:49-54, 1997.

31. West, D.C., et al. Second-hand smoke and risk of sickle cell crisis in children. *Archives of Pediatric and Adolescent Medicine* 157:1197-1201, 2003.

32. Schmidt, B.L., Tembeli, C.H., Gear, R.W., and Levine, J.D. Nicotine withdrawal hyperalgesia and opioid-mediated analgesia depend on nicotine receptors in nucleus accumbens. *Neuroscience* 106:129-36, 2001.

33. Pembrook, L. Patients taking small amounts of vitamin C experience more pain. *Pain Medicine News* January/February 2004, p. 15.

34. Flores, C.M., and Mogil, J.S. The pharmacogenetics of analgesia: toward a genetically-based approach to pain management. *Pharmacogenomics* 2:177-194, 2001.

35. Indo Y., Tsuruta Y,. Hayashida Y., Karim M.A., Ohta K., Kawano, T., Mitsubuchi H., Tonoki H., Awaya Y., and Matsuda I., Mutations in the TRKA/NGF receptor gene in patients with congenital insensitivity to pain with anhidrosis. *Nature Genetics* 13:485-488, 1996.

36. Levine J.D., Gordon N.C., Smith R., and Fields H.L. Analgesic responses to morphine and placebo in individuals with postoperative pain. *Pain* 10:379-389, 1981.

37. Zubieta, J-K., Heitzeg, M.M., Smith, Y.R., Bueller, J.A., Xu, K., Xu, Y., Koeppe, R.A., Stohler, C.S., and Goldman, D. COMT *val* 158*met* genotype affects mu-opioid neurotransmitter responses to a pain stressor. *Science* 299:1240-1243, 2003.

38. Raphael, K.G., Widom, C.S., and Lange, G. Childhood victimization and pain in childhood: a prospective investigation. *Pain* 92:283-293, 2001.

39. Strusberg, I., Mendelberg, R.C., Serra, H.A., and Strusberg, A.M. Influence of weather conditions on rheumatic pain. *Journal of Rheumatology* 29:335-338, 2002.

40. Price, D.D., Staud, R., Robinson, M.E., Mauderli, A.P., Cannon, R., and Vierck, C.J. Enhanced temporal summation of second pain and its central modulation in fibromyalgia patients. *Pain* 99:49-59, 2002.

CHAPTER THREE

1.  Portenoy, R., and Foley, K.M. Chronic use of opioid analgesics in non-malignant pain. *Pain* 25:171-186, 1986.
2.  Potter, M., Schafer, S., Gonzalez-Mendez, E., Gjeltema, K., Lopez, A., Wu, J., Pedrin, R., Cozen, M., Wilson, R., Thom, D., and Croughan-Minihane, M. Opioids for chronic nonmalignant pain: attitudes and practices of primary care physicians in the UCSF/Stanford Collaborative Research Network. University of California, San Francisco. *Journal of Family Practice* 50:145-151, 2001.
3.  Von Roenn, J.H., Cleeland, C.S., Gonin, R., Hatfield, A.K., and Pandya, K.J. Physician attitudes and practice in cancer pain management: a survey from the Eastern Cooperative Oncology Group. *Annals of Internal Medicine* 119:121-126, 1993.
4.  Lesho, E.P. When the spirit hurts: an approach to the suffering patient. *Archives of Internal Medicine* 163:2429-2432.
5.  Ferrell, B.R., Novy, D., Sullivan, M.D., Banja, J., Dubois, M.Y., Gitlin, M.C., Hamaty, D., Levovits, A., Lipman, A.G., Lippe, P.M., and Livovich, J. Ethical dilemmas in pain management. *Journal of Pain* 2:171-180, 2001.
6.  Turk, D.C. Clinicians' attitudes about prolonged use of opioids and the issue of patient heterogeneity. *Journal of Pain and Symptom Management* 11:218-230, 1996.
7.  Gianelli, D.M. Treat pain, avert suicide. *American Medical News* 39(36), Sept. 23/30, 1996, p. 1.
8.  Ganzini, L., Silveira, M.J., and Johnston, W.S. Predictors and correlates of interest in assisted suicide in the final months of life among ALS patients in Oregon and Washington. *Journal of Pain and Symptom Management* 24:312-317, 2002.
9.  Bonham, V.L. Race, ethnicity, and pain treatment: Striving to understand the causes and solutions to the disparities in pain treatment. *Journal of Law and Medical Ethics* 29:52-68, 2002.
10. Anderson, K.O., Richman, S.P., Hurley, J., et al. Cancer pain management among underserved minority outpatients: perceived needs and barriers to optimal control. *Cancer* 94:2295-2304, 2002.
11. Kutzma, E.C. Culturally competent drug administration. *American Journal of Nursing* 99:46-51, 1999.
12. Kagawa-Singer, M., and Blackall, L.J. Negotiating cross-cultural issues at the end of life. *Journal of the American Medical Association* 286:2993-3001, 2001.

CHAPTER FOUR

1.  Joint Commission on Accreditation of Health care Organizations. *Pain Assessment and Management*, 2000.
2.  Stubhaug, A., Grimstad, J., and Breivik, H. Lack of analgsic effect of 50 and 100 mg of oral tramadol after orthopaedic surgery: a randomized, double-blind, placebo and standard active drug comparison. *Pain* 62:111-118, 1995.
3.  Smith, A.J. The analgesic effects of selective serotonin reuptake inhibitors. *Journal of Psychopharmacology* 12:407-413, 1998.
4.  Jung, A.C., Staiger, T., and Sullivan, M. The efficacy of selective serotonin reuptake inhibitors for the management of chronic pain. *Journal of General Internal Medicine* 12:384-389, 1997.
5.  Staiger, T., Gaster, B., Sullivan, M., and Deyo, R. Systematic review of antidepressants for low back pain. *Spine* 22:2540-2545, 2003.
6.  Fishbain, D.A., Cutler, R., Rosomoff, H.L., and Rosomoff, R.S. Evidence-based data from animal and human experimental studies on pain relief with antidepressants: a structured review. *Pain Medicine* 1:310-316, 2000.
7.  Fishbain, D.A. Evidence-based data on pain relief with antidepressants. *Annals of Medicine* 1:310-316, 2000.
8.  Felder, M. Tizanidine in the treatment of neck and low back pain. *Adis International* 1994: Issue 1.
9.  Lavelle, T. Tizanidine in the treatment of tension-type headache. *Adis International* 1994: Issue 2.
10. Turturro, M.A., et al Cyclobenzaprine with ibuprofen versus ibuprofen alone in acute myofascial strain: a randomized, double-blind clinical trial. *Annals of Emergency Medicine* 41:818-26, 2003.
11. Krusz, J.C., Belanger, J., and Mills, C. Tizanidine: a novel effective agent for the treatment of chronic headaches. *Headache Quarterly* 11:41-45, 2000.

12. Backonja, M., Beydoun, A., Edwards, K.R., Schwartz, S.L., Fonseca, V., Hes, M., et al. Gabapentin for the symptomatic treatment of painful neuropathy in patients with diabetes mellitus: a randomized controlled trial. *Journal of the American Medical Association* 280: 1831-6, 1998

13. Rowbotham, M., Harden, N., Stacey, B., Bernstein, P., Magnus-Miller, L. Gabapentin for the treatment of postherpetic neuralgia: a randomized controlled trial. *Journal of the American Medical Association* 280: 1837-42, 1998.

14. Brandes, J.L., Saper, J.R., Diamond, M., Couch, J.R., Lewis, D.W., Schmitt, J., Neto, W., Schwabe, S., and Jacobs, D. Topiramate for migraine prevention: a randomized controlled trial. *Journal of the American Medical Association* 291:965-973, 2004.

15. Vinik, A., and Beydoun, A. Topiramate reduces pain scores in patients with diabetic neuropathy. Presentation (PO2.149) at the 2003 annual meeting of the American Academy of Neurology. Cited in *Pain Medicine News*, Nov/Dec. 2003, p. 21.

16. Dworkin, R.H., et al. Pregabalin for the treatment of postherpetic neuralgia: A randomized, placebo-controlled trial. *Neurology* 60:1274-1283, 2003.

17. Gammaitoni, A.R. and Alvarez, N.A. 24-hour application of the Lidoderm patch 5% for 3 consecutive days is safe and well tolerated in healthy adult men and women. Abstract PO6.20, Presented at the 54th Annual American Academy of Neurology Meeting, Denver, CO, April 13-20, 2002.

18. Lipman, A.G., Dalpiaz, A.S., and London, S.P. Topical lidocaine patch therapy for myofascial pain. Abstract 782. Presented at the Annual Scientific Meeting of the American Pain Society. Baltimore, MD, March 14-17, 2002.

19. Frerick, H., Keitel, W., Kuhn, U., Schmidt, S., Bredehorst, A., and Kuhlmann, M. Topical treatment of chronic low back pain with a capsicum plaster. *Pain* 106:59-64, 2003.

20. Schieszer, J. Capsaicin patches for patients with postherpetic neuralgia. *Internal Medicine World Report* Oct. 2003, p. 13.

21. O'Kane, C.J.A., and Anderson, S. Comparative efficacy of a proprietary topical ibuprofen gel and oral ibuprofen in acute soft-tissue injuries: a randomized, double-blind study. *Journal of Clinical Pharmacy and Therapeutics* 27:409-417, 2002.

22. Argoff, C.E. Targeted topical peripheral analgesics in the management of pain. *Current Pain and Headache Reports* 7:34-38, 2003.

23. Galeotti, N., DeCesare Mannelli, L., and Mazzanti, G.. Menthol: a natural analgesic compound. *Neuroscience Letters* 322:145-148, 2002.

24. Hocking, G., and Cousins, M. Ketamine in chronic pain management: an evidence-based review. *Anesthesia and Analgesia* 97:1730-1739, 2003.

25. Turturro, M.A., et al. Cyclobenzaprine with ibuprofen versus ibuprofen alone in acute myofascial strain: a randomized, double-blind clinical trial. *Annals of Emergency Medicine* 41:818-26, 2003.

26. Kolesnikov, Y., Wilson, R., and Pasternak, G. The synergistic analgesic interactions between hydrocodone and ibuprofen. *Anesthesia and Analgesia* 97:1721-1723, 2003.

27. Scharf, M.B., Baumann, and Berkowitz, D.V. The effects of sodium oxybate on clinical symptoms and sleep patterns in patients with fibromyalgia. *Journal of Rheumatology* 30:1070-74, 2003.

28. Scharf, M.B., Hauck, M., Stover, R., McDannold, R., and Berkowitz, D. Effect of gamma-hydroxybutyrate on pain, fatigue, and the alpha sleep anomaly in patients with fibromyalgia: A preliminary report. *Journal of Rheumatology* 25:1986-1990, 1998.

29. Unger, J., Cady, R., and Farmer-Cady, K. Understanding migraine: Strategies for prevention. *Emergency Medicine* October 2003, pp. 39-46.

30. Unger, J., Cady, R., and Farmer-Cady, K. Understanding migraine: Strategies for prevention. *Emergency Medicine* October 2003, pp. 39-46.

31. Unger, J., Cady, R., and Farmer-Cady, K. Understanding migraine: Strategies for prevention. *Emergency Medicine* October 2003, pp. 39-46.

32. Finn, R. "Use 'bridge therapies' for chronic daily headache." *Internal Medicine News* March 15, 2004, p. 15.

33. Spira, P.J., Beran, R.G., and Australian Gabapentin Chronic Daily Headache Group. Gabapentin in the prophylaxis of chronic daily headache: a randomized, placebo-controlled study. *Neurology* 61:1753-1759, 2003.

34. Richy, F., Bruyere, O., Ethgen, O., Cucherat, M., Henrotin, Y., and Reginster, J-Y. Structural and symptomatic efficacy of glucosamine and chondroitin in knee osteoarthritis. *Archives of Internal Medicine* 163:1514-1522, 2003.

35. Reginster, J.Y., Deroisy, R., Rovati, L.C., et al. Long-term effects of glucosamine sulphate on osteoarthritis progression: a randomised, placebo-controlled clinical trial. *Lancet* 357:251-156, 2001.

36. Pavelka, K., Gatterova, J., Oljarova, M., et al. Glucosamine sulfate use and delay or progression of knee osteoarthritis: a three-year randomized placebo-controlled, double-blind study. *Archives of Internal Medicine* 162:2113-2123, 2002.

CHAPTER FIVE

1. Rowbotham, M.C., Twilling, L., Davis, P.S., Reisner, L., Taylor, K., and Mohr, D. Oral opoid therapy for chronic peripheral and central neuropathic pain. *New England Journal of Medicine* 348:1223-32, 2003; Foley, K.M. Opioids and chronic neuropathic pain. *New England Journal of Medicine* 348:1279-81, 2003.

2. Watson, C.P., and Babul, N. Efficacy of oxycodone in neuropathic pain: A randomized trial in postherpetic neuralgia. *Neurology* 50;1837-1841, 1998.

3. Melzack, R. The tragedy of needless pain. *Scientific American* 262:2-8, 1990.

4. Andersen, G., Christrup, L., and Sjogren, P. Relationships among morphine metabolism, pain and side effects during long-term treatment: an update. *Journal of Pain and Symptom Management* 25:74-91, 2003.

5. Mercadante, S., Ferrera, P., and Villari, P. Hyperalgesia: an emerging iatrogenic syndrome. *Journal of Pain and Symptom Management* 26:769-775, 2003.

6. Staats, P., Markowitz, J., and Schein, J. Incidence of constipation with long-acting opioid therapy: a comparative study. *Southern Medical Journal* 97:129-134, 2004.

7. Payne, R., Coluzzi, P., Hart, L., Simmonds, M., Lyss, A., Rauck, R., Berris, R., Busch, M.A., Nordbrook, E., Loseth, D.B., and Portenoy, R.K. Long-term safety of oral transmucosal fentanyl citrate for breakthrough cancer pain. *Journal of Pain and Symptom Management* 22:575-583, 2001.

8. Krantz, M.I., Lewkowiez, L., Hayes, H., Woodroffe, M.A., Robertson, A.D., and Mehler, P.S. Torsade de Pointes associated with very high-dose methadone. *Annals of Internal Medicine* 2002;137:501-504.

9. Martell, B.A., Amsten, J.H., Ray, B., and Gourvitch, M.N. The impact of methadone induction on cardiac conduction in opiate users. *Annals of Internal Medicine* 139:154-155, 2003.

10. American Pain Society. *Principles of Analgesic Use in the Treatment of Acute Pain and Cancer Pain*, 4th edition. Glenview, Illinois: American Pain Society, 1999.

11. Portenoy, R.K., and Foley, K.M. Chronic use of opioid analgesics in non-malignant pain: report of 38 cases. *Pain* 25:171-186, 1986.

12. Zenz, M., Strumpf, M., and Tryba, M. Long-term oral opioid therapy in patients with chronic nonmalignant pain. *Journal of Pain and Symptom Management* 7:69-77, 1992.

13. Mystakidou, K., Parpa, E., Tsilika, E., Mavromati, A., Smyrniotis, V., Georgaki, S., and Vlahos, L. Long-term management of noncancer pain with transdermal therapeutic system-fentanyl. *Journal of Pain* 4:298-306, 2003.

14. Jamison, R.N., Raymond, S., Slawsby, E.A., Nedelijkovic, S.S., and Katz, N.P. Opioid therapy for chronic noncancer back pain: a randomized prospective study. *Spine* 23:2591-2600, 1998.

15. Roth, S.H., Fleischmann, R.M., Burch, F.X., Dietz, F., Bockow, B., Rapoport, R.J., Rutstein, J., and Lacouture, P.G. Around-the-clock, controlled-release oxycodone therapy for osteoarthritis-related pain: Placebo-controlled trial and long-term evaluation. *Archives of Internal Medicine* 160:853-860, 2000.

16. Raja, S.N., Haythornwaite, J.A., Pappagallo, M., et al. Opioids versus antidepressants in postherpetic neuralgia: a randomized placebo-controlled trial. *Neurology* 59:1015-1021, 2002.

17. Chou, R., Clark, E., and Helfand, M. Comparative efficacy and safety of long-acting oral opioids for chronic non-cancer pain: a systematic review. *Journal of Pain and Symptom Management* 26(5): 2074, 2003.

18. Galer, B.S., Coyle, N., Pasternak, G.W., and Portenoy, R.K. Individual variability in the response to different opioids: report of five cases. *Pain* 49:87-91, 1992.

19. Reuben, S.S., Connelly, N.R., and Maciolek, H. Postoperative analgesia with controlled-release oxycodone for outpatient anterior cruciate ligament surgery. *Anesthesia and Analgesia* 88:1286-1291, 1999.

20. Parris, W.C., Johnson, B.W., Jr, Croghan, M.K., Moore, M.R., Khojasteh, A., Reder, R.F., Kaiko, R.F., and Buckley, B.J. The use of controlled-release oxycodone for the treatment of chronic cancer pain: a randomized, double-blind study. *Journal of Pain and Symptom Management* 16:205-211, 1998.

21. Caldwell, J.R., Hale, M.E., Boyd, R.E., Hague, M.J., Iwan, T., Shi, M., and LaCouture, P.G. Treatment of osteoarthritis pain with controlled release oxycodone or fixed combination oxycodone plus acetaminophen added to nonsteroidal anti-inflammatory: A double blind, randomized, multicenter, placebo-controlled trial. *Journal of Rheumatology* 26:862-869, 1999.

22. Landy, S. Oral transmucosal fentanyl citrate (OTFC) for the outpatient treatment of migraine headache pain. Abstract presented at the 22nd Annual Scientific Meeting of the American Pain Society, Chicago, March 20-23, 2003.

23. Savage, S. in *Principles of Addiction Medicine*, Section 8, Chapter 3, p. 9. Chevy Chase, MD: American Society of Addiction Medicine, 1994.

24. Galer, B.S., Pasternak, G.W., and Portenoy, R.K. Individual variability in the response to different opioids: report of five cases. *Pain* 49:87-91, 1992.

25. Flores, C.M., and Mogil, J.S. The pharmacogenetics of analgesia: toward a genetically-based approach to pain management. *Pharmacogenomics* 2:177-194, 2001.

26. Maitre, P.O., Ausems, M.E., Vozeh, S., and Stanski, D.R. Evaluating the accuracy of using population pharmacokinetic data to predict plasma concentrations of alfentanil. *Anesthesiology* 68:59-67, 1988.

27. Levy, M.H. Pharmacologic treatment of cancer pain. *New England Journal of Medicine* 335:1124-1131, 1996.

28. Galer, B.S., Coyle, N., Pasternak, G.W., and Portenoy, R.K. Individual variability in the response to different opioids: report of five cases. *Pain* 49:87-91, 1992.

29. Bouckoms, A.J., Masand, P., Murray, G.B., Cassem, E.H., Stern, T.A., and Tesar, G.E. Chronic nonmalignant pain treatment with long term analgesics. *Annals of Clinical Psychiatry* 4:185-92, 1992.

30. Zenz, M., Strumpf, M., and Tryba, M. Long-term opioid therapy in patients with chronic nonmalignant pain. *Journal of Pain and Symptom Management* 7:69-77, 1992.

31. Pappagallo, M., Raja, S.N., Haythornthwaite, J.A., Clark, M., and Campbell, J.N. Oral opioids in the management of postherpetic neuralgia: a prospective survey. *Analgesia* 1:S1-S5, 1994.

32. "Doctors struggle to treat chronic pain." *The Quality Indicator Compendium on Pain,* Nov. 2002, p 9-11.

33. Keeton, W., Yuan, W., Shelby, S., and Iwan, T. Long-term, open-label efficacy and safety evaluation of Avinza (morphine sulfate extended-release capsules) in patients with chronic back pain. Presented at: Annual Meeting of the American Society of Anesthesiologists; Oct 11-15, 2003, San Francisco.

34. American Pain Society, American Society of Addiction Medicine, and American Academy of Pain Medicine. Consensus Statement on Use of Opioids, 1996.

35. Portenoy, R.K. Using opioids for chronic nonmalignant pain: current thinking. *Internal Medicine* Supplement, March 1996, pp. 25-31.

36. Mao, J., Price, D.D., and Mayer, D.J. Mechanisms of hyperalgesia and opiate tolerance: a current view of their possible interactions. *Pain* 62:259-74, 1995.

37. Mercadante, S., Ferrera, P., and Villari, P. Hyperalgesia: An emerging iatrogenic syndrome. *Journal of Pain and Symptom Management* 26:769-775, 2003.

38. Compton, P., Athanasos, P., and Elashoff, D. Withdrawal hyperalgesia after acute opioid physical dependence in nonaddicted humans: a preliminary study. *Journal of Pain* 4:511-519, 2003.

39. De Conno, F., Caraceni, A., Martini, C., Spoldi, E., Salvetti, M., and Ventafridda, V. Hyperalgesia and myoclonus with intrathecal infusion of high-dose morphine. *Pain* 47:337-339, 1991.

40. Devulder, J. Hyperalgesia induced by high-dose intrathecal sufentanil in neuropathic pain. *Journal of Neurosurgical Anesthesiology* 9:146-148, 1997.

41. Compton, P., Athanasos, P., and Elashoff, D. Withdrawal hyperalgesia after acute opioid physical dependence in nonaddicted humans: a preliminary study. *Journal of Pain* 4:511-519, 2003.

42. Pappagallo, M. The concept of pseudotolerance to opioids. *Journal of Pharm Care in Pain and Symptom Control* 6:95-98, 1998.

43. Bruera, E., Macmillan, K., Hanson, J., and Macdonald, R.N. The cognitive effects of the administration of narcotic analgesics in patients with cancer pain. *Pain* 39:13-16, 1989.

44. "The use of opioids for the treatment of chronic pain: A consensus statement from the American Academy of Pain Medicine and the American Pain Society. 1997. American Academy of Pain Medicine and American Pain Society.

45. Bruera, E., Brenneis, C., Paterson, H., and MacDonald, R.N. Use of methylphenidate as an adjuvant to narcotic analgesics in patients with advanced cancer. *Journal of Pain and Symptom Management* 4:3-6, 1989.

46. *The Medical Letter on Drugs and Therapeutics* 42:73-78, 2000.

47. Bruera, E., Strasser, F., Shen, L., Palmer, J., Willey, J., Driver, L., and Burton, A. The effect of donepezil on sedation and other symptoms in patients receiving opioids for cancer pain. *Journal of Pain and Symptom Management* 26:2103, 2003.

48. Jamison, R.N., Schein, J.R., Vallow, S., Ascher, S., Vorsanger, G.J., and Katz, N.P. Neuropsychological effects of long-term opioid use in chronic pain patients. *Journal of Pain and Symptom Management* 26:913-921, 2003.

49. *Pain Medicine News* July-Aug. 2003, p. 3.

50. Sabatowski, R., Schwalen, S., Rettig, K., Herberg, K.W., Kasper, S.M., and Radbruch, L. Driving ability under long-term treatment with transdermal fentanyl. *Journal of Pain and Symptom Management* 25:38-47, 2003.

51. Fishbain, D.A., Cutler, R.B., Rosomoff, H.L., and Rosomoff, R.L. Are opioid-dependent/tolerant patients impaired in driving-related skills? A structured evidence-based review. *Journal of Pain and Symptom Management* 25:559-577, 2003.

52. Fishbain, D.A., Cutler, R.B., Rosomoff, H.L., and Rosomoff, R.S. Can patients taking opioids drive safely? A structured evidence-based review. *Journal of Pain and Palliative Care Pharmacotherapeutics* 16:9-28, 2002.

53. Portenoy, R.K. Using opioids for chronic nonmalignant pain: Current thinking. *Internal Medicine Supplement*, March 1996, pp. 25-31.

54. American Geriatric Society Panel on Persistent Pain in Older Persons. The management of persistent pain in older persons. *Clinical Practice Guideline* 50 (supplement) S205-S224, 2002.

55. Pfeiffer, N. Tegaserod safe and effective new treatment for chronic constipation. *Internal Medicine World Report*, Nov. 2003, p.11.

56. Finch, P.M., Roberts, L.J., Hadlow, N.C., and Pullan, P.T. Hypogonadism in patients treated with intrathecal morphine. *Clinical Journal of Pain* 16:251-254,2000.

57. Rajagopal, A., Vassilopoulou-Sellin, R., Palmer, J., Kaur, G., and Bruera, E. Hypogonadism and sexual dysfunction in male cancer survivors receiving chronic opioid therapy. *Journal of Pain and Symptom Management* 26:2116, 2003.

58. Perez-Castrillon, J.L., Olmos, J.M., Gomes, J.J., et al. Expression of opioid receptors in osteoblast-like MG-63 cells, and effects of different opioid agonists on alkaline phosphatase and osteocalcin secretion by these cells. *Neuroendocrinology* 72:187-194, 2000.

59. Kolesnikov, Y., Wilson, R., and Pasternak, G. The synergistic analgesic interactions between hydrocodone and ibuprofen. *Anesthesia and Analgesia* 97:1721-1723, 2003.

60. www.deadiversion.usdoj.gov/pubs/pressrel/newsrel_102301.pdf. Accessed Nov. 30, 2003.

CHAPTER SIX

1. Roth, S.H., Fleischmann, R.M., Burch, F.X., Dietz, F., Bockow, B., Rapoport, R.J., Rutstein, J., and Lacouture, P.G. Around-the-clock, controlled-release oxycodone therapy for osteoarthritis-related pain: placebo-controlled trial and long-term evaluation. *Archives of Internal Medicine* 160:853-860, 2000.

2. American Psychiatric Association. *Diagnostic and Statistical Manual of Mental Disorders*, 4th Edition, revised Washington, DC: 1994.

3. Savage, S.R., Joranson, D.E., Covington, E.C., Schnoll, S.H., Heit, H.A., and Gilson, A.M. Definitions related to the medical use of opioids: evolution toward universal agreement. *Journal of Pain and Symptom Management* 26:655-667, 2003.

4. Weissman, D.E., and Haddox, J.D. Opioid pseudoaddiction—an iatrogenic syndrome. *Pain* 36:363-366, 1989.

5. Joranson, D.E., Ryan, K.M., Gilson, A.M., and Dahl, J.L. Trends in medical use and abuse of opioid analgesics. *Journal of the American Medical Association* 283:1710-1714, 2000.

6. Zacny J., Bigelow G., Compton P., Foley K., Iguchi M., and Sannerud C. College on Problems of Drug Dependence taskforce on prescription opioid non-medical use and abuse: position statement. *Drug and Alcohol Dependence* 69:215-232, 2003.

7. American Society of Addiction Medicine. Public policy statement on the rights and responsibilities of physicians in the use of opioids for the treatment of pain. *Journal of Addictive Diseases* 17:131-134, 1998.

8. American Academy of Pain Medicine, American Pain Society, and American Society of Addiction Medicine. Consensus Document: Definitions related to the use of opioids for the treatment of pain. AAPM, APS, and ASAM, 2001.

9. Savage, S.R., Joranson, D.E., Covington, E.C., Schnoll, S.H., Heit, H.A., and Gilson, A.M. Definitions related to the medical use of opioids: Evolution toward universal agreement. *Journal of Pain and Symptom Management* 26:655-667, 2003.

10. Federation of State Medical Boards of the United States, Inc. Model guidelines for the treatment of pain. A policy document of the Federation of State Medical Boards of the United States, Inc., May 1998.

11. www.painfoundation.org/page.asp?menu=10&item=3&file=pagepolicyopioids.htm accessed 1/16/04.

12. Porter, J., and Jick, H. Addiction rare in patients treated with narcotics. *New England Journal of Medicine* 302:123, 1980.

13. Dunbar, S.A., and Katz, N.P. Chronic opioid therapy for nonmalignant pain in patients with a history of substance abuse: report of 20 cases. *Journal of Pain and Symptom Management* 11:163-171, 1996.

14. Currie, S.R., Hodgkins, D.C., Crabtree, A., Jacovi, J., and Armstrong, S. Outcome from integrated pain management treatment for recovering substance abusers. *The Journal of Pain* 4:91-100, 2003.

15. Federation of State Medical Boards of the United States, Inc. Model guidelines for the treatment of pain. A policy document of the Federation of State Medical Boards of the United States, Inc., May 1998.

16. "The AA member – Medications & Other Drugs." New York: Alcoholics Anonymous World Services, 1984.

17. Stolberg, S.G. "FDA calls for stronger warnings on aspirin and related painkillers." *New York Times*, Sept. 21, 2002, p. A13.

## CHAPTER SEVEN

1. Nelemans, P.J., deBie, R.A., deVet, H.C.W., and Sturmans, F. Injection therapy for subacute and chronic benign low back pain. *Spine* 26:501-515, 2001.

2. Alo, K.M., and Zidan, A.R. Selective nerve root stimulation (SNRS) in the treatment of end-stage, diabetic, peripheral neuropathy: A case report. *Neuromodulation* 3:201-208, 2000.

3. Taylor, R.S., Taylor, R.J., Van Buyten, J-P., Buchser, E., North, R., and Bayliss, S. The cost effectiveness of spinal cord stimulation in the treatment of pain: a systematic review of the literature. *Journal of Pain and Symptom Management* 27:370-378, 2004.

4. Raynauld, J.P., Buckland-Wright, C., Ward, R., Choquette, D., Haraoui, B., Martel-Pelletier, J., Uthman, I., Khy, V., Tremblay, J-L., Bertrand, B. and Pelletier, J-P. Safety and efficacy of long-term intra articular steroid injections in osteoarthritis of the knee: a randomized, double-blind placebo-controlled trial. *Arthritis & Rheumatism* 48:370-377, 2003.

5.  Brandt, K.D., Smith, G.H., Jr., and Simon, L.S. Intra articular injections of hyaluronan as treatment for knee osteoarthritis: what is the evidence? *Arthritis & Rheumatism* 43:1192-1203, 2000.

6.  Lo, G.H., LaValley, M., McAlindon, T., and Felson, D.T. Intra-articular hyaluronic acid in treatment of knee osteoarthritis: A meta-analysis. *Journal of the American Medical Association* 290:3115-3121, 2003.

7.  Leopold, S.S., Redd, B.B., Warme, W.J., Wehrle, P.A., Pettis, P.D., and Shott, S. Corticosteroid compared with hyaluronic acid injections for the treatment of osteoarthritis of the knee: a prospective, randomized trial *Journal of Bone and Joint Surgery America* 85-A:1197-203, 2003.

8.  Dreyer, M., and Edwards, K. EMG guided botulinum toxin: a treatment of piriformis syndrome. Abstract. *Journal of Pain & Symptom Management* : 82, 2003.

9.  Restivo, D.A., Tinazzi, M., Patti, F., Palmeri, A., and Maimone, D. Botulinum toxin treatment of painful tonic spasms in multiple sclerosis. *Neurology* 61: 719-720, 2003.

10. Lang, A.M. Botulinum toxin type A for the management of cervicothoracic and cervicobrachial pain: treatment rational and open-label results in 25 patients. *American Journal of Pain Management* 14:13-23, 2004.

11. Oh, W., and Shim, J. A randomized controlled trial of radiofrequency denervation of the ramus communicans nerve for chronic discogenic low back pain. *The Clinical Journal of Pain* 20:55-60, 2004.

12. Bosco Vieira Duarte, J., Kux, P., and Magalhaes Duarte, D. Endoscopic thoracic sympathicotomy for the treatment of complex regional pain syndrome. *Clinic Autonomic Research* 13 suppl 1:58-62, 2003.

CHAPTER EIGHT

1.  Altman, L.K. *Who Goes First.* New York: Random House, 1986, pp.54-55.

2.  Ibid.

3.  Tverskoy, M., Cozacov, C., Ayache, M., Bradley, E.L., Kissin, I. Postoperative pain after inguinal herniorrhaphy with different types of anesthesia. *Anesthesia Analgesia* 70:29-35, 1990.

4.  Buvanendran, A., Kroin, J.S., Tuman, K.J., Elmofty, D., Moric, M., and Rosenberg, A.G. Effects of perioperative administration of a selective cyclooxygenase 2 inhibitor on pain management and recovery of knee function after knee replacement: a randomized controlled trial. *Journal of the American Medical Association* 290:2411-2418, 2003.

5.  Pandey, C., Priye, S., Singh, S., Singh, U., Singh, R., and Singh, P. Preemptive use of gabapentin significantly decreases postoperative pain and rescue analgesic requirements in laparoscopic cholecystectomy. *Canadian Journal of Anaesthesia* 51:358-363, 2004.

6.  Ibid.

7.  Ong, K.S., and Seymour, R.A. Evidence-based medicine approach to pre-emptive analgesia. *American Journal of Pain Management* 13:158-172, 2003.

8.  Bach, S., Noreng, M.F., Tjellden, N.U. Phantom limb pain in amputees during the first 12 months following limb amputation, after preoperative lumbar epidural blockade. *Pain* 33:297-301, 1988.

9.  Samad, T.A., Moore, K.A., Sapirstein, A., et al. Interleukin-1-beta-mediated induction of COX-2 in the CNS contributes to inflammatory pain hypersensitivity. *Nature* 410:471-475, 2001; Smith, C.J., Zhang, Y., Koboldt, C.M., et al. Pharmacological analysis of cyclooxygenase-1 in inflammation. *Proceedings of the National Academy of Sciences U.S.A.* 95:13313-13318, 1998.

10. Vastag, B. Knee replacement underused, says panel. *Journal of the American Medical Association* 291:413-414, 2004.

11. Brunk, D. UniSpacer insert offers limited relief in knee OA. *Internal Medicine News*, Oct. 15, 2003, p. 12.

12. Ibid.

13. Leopold, S.S. Unicompartmental; ("Mini") knee, total knee replacement, or osteotomy for knee arthritis in a young patient?"
    www.orthop.washington.edu/hip_knee/weeklyquestions/newest/01/, accessed 4/12/04.

14. Moseley, J.B., O'Malley, K., Petersen, N.J., et al. A controlled trial of arthroscopic surgery for osteoarthritis of the knee. *New England Journal of Medicine* 347:81-88, 2002.

15. Holtzman, J., Saleh, K., and Kane, R. Effect of baseline functional status and pain on outcomes or

total hip arthroplasty. *Journal of Bone and Joint Surgery* 84A:1942-1948, 2002.

16. Saal, J.A., and Saal, J.S. Intradiscal electrothermal treatment for chronic discogenic low back pain. *Spine* 25:2622-2627, 2000.

17. Davis, T., Delamarter R., Sra P., and Goldstein, T. The IDET procedure for chronic discogenic low back pain. *Spine* 29:752-756, 2004.

18. Tanner, S.B. Back pain, vertebroplasty, and kyphoplasty: treatment of osteoporotic vertebral compression fractures. *Bulletin on the Rheumatic Diseases* 52, 2003.

CHAPTER NINE

1. Biering-Sorenson, F. Physical measurements as risk indicators for low-back trouble over a one-year period. *Spine* 9:106-119, 1984.

2. Rosenfield, M., Seferiadis, A., Carlsson, J., and Gunnarsson, R. Active intervention in patients with whiplash-associated disorders improves long-term prognosis: a randomized controlled clinical trial. *Spine* 28:2491-2498, 2003.

3. King, A.C., Oman, K.F., Brassington, G.S., Bliwise, D.L., and Haskell, J.B. Moderate-intensity exercise and self-rated quality of sleep in older adults with osteoarthritis: a randomized controlled trial. *Journal of the American Medical Association* 277:32-37, 1997.

4. Ettinger, W.H., Burns, R., Messier, S.P., Applegate, W., Rejeski, W.J., Morgan, T., Shumaker, S., Berry, M.J., O'Toole, M., Monu, J., and Craven, T. A randomized trial comparing aerobic exercise and resistance exercise to a health education program on physical disability in older adults with knee osteoarthritis: the Fitness Arthritis and Seniors Trial (FAST). *Journal of the American Medical Association* 277:25-31, 1997.

5. Van Baar, M.E., Dekker, J., Oostendorp, R.A.B., Bijl, D., Voorn, T.B., Lemmens, J.A.M., and Bijlsma, J.W.J. The effectiveness of exercise therapy in patients with osteoarthritis of the hip or knee: a randomized clinical trial. *Journal of Rheumatology* 25:2432-9, 1998.

6. Melzack, R., and Wall, P.D. Pain mechanisms: a new theory. *Science* 150:971-979, 1965.

7. Sjolund, B.H., and Eriksson, M.B. The influence of naloxone on analgesia produced by peripheral conditioning stimulation. *Brain Research* 173:295-301, 1979.

8. Dawood, M.Y., and Ramos, J. Transcutaneous electrical nerve stimulation (TENS) for the treatment of primary dysmenorrhea: a randomized crossover comparison with placebo TENS and ibuprofen. *Obstetrics and Gynecology* 75:656-660, 1990.

9. Smith, H., and Younan, V. TENS in the treatment of primary dysmenorrhea. *Practical Pain Management* Nov./Dec. 2003, pp. 26-28.

10. Repice, R.M., Chu-Andrew, J., Repice, R.M., and Bilski, M.M. Wrist traction as a new method for treatment of carpal tunnel syndrome. *American Journal of Pain Management* 14:31-36, 2003.

11. Nadler, S.F., Steiner, D.J., Ersala, G.H., Hengehold, D.A., Hinkle, R.T., Toodale, M.B., Abeln, S.F., and Weingand, K.W. Continuous low-level heat wrap therapy provides more efficacy than ibuprofen and acetaminophen for acute low back pain. *Spine* 27:1012-1017, 2002.

12. Nadler, S.F., Steiner, D.J., Petty, S.R., Ersala, G.N., Hengehold, D.A., and Weingand, K.W. Overnight use of continuous low-level heat wrap therapy for relief of low back pain. *Archives of Physical Medicine and Rehabilitation* 84:335-342, 2003.

13. Hinman, R.S., Crossley, K.M., McConnell, J., and Bennell, K.L. Efficacy of knee tape in the management of osteoarthritis of the knee: blinded randomized controlled trial. *British Medical Journal* 327:135-138, 2003.

14. Wassell J.T., Gardner L.I., Landesettel D.D., Johnston J.J., and Johnston M.N. A prospective study of back belts for prevention of back pain and injury. *Journal of the American Medical Association* 284:1717-1732, 2000.

CHAPTER TEN

1. Eisenberg, D.M., Kessler, R.C., Foster, C., Norlock, F.E., Calkins, D.R., and Delbanco, T.L. Unconventional medicine in the United States—Prevalence, costs, and patterns of use. *New England Journal of Medicine* 328:246-252, 1993.

2.  Kessler, R.C., Davis, R.B., Foster, D.F., Van Rompay, M.I., Walters, E.E., Wilkey, S.A., Kaptchuk, T.J., and Eisenberg, D.M. Long-term trends in the use of complementary and alternative medical therapies in the United States. *Annals of Internal Medicine* 135:262-268, 2001.

3.  Sunshine, W., Field, T.M., Quintino, O., Fierro, K., Kuhn, C., Burman, I., and Schanberg, S. Fibromyalgia benefits from massage therapy and transcutaneous electrical stimulation. *Journal of Clinical Rheumatology* 2:18-22, 1996.

4.  Field, T.M., Diego, M., Cullen, C., Hernandez-Reif, M., Sunshine, W., and Douglas, S. Fibromyalgia pain and substance P decrease and sleep improves after massage therapy. *Journal of Clinical Rheumatology* 8:72-76, 2002.

5.  Quinn, C., Chandler, C., and Moraska, A. Massage therapy and frequency of chronic tension headaches. *American Journal of Public Health* 92:1657-1661, 2002.

6.  Cherkin, D.C., Sherman, K.J., Deyo, R.A., and Shekelle, P.G. A review of the evidence for the effectiveness, safety, and cost of acupuncture, massage therapy, and spinal manipulation for back pain. *Annals of Internal Medicine* 138:898-906, 2003.

7.  Saitz, R. *Journal Watch* July 15, 2003, p. 111.

8.  Assendelft, W.J., Morton, S.C., Yu, E.I., Suttorp, M.J., and Shekelle, P.G. Spinal manipulative therapy for low back pain: A meta-analysis of effectiveness relative to other therapies. *Annals of Internal Medicine* 138:871-881, 2003.

9.  Ernst, E. Manual therapies for pain control: chiropractic and massage. *Clinical Journal of Pain* 20:8-12, 2004.

10. Cherkin, D.C., Deyo, R.A., Battie, M., Street, J., and Barlow, W. A comparison of physical therapy, chiropractic manipulation, and provision of an educational booklet for the treatment of patients with low back pain. *New England Journal of Medicine* 339:1021-1029, 1998.

11. Andersson, B.G., Lucente, T., Davis, A.M., Kappler, R.E., Lipton, J.A., and Leurgans, S. A comparison of osteopathic spinal manipulation with standard care for patients with low back pain. *New England Journal of Medicine* 341:1426-1431, 1999.

12. Winemiller, M.H., Billow, R.G., Laskowski, E.R., and Harmsen, M.S. Effect of magnetic versus sham-magnetic insoles on plantar heel pain: a randomized controlled trial. *Journal of the American Medical Association* 290:1474-1478, 2003.

13. Weintraub, A. *Yoga for Depression.* New York: Broadway Books, 2004, p. 7.

14. Weintraub A. Personal communication, 4/19/04.

15. van der Kolk, B. In terror's grip: healing the ravages of trauma. *Cerebrum* 4:34-50, 2002.

16. Wang, C.C., Lau, J., and Collet, J.P. Efficacy of tai chi in rheumatoid arthritis. A pilot study. *Archives of Internal Medicine,* March 2004.

17. Pomeranz, B. Scientific research into acupuncture for the relief of pain. *Journal of Alternative and Complementary Medicine* 2:53-60, 1996.

18. Mayer, D.J., Price, D.D., and Rafii, A. Antagonism of acupuncture analgesia in man by the narcotic antagonist naloxone. *Brain Research* 121:368-372, 1977.

19. Sjolund, B.H., and Eriksson M.B.E. The influence of naloxone on analgesia produced by peripheral conditional stimulation. *Brain Research* 173:295-301, 1979.

20. Ha, H., Tan, E., Fukunaga, H., and Aochi, O. Naloxone reversal of acupuncture analgesia in the monkey. *Experimental Neurology* 73:298-303, 1981.

21. Clement-Jones, V., McLoughlin, L., Tomlin, S., Besser, G.M., Rees, L.H., and Wen, L. Increased beta-endorphin but not met-enkephalin levels in human cerebrospinal fluid after acupuncture for recurrent pain. *Lancet* 2:946-949, 1980.

22. Acupuncture. NIH Consensus Statement 15(5), Nov. 3-5, 1997: 1-34.

23. Kim, Y., Kim, C.W., and Kim, K.S. Clinical observations on postoperative vomiting treated by auricular acupuncture. *American Journal of Chinese Medicine* 31:475-480, 2003.

24. Gilbertson, B., Wenner, K., and Russell, L.C. Acupuncture and arthroscopic acromioplasty. *Journal of Orthopaedic Research* 21:752-758, 2003.

25. Edwards, J., and Knowles, N. Superficial dry needling and active stretching in the treatment of myofascial pain: a randomized controlled group. *Acupuncture in Medicine* 21:80-86, 2003.

26. Alimi D., Rubino C., Pichard-Leandri E., Fermand-Brule S., Dubreuil-Lemaire M.L., and Hill C. Analgesic effect of auricular acupuncture for cancer pain: A randomized, blinded, controlled trial. *Journal of Clinical Oncology* 21:4120-4126, 2003.

27. Gilbertson, B., Wenner, K., and Russell, L.C. Acupuncture and arthroscopic acromioplasty. *Journal of Orthopedic Research* 21:752-758, 2003.

28. Meng, C.F., Wang, D., Ngeow, J., Lao, L., Peterson, M., and Paget, S. Acupuncture for chronic low back pain in older patients: a randomized, controlled trial. *Rheumatology* 42:1508-1517, 2003.

29. Vickers A.J., Rees R.W., Zollman, C.E., McCarney R., Smith C.M., Ellis N., Fisher P., and Van Haselen R. Acupuncture for chronic headache in primary care: large, pragmatic, randomised trial. *British Medical Journal*, doi:10.1136/bmj.38029.421863.EB (published 16 March 2004).

30. McCaffery, A.M., Eisenberg, D.M., Legedza, A.T.R. Davis, R.B., and Phillips, R.S. Prayer for health concerns: Results of a national survey on prevalence and patterns of use. *Archives of Internal Medicine* 164:858-862, 2004.

31. Harris, W.S., Gowda, M., Kolb, J.W., Strychacz, C.P., Vacek, J.L., Jones, P.G., et al. Effect of intercessory prayer on cardiac care unit patients. *Archives of Internal Medicine* 159:2273-, 1999.

32. Aviles, J., and Kopecky, S.L., Intercessory prayer and cardiovascular disease progression in a coronary care unit population: A randomized controlled trial. Mayo Clinic Proceedings, 12/01.

33. www.pueblo.gsa.gov/cic_text/food/food-pyramid/main.htm/

34. Choi, H. K., Atkinson, K., Karlson, E.W., Willet, W., and Curhan, G. Purine-rich foods, dairy and protein intake, and the risk of gout in men. *New England Journal of Medicine*;350; 093-1103.

35. Choi, H. Gout and alcohol. *Lancet* March 2004.

36. Vivekananthan, D.P., Penn, M.S., Sapp, S.K., Hsu, A., and Topol, E.J. Use of antioxidant vitamins for the prevention of cardiovascular disease: meta-analysis of randomized trials. *Lancet* 361:2017-2023, 2003.

37. Kirn, T.F. Group rates efficacy of herbal treatments, compiles safety date. *Internal Medicine News* April 1, 2004, p. 15.

38. Lynch, M.E., and Clark, A.J. Cannabis reduces opioid dose in the treatment of chronic non-cancer pain. *Journal of Pain and Symptom Management* 25:496-498, 2003.

39. DiPaula, R.S., Zhang, H., Lambert, G.H., et al. Clinical and biologic activity of an estrogenic herbal combination (PC-SPES) in prostate cancer. *New England Journal of Medicine* 339:785-791, 1998.

40. Dangerous Supplements, *Consumer Reports* May 2004, pp. 12-17.

41. Winslow, L.C., and Kroll, D.J. Herbs as medicines. *Archives of Internal Medicine* 158:2192-2199,1998.

42. Miller, L.G. Selected clinical considerations focusing on known or potential drug-herb interactions. *Archives of Internal Medicine* 158:2200-2211, 1998.

43. Cui, J., Garle, M., Eneroth, P., and Bjorkhem, I. What do commercial ginseng preparations contain? *Lancet* 344:134-144, 1994.

44. Harkey, M. R., Henderson, G. L., Gershwin, M. E., Stern, J. S., and Hackman, R. M. Variability in commercial ginseng products. *American Journal of Clinical Nutrition* 73:1101-1106, 2001.

45. Kaufman, D.W., Kelly, J.P., Rosenberg, L., Anderson, T.E., and Mitchell, A.A. Recent patterns of medication use in the ambulatory adult population of the United States: the Slone survey. *Journal of the American Medical Association* 287:337-344, 2002.

46. De Smet, P.A.G.M. Herbal remedies. *New England Journal of Medicine* 347:2046-2056, 2002.

CHAPTER ELEVEN

1. Vastag, B. Scientists find connections in the brain between physical and emotional pain. *JAMA* 290:2389-2390, 2003.

2. Eisenberger, N.I., Lieberman, M.D., and Williams, K.D. Does rejection hurt? An MRI sudy of social exclusion. *Science* 302:290-292, 2003.

3. Panksepp, J. Feeling the pain of social loss. *Science* 302:237-238, 2003.

4. Fishbain, D.A., Arnold, L.M., and Gallagher, R.M. Pain and depression – the clinical conundrum: What comes first? Special report by the publishers of *Pain Medicine News*, July 2003.

5.   Mossey, J.M., Gallagher, R.M., and Tirumalasetti, F. The effects of pain and depression on physical function in elderly residents of a continuing care retirement community. *Pain Medicine* 1:340-350, 2001.

6.   Verma, S., and Gallagher, R.M. Evaluating and treating co-morbid pain and depression *International Review of Psychiatry* 12:103-114, 2002.

7.   Fishbain, D.A., Goldberg, M., Meagher, B.R., Steele, R., Rosomoff, H. Male and female chronic pain patients categorized by DSM-III psychiatric diagnostic criteria. *Pain* 26:181-197, 1986.

8.   Lin, E.H.B., Katon, W., Von Korff, M., Tang, L., Williams, J.W., Kroenke, K., Hunkeler, E., Harpole, L., Hegel, M., Arean, P., Hoffing, M., Della Penna, R., Langston, C., and Unutzer, J. Effect of improving depression care on pain and functional outcomes among older adults with arthritis: a randomized controlled trial. *Journal of the American Medical Association* 290:2428-2434, 2003.

9.   Dickens, C., McGowan, L., Clark-Carter, D., and Creed, F. Depression in rheumatoid arthritis: a systematic review of the literature with meta-analysis. *Psychosomatic Medicine* 64:52-60, 2002.

10.  Bair, M.J., Robinson, R.L., Katon, W., and Kroenke, K. Depression and pain comorbidity: a literature review. *Archives of Internal Medicine* 163:2433-2445, 2003.

11.  Kerns, R.D., and Haythornthwaite, J.A. Depression among chronic pain patients: cognitive-behavioral analysis and effect on rehabilitation outcome. *Journal of Consulting Clinical Psychology* 56:870-876, 1988.

12.  Asmundson, G.J., Jacobson, S.J., Allerdings, M.D., and Newton, G.R. Social phobia in disabled workers with chronic musculoskeletal pain. *Behavior Research and Therapy* 34:939-943, 1996.

13.  Lynch, M.R. Antidepressants as analgesics: a review of randomized controlled studies. *Journal of Psychiatry and Neuroscience* 26:30-36, 2001.

14.  Talbot, J.D., Marrett, S., and Evans, A.C. Multiple representations of pain in human cerebral cortex. *Science* 251:1355-1358, 1991.

15.  Nicassio, P.M., Wallston, K.A., Callahan, L.F., Herbert, M., and Pincus, T. The measurement of helplessness in rheumatoid arthritis: The development of the arthritis helplessness index. *Journal of Rheumatology* 12:462-467, 1985.

16.  Keefe, F.J., Caldwell, D.S., Queen, K.T., Gil, K.M., Martinez, S., Crisson, J.E., Ogden, W., and Nunley, J. Pain coping strategies in osteoarthritis patients. *Journal of Consulting and Clinical Psychology* 55:208-212, 1987.

17.  Keefe, F.J., Caldwell, D.S., Queen, K.T., Gil, K.M., Martinez, S., Crisson, J.E., Ogden, W., and Nunley, J. Pain coping strategies in osteoarthritis patients. *Journal of Consulting and Clinical Psychology* 55:208-212, 1987.

18.  Haythornthwaite, J., Clark, M., Pappagallo, M., and Raja, S. Pain coping strategies play a role in the persistence of pain in post-herpetic neuralgia. *Pain* 106:453-460, 2003.

19.  Koenke, K., and Swindle, R. Cognitive-behavioral therapy for somatization and symptom syndromes: a critical review of controlled clinical trials. *Psychotherapy and Psychosomatics* 69:205-215, 2000.

20.  Morley, S., Eccleston, C., and Williams, A. Systematic review and meta-analysis of randomized controlled trials of CBT for chronic pain in adults, excluding headache. *Pain* 80:1-13, 1999.

21.  Corrado, P., and Gottlieb, H. The effect of biofeedback and relaxation training on depression in chronic pain patients. *American Journal of Pain Management* 9:18-21, 1999.

22.  Corrado, P., Gottlieb, H., and Abdelhamid, M.H. The effect of biofeedback and relaxation training on anxiety and somatic complaints in chronic pain patients. *American Journal of Pain Management* 13:133-139, 2003.

23.  Kabat-Zinn, J., Lipworth, L., and Burney, R. The clinical use of mindful meditation for the self-regulation of chronic pain. *Journal of Behavioral Medicine* 8:163-190, 1985.

24.  Hammond, C. Hypnosis. Presentation at Frontiers in Pain Conference, Phoenix, AZ, April 12, 1996.

25.  Montgomery, G.H., David, D., Winkel, G., Silverstein, J.H., and Bovbjerg, D.H. The effectiveness of adjunctive hypnosis with surgical patients: a meta-analysis. *Anesthesia and Analgesia* 94:1639-1645, 2002.

26. Montgomery, G.H., DuHamel, K.N., and Redd, W.N. A meta-analysis of hypnotically induced analgesia: how effective is hypnosis? *International Journal of Clinical and Experimental Hypnosis* 48:138-153, 2000.

27. Mauer, M.G., Burnett, K.F., Ouellette, E.A., Ironson, G.H., and Dandes, H.M. Medical hypnosis and orthopedic hand surgery: pain perception, postoperative recovery, and therapeutic comfort. *International Journal of Clinical and Experimental Hypnosis* 47:144-161, 1999.

28. Defechereux, T., Meurisse, M., Hamoir, E., Gollogly, L., Joris, J., and Faymonville, M.E. Hypnoanesthesia for endocrine cervical surgery: a statement of practice. *Journal of Alternative and Complementary Medicine* 5:509-520, 1999.

29. Lang, E.V., Benotsch, E.G., Fick, L.J., Lutgendorf, S., Berbaum, M.L., Berbaum, K.S., Logan, H., and Spiegel, D. Adjunctive non-pharmacological analgesia for invasive medical procedures: a randomized trial. *Lancet* 355:1486-1490, 2000.

30. Lambert, S.A. The effects of hypnosis/guided imagery on the postoperative course in children. *Developmental and Behavioral Pediatrics* 17:307-310,1996.

31. Lynn, S.J., Kirsch, I., Barabasz, A., Cardena, E., and Patterson, D. Hypnosis as an empirically supported clinical intervention: the state of the evidence and a look to the future. *International Journal of Clinical and Experimental Hypnosis* 48:239-259, 2000.

32. Rainville, P., Duncan, G.H., Price, D.D., Carrier, B., and Bushnell, M.C. Pain affect encoded in human anterior cingulate but not somatosensory cortex. *Science* 277:968-971, 1997.

33. Petrovic, P., Kalso, E., Petersson, K.M., and Ingvar, M. Placebo and opioid analgesia—imaging a shared neuronal network. *Science* 295:1737-1740, 2002.

34. Shapiro, F. *Eye Movement Desensitization and Reprocessing: Basic Principles, Protocols, and Procedures.* New York: Guilford Press, 1995.

CHAPTER TWELVE

1. Palmer, H. *The Enneagram.* San Francisco: Harper San Francisco, 1988.

2. Palmer, H. *The Enneagram in Love and Work.* San Francisco: Harper San Francisco, 1995.

3. Barron, R., and Wagelie, E. *The Enneagram Made Easy.* San Francisco: Harper San Francisco, 1994.

4. Goldberg, M. *The Nine Ways of Working.* New York: Marlowe & Company, 1999.

5. Riso, D., and Hudson, R. *Personality Types.* New York: Houghton Mifflin, 1996.

6. Condon, T. *The Enneagram Movie & Video Guide,* 2nd Edition. Portland, Oregon: Metamorphous Press, 1999.

CHAPTER FIFTEEN

1. Lear, M.W. *Heartsounds.* New York: Simon and Schuster, 1980.

2. Dillard, J. *The Chronic Pain Solution.* New York: Bantam, 2002, p. 382.

CHAPTER SIXTEEN

1. Viscusi, E.R., Reynolds, L., Chung, F., Atkinson, L.E., and Khanna, S. Patient-controlled transdermal fentanyl hydrochloride vs intravenous morphine pump for postoperative pain: A randomized controlled trial. *Journal of the American Medical Association* 291:1333-1341, 2004.

# ACKNOWLEDGEMENTS

*I wish to give thanks to the following people for their assistance in preparation of this book:*

**Marni Dittmar**, *Librarian at Tucson Medical Center Medical Library, Tucson, for obtaining dozens of journal articles and references for me. Her help was immense.*

**Steve Gurgevich, Ph.D.** *for providing information about mind-body therapies.*

**Jeri Hassman, M.D.** *for reviewing the material and sharing her expertise in physical medicine and rehabilitation.*

**Katherine Norgard, Ph.D.** *for reminding me of the importance of including the family.*

**Russell Portenoy, M.D.** *for reviewing the chapters on opioids.*

**Audrey Russell-Kibble, N.P.** *for reviewing the chapter on alternative medicine.*

**Paul Steenhoek** *for reviewing the chapters on opioids.*

**Amy Weintraub** *for contributing to the section on yoga.*

*My editor,* **Andrea Au**, *at Hatherleigh Press, for her suggestions, and publisher* **Kevin Moran** *for proposing that I write this book.*

*All the patients, friends, and family who bared their souls and told me about their pain experiences.*

# INDEX